Sexual Mutilations
A Human Tragedy

Sexual Mutilations
A Human Tragedy

Edited by

George C. Denniston
University of Washington
Seattle, Washington

and

Marilyn Fayre Milos
National Organization of Circumcision
Information Resource Centers
San Anselmo, California

Plenum Press • New York and London

Library of Congress Cataloging in Publication Data

Sexual mutilations: a human tragedy / edited by George C. Denniston and Marilyn
Fayre Milos.
    p.   cm.
Includes bibliographical references and index.
ISBN 0-306-45589-7
    1. Female circumcision—Congresses. 2. Circumcision—Congresses. 3. Mutilation—
Congresses. I. Denniston, George C. II. Milos, Marilyn Fayre. III. International Sympo-
sium on Sexual Mutilations (4th: 1996: Lausanne, Switzerland)
GN484.S48   1997   97-9243
392.1′4—dc21   CIP

Proceedings of the Fourth International Symposium on Sexual Mutilations,
held August 9–11, 1996, in Lausanne, Switzerland

ISBN 0-306-45589-7

© 1997 Plenum Press, New York
A Division of Plenum Publishing Corporation
233 Spring Street, New York, N. Y. 10013

http://www.plenum.com

10 9 8 7 6 5 4 3 2

Printed in the United States of America

PREFACE

Sexual mutilation is a global problem that affects 15.3 million children and young adults annually. In terms of gender, 13.3 million boys and 2 million girls are involuntarily subjected to sexual mutilation every year. While it is tempting to quantify and compare the amount of tissue removed from either gender, no ethical justification can be made for removing any amount of flesh from the body of another person. The violation of human rights implicit in sexual mutilation is identical for any gender. The violation occurs with the first cut into another person's body.

Although mutilation is a strong term, it precisely and accurately describes a condition denoting "any disfigurement or injury by removal or destruction of any conspicuous or essential part of the body." While such terms as "circumcision" and "genital cutting" are less threatening to our sensitivities, they ultimately do a disservice by masking the fact of what is actually being done to babies and children. Although the courageous example of the survivors of sexual mutilation indicates that humans can certainly live and even reproduce without all of their external sexual organs, this biological phenomenon does not, however, justify subjecting a person to sexual mutilation. The remarkable resilience of the human body is a testament to the importance nature places on reproduction rather than a vindication for surgical practices that compromise this function.

According to the belief systems of those cultures that practice the sexual mutilation of children, the sexual organs do not belong to the person to whom they are attached: Instead, they are regarded as community property, under the immediate control of physicians, witch doctors, religious figures, tribal elders, relatives, or their agents. Sexual mutilations are generally perpetrated against defenseless babies and children by operators who themselves were mutilated. While young adults in these cultures are potentially capable of defending themselves against sexual mutilation, powerful cultural taboos and, often, real threats of social, economic, and political discrimination, banishment, or death, prevent escape.

The number of children who die as a direct result of traditional sexual mutilations is high. The number of children who *almost* die is higher. In one study of the penile mutilation practice (foreskin amputation in this instance) of the Xhosa tribe of Southern Africa, 9% of the mutilated boys died; 52% lost all or most of their penile shaft skin; 14% developed severe infectious lesions; 10% lost their glans penis; and 5% lost their entire penis.[1] This represents only those boys who made it to the hospital. The true complication rate is likely to be much higher. In the United States, it is estimated that 229 babies die each year as a result of the complications of the sexual mutilation of routine foreskin amputation.[2] Additionally, 1 in 500 suffer serious complications requiring emergency medical attention.[3] Regardless of the number that die or are forced to spend the rest of their lives as genital cripples, the death or injury of even one child during the course of sexual mutilation is unjustifiable. Even when there are no officially recognized complications, the survivors are left with semifunctional, scarred, and desensitized sex organs. Sexual mutilations to any degree, to any gender, wherever they occur, and for whatever reason are always prejudicial to the health of the individual.

Traditional sexual mutilations occur primarily in two parts of the world: Saharasia, the great swath of desert extending across Saharan Africa to the deserts of Saudi Arabia; and Melanesia, the scattered islands in the South Pacific extending from Australia to New Guinea. Dr. James DeMeo speculates that sexual mutilations of all kinds arose in Saharasia at approximately 4000 BCE as a result of drastic climatic changes. These changes resulted in an ecologically devastating, irreversible process of desertification and resulted in mass migrations. Previously peaceful cultures were transformed into cultures with strong tendencies toward male dominance, despotism, sexual and economic repression of women and children, sadistic violence, and warfare. In modern times, civil and religious warfare and conquests have spread sexual mutilations from these areas and imposed them on neighboring cultures. Migrating peoples from expansionist mutilating cultures have imposed ritual penile mutilations on the peoples of newly conquered territories. This can be seen in the southerly and easterly political and military expansion of Islamic regimes into sub-Saharan Africa and Asia. Historian Frederick Hodges documents the almost spontaneous genesis of sexual mutilation in historic times in the United States at the hands of physicians, providing insightful clues about the earlier origins of sexual mutilation in prehistory.

As documented in the papers of Berhane Ras-Work, Jeannine Parvati Baker, and Hanny Lightfoot-Klein, the perpetrators of sexual mutilations today generally believe that they are acting in the best interest of the victim. Parents who hand over their children to sexual mutilators generally do so because they believe that mutilation will improve the lives of their children. Powerful mythologies support these practices. Powerful taboos prevent dissent. Some cultures use sexual mutilations as a tribal mark. Some cultures use sexual mutilations as an involuntary initiation into a larger community of similarly mutilated individuals. Others use sexual mutilations as sympathetic magic or for alleged medical purposes imagined to protect the child. Some cultures do not know why they mutilate their children's sexual organs and do so only from force of habit. Some cultures mutilate their children's sexual organs for purely superstitious reasons: to appease angry deities or to ward off evil spirits. The majority of sexually mutilating cultures, however, use sexual mutilations either as a deliberately frightening test of pain endurance intended to strengthen the character of the victim or as a deliberate destruction of erogenous function.

Older victims of sexual mutilation are likely to be mutilated as part of an initiation ceremony for which they are only partially prepared. They are generally unaware that their sexual organs will be cut until the actual cutting begins. In those few cultures that do prepare the initiates, the operator generally gives the victims little accurate information about what will happen, or he deliberately gives them inaccurate information. In such ceremonies, the infliction of terror plays an important supplementary role. Over time, many of the victims can become reconciled to what has happened to their sexual organs and are often accepting of the fact that, when the time comes, they will, without protest, hand over their own children to the mutilators.

What the young victims of penile mutilation themselves understand about what is happening to them is not documented. The younger the victim, the less likely he or she will be able to understand the stated reasons for the mutilation. Clearly, when infants are sexually mutilated, they have no way of comprehending the motives of their mutilators.

For the younger victim, the experience is one of terror and of betrayal at the hands of his or her supposed protectors. Whatever the age of the victim, sexual mutilation results in the destruction of self-confidence, the infliction of excruciating pain, and the creation of massive tissue damage.

The functional consequences of sexual mutilation are well documented in this volume by such contributors as Tim Hammond and Dr. Gérard Zwang. Studies have found that flooding the neonatal brain with massive trauma creates detrimental physiological changes in brain structure. Boys who have been subjected to circumcision have a lower threshold for pain than intact boys or girls.[4] One study, published in the *British Journal of Medical Psychology*, found that circumcision of children causes a remarkable decrease in IQ and has a detrimental effect on the child's functioning and adaptation, particularly on his ego strength, resulting in behavioral and personality disorders.[5] As Miriam Pollack asks in this volume, what does it mean when society holds a knife to the genitals of its children and inflicts such psychological and physical harm?

The Fourth International Symposium on Sexual Mutilations brought together representatives of various academic disciplines and members of ad hoc human rights organizations dedicated to safeguarding the human right to physical security and integrity and preserving all children from sexual mutilation. At the First International Symposium on Sexual Mutilations, held in Anaheim, California, in 1989, delegates unanimously ratified the *Declaration of Genital Integrity* (initially entitled *The Declaration of the First International Symposium on Circumcision*). Because of the historic nature of this document, and because several of the contributors of this volume refer to it, it is reprinted here for the benefit of the reader. Delegates at the Fourth International Symposium on Sexual Mutilations unanimously ratified *The Ashley Montagu Resolution to End the Genital Mutilation of Children Worldwide*. This document, named in honor of Dr. Ashley Montagu, distinguished scientist, scholar, and humanist, at the time of this writing has been sent to the Secretary General of the United Nations and to the World Court, the Hague, for a de jure ruling that the sexual mutilation of children violates the *Universal Declaration of Human Rights* and the *United Nations Convention on the Rights of the Child*.

Humanity has faced many hurdles as it has moved from superstition and tyranny toward enlightment and freedom. The hurdle of sexual mutilation, though daunting, can be overcome. Education, cooperation, dialogue, and understanding are the first steps to raising global consciousness about the problem of sexual mutilation. Until the most vulnerable among us are safe from the threat of sexual mutilation, no one is safe. The contributors to this volume bring their unique talents and perspectives to the global problem of sexual mutilation and suggest strategies for safeguarding the world's children and the adults they will become from these mutilations. While the study of sexual mutilations paints an unfavorable picture of human frailty and error, it also brings fascinating insight into human culture and hope for future progress. We think you will agree with us.

REFERENCES

1. Crowley IP, Kesner KM. Ritual Circumcision (Umkhwetha) amongst the Xhosa of the Ciskei. British Journal of Urology 1990;66:318–21.
2. Baker RB. Newborn male circumcision: needless and dangerous. Sexual Medicine Today 1979;3.
3. Gee WF, Ansell JS. Neonatal circumcision: a ten-year overview: with comparison of the gomco clamp and the plastibell device. Pediatrics 1976;58:824–7.

4. Taddio A, Goldbach M, Ipp M, Stevens B, Koren G. Effect of Neonatal Circumcision on Pain Responses During Vaccination in Boys. Lancet 1995;345:291–2.
5. Cansever G. Psychological Effects of Circumcision. British Journal of Medical Psychology 1965;38:321–31.

ACKNOWLEDGMENTS

At the invitation of Sami Aldeeb of the Swiss Institute of Comparative Law, the papers in this book were first presented at the Fourth International Symposium on Sexual Mutilations, held at the University of Lausanne in 1996. We owe a tremendous debt of gratitude to Dr. Aldeeb for organizing the symposium and bringing together such a powerful body of research from such diverse disciplines as medicine, law, history, religion, and political science.

Among the numerous people who have encouraged and helped us in this project, we would like to express our sincere gratitude to Miriam Pollack, whose brilliant keynote address set the theme of the symposium and created an environment in which many voices could come together in unity for the sake of the children. We would like to thank Ken Brierley, John A. Erickson, Marianne Sarkis, and especially Matthew Orlando for their helpful and constructive criticisms and suggestions. We are grateful to Michel Odent, who has influenced our thinking considerably and given us helpful suggestions for individual chapters. We are indebted to John Money, John R. Taylor, Shaun Mather, Hanny Lightfoot-Klein, the Saturday Evening Post Society, and the ubiquitous John A. Erickson for permission to reprint the photographs used to illustrate the book. Most particularly, we are grateful to Frederick Hodges for his usual wise counsel and cheerful support. Finally, we would like to express our deepest appreciation to the contributors for allowing us to publish their work.

VOICES IN SUPPORT OF *THE ASHLEY MONTAGU RESOLUTION TO END THE GENITAL MUTILATIONS OF CHILDREN WORLDWIDE: A PETITION TO THE WORLD COURT, THE HAGUE*

Add my name to those opposed to the genital mutilations of children worldwide and supportive of the Montagu Resolution.
> —**Francis H. C. Crick,** Ph.D., Humanist Distinguished Service Award, 1986; Nobel Laureate in Physiology or Medicine, 1962; President, The Salk Institute for Biological Studies

Throughout history and to the present day, patriarchal societies have circumcised females to repress their sexuality and status. . . . Today, an estimated 110 million African women are suffering the medical, social, and psychological complications of genital mutilation. . . . A collective international effort is necessary to support the indigenous organizations and national governmental agencies devoted to the eradication of this custom.
> —**Asha Mohamud,** M.D., M.P.H., Physician/consultant in maternal/child health

Circumcision is a brutal ritual rooted in superstition and should be abandoned. . . . What is called for is a well-thought-out approach to the eradication of antiquated beliefs and practices that cause so much needless suffering, mutilation, tragedy, and death. [We need] an approach that takes into consideration all those factors I have mentioned, and more. We can begin with carefully designed programs, possibly under the auspices of the United Nations or a similar body, with the purpose of rendering obsolete the practice of circumcision, an archaic ritual mutilation that has no justification whatever, and no place in a civilized society.
> —**Ashley Montagu,** Ph.D., Anthropologist; Humanist of the Year, 1995

The confounding of pain and pleasure in the developing brain provides the neuropsychological foundation for individuals who must experience pain to experience pleasure, or who derive pleasure from the experience of pain (sado-masochism). . . . These developmental experiences of genital pain and affectional deprivation preclude the possibility of realizing the spiritual dimensions of human sexuality.
> —**James W. Prescott,** Ph.D., Director, Institute of Humanistic Science

You may add my name to those in support of the Montagu Resolution expressing opposition to the genital mutilation of children.
        —**Jonas Salk,** M.D., Humanist of the Year, 1976

When slavery was a custom, every right-minded person supported it. Nothing is as powerful a legitimizer as social custom, even more powerful than law.
        —**Thomas Szasz,** M.D., Humanist of the Year, 1973

I recognize and acknowledge the growing consciousness within the Jewish community, which has been struggling with bris milah for the last 150 years. As the son of a Reform rabbi, I know that Judaism will survive and prosper without bris milah. The covenant between God and the Jewish people will continue after the symbolic token—the physical mutilation—is abandoned. No one who truly understands the depth of Judaism can say otherwise. . . . Jews like myself have taken a leadership role in groups working to end all circumcisions. . . . Passage of The Ashley Montagu Resolution To End The Genital Mutilation of Children Worldwide would provide reassuring support to those Jews who already privately agree that the practice of circumcision should end.
        —**Norm Cohen,** Director, NOCIRC of Michigan

Understanding the pain and loss of function I have caused my son has been one of the greatest sources of grief I carry as a parent. One of my greatest joys in life is that I was able to educate my son and his wife about circumcision, which enabled them to break the cycle of abuse and prevent the circumcision of my twin baby grandsons. . . . I believe with my heart and soul that ending circumcision is one of the most important things I can do as a Jewish man. I am proud to join with others who feel as I do.
        —**Jed Diamond,** Author; Psychotherapist

As a proud Jew and a critic of genital mutilation, I am disheartened when people condone circumcision in deference to the Jewish community. A desire to protect millions of Jewish boys from physical and emotional trauma is as far from anti-Semitism as you can get. . . . Fact is, even if a Christian fundamentalist were whipping his or her child with the best of intentions ("The Bible says, 'spare the rod'"), I would still call it child abuse. I doubt that there is a parent alive who chooses circumcision with sadistic intention. Nevertheless, what the child experiences is child abuse, pure and simple.
        —**Fredric Hayward,** Executive Director, Men's Rights, Inc.

Judaism is not a monolithic, unchanging institution, but is instead an ever-evolving humanistic religion. . . . The move away from circumcision is not a departure from the core tenants of Judaism, but is instead a reaffirmation of the very values that form the foundation of Judaism.
        —**Moshe Rothenberg,** C.S.W., Educator; Teacher; Counselor

CONTENTS

THE GEOGRAPHY OF MALE AND FEMALE GENITAL MUTILATIONS

James DeMeo

The desire by adults to attack the genitals of their infants and young children with sharp knives is a subject about which a tremendous amount has been written, the majority of which attempts to justify and "explain" it, but in a manner which leaves the larger cultural-social backdrop uncriticized. This paper will take a different approach, not only to criticize that "backdrop" but to lift it up, and get a good look at what's going on "behind the curtain" of this deeply emotional and brutal human drama. Genital mutilations were originally studied by the author as part of a larger investigation of the geographical and cross-cultural aspects of human behavior among subsistence-level, aboriginal peoples.[1-3] The focus in this paper will be restricted mainly to the phenomenon of male and female genital mutilations, but the larger cross-cultural and psychological-emotional aspects will be exposed and discussed as well.

Genital mutilations are often classified as a "cultural practice," but there is growing evidence that this benign-sounding label merely serves to dismiss or evade the painful and contractive effects the mutilations have upon the psyche and soma of the child. The practices elicit severe pain and terror in infants and children subject to them, and are often very dangerous to health, which raises important questions about how they could have gotten started in the first instance. People who do not engage in such practices view them almost always with horror and disbelief, while people who do them often have difficulty imagining life without the practices. Oftentimes, the presence or the absence of the rites are seen as important requirements for the selection of a marriageable partner, and very powerful emotions focus upon them. They are among the most strongly defended, or defended against, of all cultural practices. Among the various theories developed to account for the mutilations, their geographical distribution has rarely been determined or discussed in detail with few exceptions.[4-7]

Figures 1 and 2 show the overlapping distributions of various types of male and female genital mutilations, respectively, as they existed among aboriginal, subsistence-level peoples within the last several hundred years. As such, the maps greatly minimize or eliminate the more recent diffusion of male genital mutilation (circumcision) as adopted in the United States, Canada, Australia and Britain over the last 100 years. For North and

Sexual Mutilations: A Human Tragedy, edited by Denniston and Milos
Plenum Press, New York, 1997

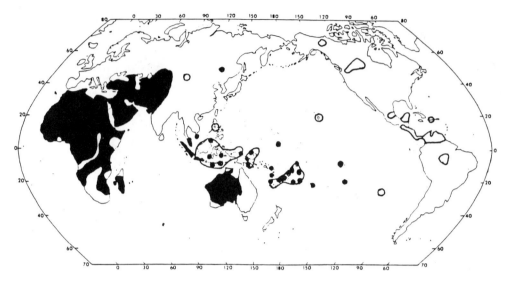

Figure 1. Male Genital Mutilations. Data from aboriginal, native peoples only. Does not include the more recent historical adoption within the United States, Canada, Australia and Britain. Black areas: extremely severe forms (e.g. flaying circumcision, subincision); outlined areas: forms of lesser severity (e.g. incision).

South America, for example, the maps reflect the existence of the practices among various native "Indian" cultures, and also among the Mesoamerican empires of the Maya, Aztec and Inca. Other authors in this book will address the more recent historical adoption of male circumcision in the United States and a few other English-speaking nations, and the reasons behind it. Our attempt here is to identify the global-historical and cross-cultural dynamics of the practices, in an attempt to better understand their ultimate origins, and the

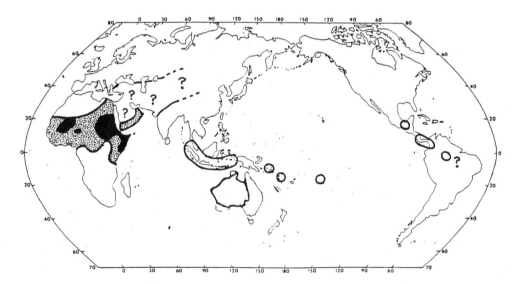

Figure 2. Female Genital Mutilations (5, 6, 22, 25). Black areas: extremely severe forms (e.g. Infibulation); shaded areas: severe forms (e.g. clitoridectomy, excision); outlined areas: present, but form and incidence unknown.

nature of the strong emotional push which has kept the practices alive, in spite of their obviously painful and even horrific, life-threatening qualities.

1. MALE GENITAL MUTILATIONS

Incision, the least harsh of the male genital mutilations, consists of either a simple cut on the foreskin to draw blood, or a complete cutting through of the foreskin in a single place so as to partly expose the glans. Incision existed primarily among peoples of the East African coast, in Island Asia and Oceania, and among a few peoples of the New World. Circumcision, a harsher mutilation where the foreskin of the penis is cut or torn away, was and is practiced across much of the Old World desert belt, and in a number of Sub-Saharan, Central Asian, and Pacific Ocean groups. When performed during puberty, circumcision was largely a premarital rite of pain endurance.

Circumcision only gained the status of being an "hygienic operation" in relatively recent times, although the most recent and best medical evidence has in fact shown that routine circumcision has neither short- nor long-term hygienic benefits; indeed, it has mild to severe negative psychological and physiological effects.[8-19] Particularly in the bush, under less than sanitary conditions, the circumcised boy infant or child would have been at greater risk than the uncircumcised boy.[20]

The most severe male genital mutilation, which is called, simply, genital skin stripping, was practiced along the Red Sea coast in Arabia and Yemen, at least into the 1800s. Here, in an endurance ritual performed on a potential marriage candidate, skin was completely flayed from the entire penile shaft as well as from a region of pubis. The community blessing would only be bestowed upon the young man who could refrain from expressing emotion during the event.[21-32]

Another harsh ritual, subincision, was practiced primarily among Australian aborigines and on a few Pacific islands. It consisted of a cutting open of the urethra on the underside of the penis down to near the scrotum; the subincision ritual was generally preceded by a circumcision ritual.[33-34] The practice did not confer any contraceptive advantage, and no claims as such were made for it by the Australian aborigines. The geographical aspects of the Australian genital mutilations have been studied previously, and two competing theories were developed. Northwest Australia, specifically the Kimberly region, was identified as a location where genital skin stripping was performed,[35] and some believed that circumcision and subincision spread into Australia from that region, diffusing to the east and south. On the other hand, independent development of the traits within Australia has been argued, based upon the observation that the most intense forms of subincision occurred in the desert center of the continent, being absent in a few border regions where only circumcision was practiced.[36]

The Ethnographic Atlas of G.P. Murdock,[37] plus the various works of Montagu and others,[38-44] provided the basic data for Figure 1. Murdock's Atlas also contains raw data on the age at which the mutilations were customarily done among a globally-balanced sample of 350 cultures. A map of that data which I constructed indicated that the mutilations possessed a widespread distribution, centered on Northeast Africa and Arabia. Furthermore, as demonstrated in Figure 3, the greater the distance from those central regions, the older was the male at the time of the mutilation.[45] As one moves farther and farther east from Africa and the Near East, the males are progressively older at the time of the mutilation. Furthermore, the practices occur less frequently, and undergo a gradual dilution of harshness as distance from those central regions increases. Genital skin stripping,

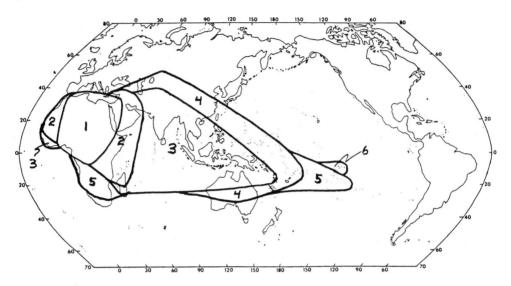

Figure 3. Age Distribution of Male Genital Mutilations. 1 = Performed within the first 2 months, 2 = Performed from 2 months to 2 years, 3 = Performed from 2 - 5 years, 4 = Performed from 6 - 10 years, 5 = Performed from 11 - 25 years, 6 = Performed after 25 years.

the harshest mutilation, was centered on the Red Sea region, and was surrounded by a region practicing only male circumcision. Circumcision, in turn, gives way to the less-harsh practice of incision as one moves eastward across the Pacific. Genital mutilations were not practiced at all among most of the aboriginal peoples of the Americas or Eastern Oceania. It was precisely in these regions of mutilation absence where the decorative "penis tops" were most frequently found among native peoples, indicating a similar interest in the genitalia, but only in a decorative and pleasurable sense.

From the standpoint of the pain involved in circumcision as a puberty or premarital rite, the easterly decline in mutilation frequency and dilution of the rite towards less painful methods, and to older ages, makes perfect sense if we also assume that the emotional attitudes, beliefs, and cultural institutions which originally mandated the painful ritual were likewise diluted as they were carried eastward from a Northeast African or Arabian point of origin.[46] With the social and emotional root reasons for the rituals becoming diluted with time and distance, less painful methods such as incision were substituted, or it was put off as long as possible, certainly well past the period just before marriage, preferably into the period of old age. Or it was relinquished altogether. In the Near Eastern desert regions where the social institutions and emotional roots for the ritual remained, but where the pain of the mutilation was feared as a puberty/premarital rite, it was occasionally shifted into infancy, or adopted as such from the start.

There have been several phases of diffusion of the mutilations. Egyptian bas-reliefs give the earliest known unambiguous evidence of male genital mutilations, performed as a puberty rite during the early Dynastic era (by c.2300 BC).[47] It seems probable, however, that the mutilations were introduced beforehand, when the Nile Valley was invaded by militant pastoral nomads, and culturally transformed around c.3100 BC. These invaders, who possessed Asian and Semitic characteristics, ushered in an era of divine kings, ritual widow murder, a military and priestly caste, massive graves and fabulous grave wealth, temple architecture, and other trappings of extreme patriarchal authoritarian culture.[48] As discussed below, cultural tendencies of a similar direction, but of lesser intensity, are positively correlated with genital mutilating cultures of more recent times.

According to Hebrew scripture, the Hebrews institutionalized the mutilations after the Exodus from Egypt, and it thereafter became a special mark of the tribe. The mutilations appeared widely across the Near East prior to the irruptions of Moslem armies in the 600s AD, but were subsequently spread wherever Moslem armies ventured. While neither male nor female genital mutilations have any specific Koranic mandate, Mohammed thought them to be "desirable," and they predominate in Moslem areas. Still, there are regions of non-Moslem Africa and Oceania that possess the mutilations as a probable diffusion from ancient, pre-Moslem times. Diffusion from these earlier Pre-Moslem and Pre-Columbian periods may also yet account for isolated, rare examples of the traits in the far reaches of Oceania, and the New World.[49–53] Figure 4 identifies the maximum geographical extent of various Islamic Empires after 632 AD, demonstrating a good spatial agreement with the map in Figure 1, of male genital mutilations, underscoring the role of Islam in spreading and/or reinforcing the mutilations in many world regions.[54]

Male genital mutilations were never adopted widely in Europe, Central America, French Canada, Latin America, in the Orient, or by Hindus, Southeast Asians, or Native Americans. The spread of the rite of infant circumcision to the United States during the late 1800s and early 1900s is a most recent phenomenon not reflected on the maps. Circumcision gained validity and became more widespread in the United States only after allopathic medical doctors, playing upon prevailing sexual anxieties, urged it as a "cure" for a long list of childhood diseases and "disorders," to include polio, tuberculosis, bedwetting, and a new syndrome which appeared widely in the medical literature known as "masturbatory insanity." Circumcision was then advocated along with a host of exceedingly harsh, pain-inducing devices and practices designed to thwart any vestige of genital pleasure in children.[55]

Freud and other psychoanalysts have discussed male genital mutilations as inducing a form of "castration anxiety" in the child by which the taboo against incest and patricide is pathologically strengthened.[56–59] Montagu, Lewis, and Bettleheim have discussed their

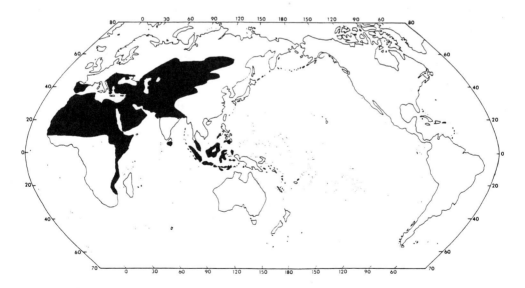

Figure 4. Areas Influenced or Occupied by Arab Armies Since 632 AD.

connections to the male fear of vaginal blood, where menstruation is imitated (subincision), or where the male must be ritually absolved of contact with poisonous childbirth blood (infant circumcision), or hymenal blood (pubertal circumcision).[60–62] Reich identified genital mutilations as but one, albeit a major one, of a series of brutal and cruel acts directed toward infants and children which possess hidden motives designed to cause a painful, permanent contraction of the child's physical and emotional self. He saw the real purpose of circumcision, and other assaults upon the child's sexuality, to be the reduction of the child's emotional fluidity and energy level, and of their ability to experience maximal pleasurable genital excitation later in life, a major step in, as he put it, transmuting Homo sapiens into armored Homo normalis. Reich argued that parents and doctors blindly advocated or performed the mutilations, and other painful shamanistic medical procedures, in proportion to their own emotional armoring and pleasure-anxiety, to render children more like themselves: obedient, docile, and reduced in sexual vigor and emotional vitality. From his research with many patients expressing mild to severe sexual problems, Reich concluded: A person who had suffered through a severe trauma, and learned to suppress the emotions associated with it, could not later on recognize the expression of those same emotions in another person. Moreover, the child who suffered from the destruction of capacity for strong sexual pleasure, would later in life be made highly anxious by the mere presence of others who retained such a capacity.[63–64] Through such mechanisms of emotional armoring and severe pleasure-anxiety, the traumatized and mutilated later on become enthusiastic mutilators. The parent and physician, having suffered from abusive trauma during their own childhoods, blindly and compulsively heap a similar sadistic abuse upon the defenseless young, as it was done to them. The intact genitalia of the young literally provoke an "urge to mutilate," which is carried out during the time when the victim is most defenseless — in childhood. Culture and law generally support the mutilators in their practices.

These ideas, as disturbing as they may be, find support in cross-cultural comparisons of cultures which mutilate the genitals of their males. Textor's *Cross-Cultural Summary* demonstrates positive correlations between male genital mutilations and the following other cultural characteristics:[65–68]

High narcissism index
Slavery and castes are present
Class stratification is high
Land inheritance favors male line
Cognatic kin groups are absent
Patrilineal descent is present
Female barrenness penalty is high
Bride price is present
Father has family authority
Polygamy is present
Marital residence near male kin
Painful female initiation rites are present
Segregation of adolescent boys is high
Oral anxiety potential is high
Average satisfaction potential is low
Speed of attention to infant needs is low
High God present, active, supportive of human morality

One cannot extract a list of correlated pro-child, pro-female, or sex-positive traits from the cross-cultural literature, as cultures which mutilate the male genitalia do not significantly possess such characteristics. Male genital mutilations are found present in a cultural complex where children, females, and weaker social or ethnic groups are subordinated to elder, dominant males in rigid social hierarchies of one form or another. While the cross-cultural analysis contrasted only aboriginal, subsistence-level cultures, many of the factors identified in the above list are or once were applicable to the United States, where male circumcision predominates. It must be noted, however, that many or most of these characteristics may be present in cultures where genital mutilations are absent, but where other severe forms of painful trauma and pleasure deprivation exist in their place.[69–73] There were many positive, but no negative correlations between male genital mutilations and other harsh, traumatic treatments of infants, children, and women, indicating that cultures which mutilate the genitals of their children also engage in a host of other painful and trauma-inducing behaviors.

Both Hindu India and Dynastic China engaged in ritual widow murder, strict child obedience training, and were patriarchal with strict forms of social hierarchy, though to my knowledge neither ever practiced the genital mutilations. German and Asian despotic cultures also did not mutilate the genitals, but did practice other severe practices aimed at their children, such as prolonged swaddling and even infant cranial deformation in earlier times. All such patriarchal authoritarian cultures had one or another method for destroying the natural spontaneous and self-regulatory qualities of their children. Some engaged in genital mutilations, while others had different harsh practices.

2. FEMALE GENITAL MUTILATIONS

There are many different varieties of female genital mutilation, and they tend to occur in the same regions and among the same peoples where male genital mutilations are practiced. The central region of female genital mutilations is North and North Central Africa, as demonstrated in Figure 2, which was largely derived from prior maps by Hosken,[74–76] with additional data from Montagu and others.[77–84] Their distribution, however, is not as widespread as the male mutilations.

Most of the female mutilations are harsher, more painful, and more life-threatening than those performed upon the male. While the ritual may be a doorway for the young boy into the world of adult privileges, including sexual activity, the female mutilations generally do not have such a social significance; indeed, the more severe forms may destroy entirely any capacity to obtain sexual pleasure whatsoever. Often they are specifically and consciously designed to do this, with such as a stated, explicit goal. The grandmother or daya (unskilled midwife) will, with help from other village women, perform the operation without anesthetic. Unlike the male circumcision ritual, there is generally no ceremony or "coming out" ritual involved. The women of the cultural unit gather about the poor girl to chant and beat drums and tambourines, largely to drown out her hysterical screaming. The girl is held down while her grandmother or the *daya*, razor in hand, sets to work upon the child's genitals.[85–87]

With female incision, only a small cut may be made on the external genitalia, or into the skin covering the clitoris. With female circumcision, the skin hood of the clitoris may be entirely removed, but it is usual for the clitoris to also be cut out, which is called clitoridectomy or excision. Accounts from the literature indicate that the distinctions between simple circumcision and excision are blurred, and a good deal of cutting may be done depending upon the "moral" inclinations of the operator. With infibulation, the severest female genital mutilation, the clitoris, labia majora and labia minora are cut away with the razor, following which much soft tissue may be randomly sliced away from the exterior vaginal opening. After this, the young girl's legs are bound together with rope. She is left immobilized for months, with a hollow reed inserted for micturition, until the vaginal walls grow together to form a sheaf of skin which thereafter covers the vaginal opening. In this way the girl's virginity is insured. She is thereafter deemed more socially fit, due to the severe reduction in her ability to become sexually excited. After marriage, the infibulation is cut open (defibulation) just enough for intercourse; this is usually done on the wedding night when a husband's intercourse with the new bride is mandated. Subsequent sexual relations are impeded by scar tissue, a generally too-small vaginal opening, the defibulation wound, and by psychological traumata on the part of both husband and wife who in any case may have met each other via an arranged marriage, just prior to the wedding night.[88]

Childbirth for the infibulated woman is very difficult, given the amount of inelastic scar tissue which forms in the vagina. The infibulated woman in labor needs to be cut open even more to provide an adequate passageway for the child; after childbirth, her vagina may again be lacerated and her legs once again bound up to reform the infibulation. Women in such cultures are not only usually denied contraceptive information and devices, but also basic education on matters of sexual hygiene. Deprived of legal rights and social status, these women live a life oscillating between horrifying rituals of infibulation-defibulation-infibulation. Mortality and morbidity of girls and women, immediately after the mutilations and during childbirth, are thereby significantly increased. Infections, hemorrhage, shock, fistulas, and even death are not uncommon results of such mutilations.[89-91]

Female genital mutilations have been observed in North Africa, parts of the Near East, in aboriginal Australia, and in parts of Oceania and the Amazon Basin. Not all cultures that mutilated the genitals of their males also mutilated the genitals of their females, but many did. Where clitoridectomy or infibulation exist, male circumcision also prevails. Cultures that practiced male subincision also tended to introcise women, that is, they made a cut into the vaginal wall, similar to an episiotomy. Cultures which incised the penis of the male also sometimes incised the external genitalia of the female, as was the case in Mesoamerica. These rites are similar to but not as severe as excision, where the entire clitoris is cut out down to the root, and infibulation, where portions of the female's external genitalia are entirely cut away, and the outer vaginal lips sewn shut. These latter harsh practices continue to be found predominantly in North Africa and the Near East, but a few isolated examples were also found in the Amazon region.[92-96] The harshness of male genital mutilations diminishes and their frequency declines as the distance from North Africa increases. This is also true of female genital mutilations.

Disturbances of the maternal-infant bond, and trauma to babies and children are significant factors in the genesis and perpetuation of social violence and patriarchy. Both males and females participate in and defend such activities as genital mutilations, abusive hospital obstetrics, the compulsory school system, and the sexual repression of children. These factors have deeper influences upon the psyche and soma of the child than subtle "role model" influences or economic factors. Historical examples clearly demonstrate that socio-economic restructuring alone, without reference to the real traumas enacted upon both male and female babies and children, will not bring about a change in national character structure, or a significant reduction in violent patriarchy.

The map of female genital mutilations in Figure 2 was constructed primarily from the works of Hosken,[97-99] with a few additional regions added from Montagu.[100] The *Cross*

Cultural Summary did not contain any data specifically addressing female genital mutilations, but did contain a variable identified as "painful female initiation rites;" this variable was found to have a positive cross-cultural association with the following other cultural variables:[101]

> Protection of infants from the environment is low
> Segregation of adolescent boys is high
> Male genital mutilations are present
> Patrilineal descent is present
> Killing, torturing, mutilation of the enemy is high

As was the case with male genital mutilations, the female mutilations exist within an hierarchical, sex-repressive and child-repressive cultural complex. In the case of the female mutilations, however, it is the older females who enthusiastically perform the mutilations on the younger girls, and who are its primary defenders. The men generally do not participate in the actual mutilations of the female, except to endorse it, or demand it. The older women themselves are the primary mutilators of the young girls, underscoring the same emotional pattern as seen in the male mutilations, which are done by older men. The mutilated become the mutilators. The overall problem is therefore one in which females play a role of equal importance to that of males; both are generally enthusiastic supporters of the established patriarchal authoritarian social order.[102–108]

A girl who attempts to avoid the mutilation is socially ostracized, the stigma of possessing a clitoris and intact genitalia being enormous. Prevailing sexual anxieties dictate that few village men of these regions will agree to marry an uncircumcised woman, just as women of male mutilating cultures will usually be anxious about marrying an uncircumcised man.[109]

Popular myths of the greater potency and cleanliness of the circumcised man prevail in the Near East, and to a lesser extent in the United States. Myths of the greater cleanliness of the circumcised woman likewise prevail where women are subject to the operation. There is no evidence to support any of these myths. The evidence, cited above, demonstrates that circumcision of men or women results in clearly negative health effects. Effects upon potency would also be negative in character as inferred from the antipleasure sexual attitudes correlated with the desire to mutilate.

Where the mutilations are mandated by custom, few girls can escape, as prevailing laws usually empower her relatives to have the operation done against her will, and to retrieve runaways. The practices, after all, exist only where the legal rights of the female are subordinate to the family elders.[110–111] In the regions where the female mutilations prevail, to call a woman "uncircumcised one," or a man the "son of an uncircumcised woman" is an insult of the most extreme proportions. So entrenched and emotionally-charged are the female mutilations that opposition to them in the past by Western colonials has triggered popular uprisings and revolts.[112–113]

The descriptions of female genital mutilations collected by Hosken indicate that the older women as well as men demand the mutilations, the elder grandmothers often cited as being its most enthusiastic supporters; they may express concerns that the mutilations be extensive enough, such that the clitoris is completely and not only partly removed. Here it can be seen that the character structure of both men and women possess powerful attitudes of denigration and horror toward female reproductive functions, anatomy, and sexual pleasure. These concerns echo back to Reich's claim that the mutilations are designed to kill sexual vitality of children, to make them sexually weakened or crippled, just like their parents.

3. SUMMARY

The descriptions of the infibulation of young women in North Africa are similar in character and severity to the nineteenth-century descriptions of forcible castration of young African boys for the eunuch trade.[114-115] Girls were once infibulated to insure their virginity when presented for the Near Eastern harem slave trade. The regions that today practice infibulation were once primary "capture zones" in the Turk and Arab slave trade for young African girls and boys. This suggests that some severe forms of genital mutilation may have originated with, or were at the very least intensified by, the institutions of slavery and the harem system.

The underlying psychology of both male and female genital mutilations is anxiety regarding sexual pleasure, mainly heterosexual genital intercourse, as indicated by the associated virginity taboos and ritual absolutions against vaginal blood. In the final analysis, these mutilations say more about predominant sexual attitudes than anything else.

Given their similar distributions, similar cross-cultural aspects, and similar psychological motifs, the time and location of origins of male and female genital mutilations are probably identical, the use of each being mandated and widely expanded by groups where dominance of the sexual lives of children by adults, and of females by males, was most extreme. The use of eunuchs has died out over the last 100 years with the decline of the harem system, but female infibulation and other forms of female genital mutilation persist in accordance with the arranged marriage system, and other vestiges of a powerful and hysterical virginity taboo.

Based upon the geographical distributions of the mutilations, it seems reasonable to assume that they began somewhere in the eastern part of North Africa, or possibly even in Arabia, prior to the Dynastic period in Egypt (c.4000–3500 BC) in association with a major climatic change which affected North Africa and the Near East at this same period. Thereafter, the mutilations were spread by the inhabitants of these regions, in accordance with their customs and beliefs, following historically-recorded migratory pathways. Nearly every male-dominated patriarchy which developed within North Africa and the Near East, up to and including more recent Moslem Empires and later Moslem nation-states, adopted and further spread the mutilations. Over the centuries, ocean-navigating peoples from these same regions spread the practices out from the Red Sea and Persian Gulf regions to places as far removed as Indonesia, New Guinea, Borneo, and other areas now inhabited by Moslem peoples. Genital mutilations in Australia, central and eastern Oceania and the Americas may have arisen independently; but even here, as discussed above, Pre-Moslem and Pre-Columbian diffusion of the traits is strongly suggested by the mapped geographical characteristics, and cannot be ruled out.

The genital mutilations of young males and females are major examples of cultural "traits" or "practices" which, on deeper analysis, reveal roots in severe pleasure-anxiety, with sadistic overtones. The older woman who cuts the genitals of the young girls was subject to the rite herself as a child, just as, in our own culture, the violent, child-abusing parent was subject to a general pattern of abuse and neglect in his or her own childhood.[116-118] Harlow demonstrated a similar principle for transmission of disturbed, anti-child and antisexual behaviors in monkeys deprived of maternal love,[119-121] a principle first identified for Homo sapiens by Reich, who, as mentioned above, also identified the role that social institutions play in recreating the trauma and damage.[122-126] Prescott was the first to confirm many of these relationships in a cross-cultural manner, gathering additional evidence of neurological damage from such trauma and pleasure-deprivation.[127-129] The cross-cultural materials summarized here further confirm these processes, which possess historically-identifiable roots in specific geographical regions.[130–131] Seen from this perspective, the urge to mutilate the genitals of children stems from deeply ingrained adult anxieties regarding sexual pleasure and happiness. Genital mutilations always exist within a complex of other social institutions that provide for the socially-sanctioned expression of adult sadism and destructive aggression towards the infant and child, with unconscious motivations aimed at destroying or damaging the capacity for pleasurable emotional/sexual bonding between mothers and babies, and between young males and females.

This discomforting view of the mutilations is further reinforced by reviewing Figure 5, a map which summarizes other abusive and neglectful "cultural traditions" aimed at infants and children, and related anti-sexual, anti-female, hierarchical, obedience-demanding, patriarchal authoritarian characteristics.

Figure 5, a World Behavior Map previously developed by the author in a comprehensive global review of cross-cultural data from over 1,000 different social groups,[132] shows a very clear spatial correlation to all the previously-presented maps focused more exclusively on genital mutilations. This profound geographical similarity once again demonstrates the intimate relationship between the urge to mutilate the genitals of children, and much broader antisexual, anti-female, and authoritarian social customs and attitudes. These customs and attitudes are what is revealed when one takes a look "behind the backdrop curtain" of the social theater, which sanctifies and demands the mutilation of children's genitals. It appears certain that genital mutilations will stubbornly persist so long as these broader customs and attitudes remain unmasked, unchallenged and uncriticized.

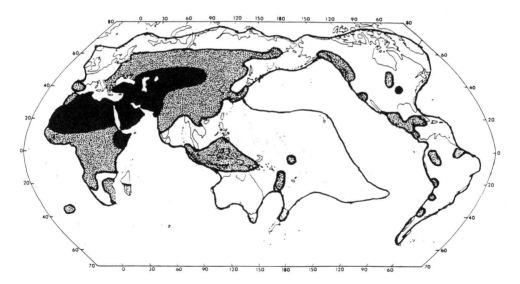

Figure 5. The World Behavior Map. **Black areas**: extreme patrist-dominator culture, abusive/neglectful treatments of infants, children, harsh treatment of women, sex-repressive, hierarchical, authoritarian, high religiosity; **shaded areas**: intermediate, moderate cultural conditions; **outlined areas**: extreme matrist-partnership culture, gentle/attentive treatment of infants, children, female equality predominates, sex-positive, egalitarian, democratic, low religiosity. For the period roughly between 1840 and 1960, as reconstructed from aboriginal, native cultural data, from over a thousand different distinct cultural groups. As with the maps on genital mutilations, data for North and South America reflect non-European, native peoples only. Data for Europe composed from culturally-isolated groups, thereby minimizing feudalistic and repressive influences.

4. REFERENCES

1. DeMeo J. On The Origins and Diffusion of Patrism: The Saharasian Connection, Dissertation, U. of Kansas, Geography Department, 1986. (Xerox available from Natural Energy Works, P.O. Box 1148, Ashland, Oregon 97520. Book version under preparation, 1997.)
2. DeMeo J. The Origins and Diffusion of Patrism in Saharasia, 4000 BCE: Evidence for a Worldwide, Climate-Linked Geographical Pattern in Human Behavior. World Futures March-May 1991;30:247–71.
3. DeMeo J. The Origins and Diffusion of Patrism in Saharasia, 4000 BCE: Evidence for a Worldwide, Climate-Linked Geographical Pattern in Human Behavior. Pulse of the Planet 1991;3:3–16.
4. Davidson D. The Chronological Aspects of Certain Australian Social Institutions, As Inferred from Geographical Distribution (Thesis, U. Pennsylvania), Philadelphia, 1928.
5. Loeb E. The Blood Sacrifice Complex. Memoirs, Am. Anthropological Assn. 1923;30:1–40.
6. Smith GE. The Diffusion of Culture, New York: Kennikat Press (1933); reprinted 1971.
7. Smith GE. The Migrations of Early Culture, London: Manchester U. Press, 1915.
8. Brackbill Y. Continuous Stimulation and Arousal Level in Infancy: Effects of Stimulus Intensity and Stress. Child Development 1975;46:364–9.
9. Ozturk O. Ritual Circumcision and Castration Anxiety. Psychiatry 1973;36:49–60.
10. Marshall R, et al. Circumcision: Effects Upon Newborn Behavior, Infant Behavior and Development 1980;3:1–14.
11. Emde R, et al. Stress and Neonatal Sleep. Psychosomatic Medicine 1971;33(6):491–7.
12. Anders T. The Effects of Circumcision on Sleep-Wake States in Human Neonates. Psychosomatic Medicine 1974;36:174–9.
13. Carter N. Routine Circumcision: the Tragic Myth, London: Londinium Press, 1979:85–93.
14. Cansever G. Psychological Effects of Circumcision. British Journal of Medical Psychology 1965;38:328–9.
15. Richards M, et al. Early Behavioral Differences: Gender or Circumcision? Developmental Psychobiology 1976;9:89–95.
16. Thompson H, et al. Report on the Ad Hoc Task Force on Circumcision. Pediatrics 1975;56:610–11.
17. Wallerstein E. Circumcision, An American Health Fallacy; Springer, 1980.
18. Zimmer P. Modern Ritualistic Surgery.Clinical Pediatrics June 1977;16:503–6.
19. Klauber G. Circumcision and Phallic Fallacies, or The Case Against Routine Circumcision. Connecticut Medicine 1973;37:445–8.
20. Theisenger W. The Marsh Arabs. NY: E.P.Dutton, 1964:101–2.
21. Burton R. Personal Pilgrimage to Al-Medinah and Mecca, Vol. 2. Dover, 1962:110.
22. Doughty C. Travels in Arabia Deserta. Random House, 1920:170.
23. Byrk F. Circumcision in Man and Woman. New York: American Ethnological Press, 1934:137.
24. Remondino P. History of Circumcision, Philadelphia: FA. Davis, 1891:55.
25. Montagu A. Ritual Mutilation Among Primitive Peoples. Ciba Symposium, October 1946;424.
26. Montagu A. The Origins of Subincision in Australia. Oceania 1937;8:193–207.
27. Montagu A. Coming into Being Among the Australian Aborigines. London: Routledge & Kegan Paul, 1974:312–25.
28. Burton R. Personal Pilgrimage to Al-Medinah and Mecca, Vol. 2. Dover, 1962:110.
29. Doughty C. Travels in Arabia Deserta. Random House, 1920:170.
30. Byrk F. Circumcision in Man and Woman. New York: American Ethnological Press, 1934:137.
31. Remondino P. History of Circumcision, Philadelphia: FA. Davis, 1891:55.
32. Montagu A. Ritual Mutilation Among Primitive Peoples. Ciba Symposium, October 1946;424.
33. Montagu A. The Origins of Subincision in Australia. Oceania 1937;8:193–207.
34. Montagu A. Coming into Being Among the Australian Aborigines. London: Routledge & Kegan Paul, 1974:312–25.
35. Montagu A. The origins of subincision in Australia. Oceania 1937;8:203.
36. Davidson D. The Chronological Aspects of Certain Australian Social Institutions, As Inferred from Geographical Distribution (Thesis, U. Pennsylvania), Philadelphia, 1928.
37. Murdock GP. Ethnographic Atlas. Pittsburg: HRAF Press, 1967.
38. Burton R. Personal Pilgrimage to Al-Medinah and Mecca, Vol. 2. Dover, 1962:110.
39. Doughty C. Travels in Arabia Deserta. Random House, 1920:170.
40. Byrk F. Circumcision in Man and Woman. New York: American Ethnological Press, 1934:137.
41. Remondino P. History of Circumcision, Philadelphia: FA. Davis, 1891:55.
42. Montagu A. Ritual Mutilation Among Primitive Peoples. Ciba Symposium, October 1946;424.

43. Montagu A. The Origins of Subincision in Australia. Oceania 1937;8:193–207.
44. Montagu A. Coming into Being Among the Australian Aborigines. London: Routledge & Kegan Paul,
     1974:312–25.
45. DeMeo J. On The Origins and Diffusion of Patrism: The Saharasian Connection, Dissertation, U. of Kan-
     sas, Geography Department, 1986:159.
46. DeMeo J. On The Origins and Diffusion of Patrism: The Saharasian Connection, Dissertation, U. of Kan-
     sas, Geography Department, 1986:153–70, 398–426.
47. Paige K. The Ritual of Circumcision. Human Nature 1978;(May):40–8.
48. DeMeo J. On The Origins and Diffusion of Patrism: The Saharasian Connection, Dissertation, U. of Kan-
     sas, Geography Department, 1986:281–94.
49. MacDonald D. Oceanic Languages: Their Grammatical Structure, Vocabulary, and Origin. London: Henry
     Frowde, 1907.
50. Murdock G. Genetic Classification of the Austronesian Languages: A Key to Oceanic Culture History. Eth-
     nology; 1907;3:124–6.
51. Fell B. America BC. New York: Demeter Press, 1977:180–7.
52. Jett S. Precolumbian Transoceanic Contacts. In: Jennings J. ed. Ancient North Americans. W.H.Freeman,
     1983.
53. DeMeo J. On The Origins and Diffusion of Patrism: The Saharasian Connection, Dissertation, U. of Kan-
     sas, Geography Department, 1986:398–426.
54. Jordan T, Rowntree L. The Human Mosaic. New York: Harper & Row, 1979:187.
55. Paige K. The Ritual of Circumcision. Human Nature 1978;(May):40–8.
56. Schlossman H. Circumcision as Defense: Study in Psychoanalysis and Religion. Psychoanalytic Quarterly
     1966;35:340–56.
57. Zimmerman F. Origin and Significance of the Jewish Rite of Circumcision. Psychoanalytic Review
     1951;38:103–12.
58. Nunberg H. Problems of Bisexuality as Reflected in Circumcision. London: Imago, 1949.
59. Ozturk O. Ritual Circumcision and Castration Anxiety. Psychiatry 1973;36:49–60.
60. Bettleheim B. Symbolic Wounds. New York: Collier Books, 1962.
61. Lewis J. In the Name of Humanity. New York: Freethought Press, 1967.
62. Montagu A. Ritual Mutilation Among Primitive Peoples. Ciba Symposium, October 1946.
63. Reich W. Reich Speaks of Freud. New York: Farrar, Straus & Giroux, 1967:27–31.
64. Reich W. Ether, God & Devil. New York: Farrar, Straus & Giroux, 1973:67–70.
65. Textor R. A Cross-Cultural Summary. New Haven: HRAF Press, 1967.
66. DeMeo J. On The Origins and Diffusion of Patrism: The Saharasian Connection, Dissertation, U. of Kan-
     sas, Geography Department, 1986.
67. DeMeo J. The Origins and Diffusion of Patrism in Saharasia, 4000 BCE: Evidence for a Worldwide, Cli-
     mate-Linked Geographical Pattern in Human Behavior. World Futures March-May 1991;30:247–71.
68. Prescott J. Body Pleasure and the Origins of Violence. Futurist April 1975;64–74.
69. DeMeo J. On The Origins and Diffusion of Patrism: The Saharasian Connection, Dissertation, U. of Kan-
     sas, Geography Department, 1986.
70. DeMeo J. The Origins and Diffusion of Patrism in Saharasia, 4000 BCE: Evidence for a Worldwide, Cli-
     mate-Linked Geographical Pattern in Human Behavior. World Futures March-May 1991;30:247–71.
71. Prescott J. Body Pleasure and the Origins of Violence. Futurist April 1975;64–74.
72. Prescott J. Deprivation of Physical Affection as a Primary Process in the Development of Physical Vio-
     lence. In: Gil D. ed. Child Abuse and Violence. New York: AMS Press, 1979:66–137.
73. Prescott J. Affectional Bonding for the Prevention of Violent Behaviors. In: Hertzberg LJ, et al. eds. Vio-
     lent Behavior: Assessment and Intervention (Vol.1). New York: PMA Publishing, 1989:109–142.
74. Hosken F. The Hosken Report on Genital and Sexual Mutilation of Females, 2nd Edition. Lexington,
     Mass.: Women's International Network News, 1979.
75. Hosken F. Genital Mutilation of Women in Africa. Munger Africana Library Notes October 1976;36.
76. Morgan R, Steinem G. The International Crime of Genital Mutilation. Ms Magazine March
     1980;65–7,98,110.
77. Burton R. Personal Pilgrimage to Al-Medinah and Mecca, Vol. 2. Dover, 1962:110.
78. Doughty C. Travels in Arabia Deserta. Random House, 1920:170.
79. Byrk F. Circumcision in Man and Woman. New York: American Ethnological Press, 1934:137.
80. Remondino P. History of Circumcision, Philadelphia: FA. Davis, 1891:55.
81. Montagu A. Ritual Mutilation Among Primitive Peoples. Ciba Symposium, October 1946;424.
82. Montagu A. The Origins of Subincision in Australia. Oceania 1937;8:193–207.

83. Montagu A. Coming into Being Among the Australian Aborigines. London: Routledge & Kegan Paul, 1974:312–25.
84. Montagu A. Infibulation and Defibulation in the Old and New Worlds. Am. Anthropologist 1945;47:464–7.
85. Hosken F. The Hosken Report on Genital and Sexual Mutilation of Females, 2nd Edition. Lexington, Mass.: Women's International Network News, 1979.
86. Hosken F. Genital Mutilation of Women in Africa. Munger Africana Library Notes October 1976;36.
87. Morgan R, Steinem G. The International Crime of Genital Mutilation. Ms Magazine March 1980;65–7,98,110.
88. Hosken F. The Hosken Report on Genital and Sexual Mutilation of Females, 2nd Edition. Lexington, Mass.: Women's International Network News, 1979.
89. Widstrand C. Female Infibulation. Studia Ethnographica Upsaliensa 1965;20:95–122.
90. Mustafa A. J. Obstet. Gynaec. Brit. Cwlth. 1966;73:302–6.
91. Hosken F. The Hosken Report on Genital and Sexual Mutilation of Females, 2nd Edition. Lexington, Mass.: Women's International Network News, 1979.
92. Montagu A. Infibulation and Defibulation in the Old and New Worlds. Am. Anthropologist 1945;47:464–7.
93. Montagu A. The Origins of Subincision in Australia. Oceania 1937;8:193–207.
94. Montagu A. Ritual Mutilation Among Primitive Peoples. Ciba Symposium, October 1946.
95. Montagu A. Coming into Being Among the Australian Aborigines. London: Routledge & Kegan Paul, 1974:312–25.
96. Byrk F. Circumcision in Man and Woman. New York: American Ethnological Press, 1934:137.
97. Hosken F. The Hosken Report on Genital and Sexual Mutilation of Females, 2nd Edition. Lexington, Mass.: Women's International Network News, 1979.
98. Hosken F. Genital Mutilation of Women in Africa. Munger Africana Library Notes October 1976;36.
99. Morgan R, Steinem G. The International Crime of Genital Mutilation. Ms Magazine March 1980;65–7,98,110.
100. Montagu A. Infibulation and Defibulation in the Old and New Worlds. Am. Anthropologist 1945;47:464–7.
101. Textor R. A Cross-Cultural Summary. New Haven: HRAF Press, 1967.
102. Reich W. The Mass Psychology of Fascism. New York: Farrar, Straus & Giroux, 1970.
103. Reich W. The Sexual Revolution. New York: Octagon Books, 1971.
104. Reich W. People in Trouble. New York: Farrar, Straus & Giroux, 1976.
105. Frankl G. Failure of the Sexual Revolution. London: Khan & Averill, 1974.
106. Stern M. Sex in the USSR. New York: Times Books, 1979.
107. Hansson C, Liden K. Moscow Women: Thirteen Interviews. Pantheon, 1983.
108. Stafford P. Sexual Behavior in the Communist World. New York: Julian Press, 1967.
109. Accad E. The Social Position of Women in North Africa and the Arab World. in: Veil of Shame. Sherbrooke, Quebec: Editions Naaman, 1978.
110. Beck L, Keddie N. Women in the Muslim World. Cambridge: Harvard U. Press, 1978.
111. Accad E. The Social Position of Women in North Africa and the Arab World. in: Veil of Shame. Sherbrooke, Quebec: Editions Naaman, 1978.
112. Murray J. The Kikuyu Female Circumcision Controversy. Dissertation, UCLA, 1974.
113. Kenyata J. Facing Mt. Kenya. New York: Vintage, 1965:125–48.
114. Remondino P. History of Circumcision, Philadelphia: FA. Davis, 1891:98–9.
115. Hosken F. The Hosken Report on Genital and Sexual Mutilation of Females, 2nd Edition. Lexington, Mass.: Women's International Network News, 1979.
116. Leavitt JE, ed. The Battered Child: Selected Readings. General Learning, 1974.
117. Helfer RE, Kempe CH, eds. The Battered Child. U. Chicago Press, 1974.
118. Herbruck CC. Breaking the Cycle of Child Abuse. Winston Press, 1979.
119. Harlow H. Love in Infant Monkeys. San Francisco, 1959 (reprinted in Scientific American, June 1959;200:68.
120. Harlow H. The Human Model: Primate Perspectives. Washington DC: V.H. Winston, 1979.
121. Mitchell G. What Monkeys Can Tell Us About Human Violence. Futurist April 1975;75–80.
122. Reich W. Reich Speaks of Freud. New York: Farrar, Straus & Giroux, 1967:27–31.
123. Reich W. The Mass Psychology of Fascism. New York: Farrar, Straus & Giroux, 1970.
124. Reich W. The Sexual Revolution. New York: Octagon Books, 1971.
125. Reich W. Ether, God & Devil. New York: Farrar, Straus & Giroux, 1973:67–70.
126. Reich W. People in Trouble. New York: Farrar, Straus & Giroux, 1976.
127. Prescott J. Body Pleasure and the Origins of Violence. Futurist April 1975;64–74.
128. Prescott J. Deprivation of Physical Affection as a Primary Process in the Development of Physical Violence. In: Gil D. ed. Child Abuse and Violence. New York: AMS Press, 1979:66–137.

129. Prescott J. Affectional Bonding for the Prevention of Violent Behaviors. In: Hertzberg LJ, et al. eds. Violent Behavior: Assessment and Intervention (Vol.1). New York: PMA Publishing, 1989:109–142.
130. DeMeo J. On The Origins and Diffusion of Patrism: The Saharasian Connection, Dissertation, U. of Kansas, Geography Department, 1986.
131. DeMeo J. The Origins and Diffusion of Patrism in Saharasia, 4000 BCE: Evidence for a Worldwide, Climate-Linked Geographical Pattern in Human Behavior. World Futures March-May 1991;30:247–71.
132. DeMeo J. On the Origins and Diffusion of Patrism: The Saharasian Connection, Dissertation, U. of Kansas, Geography Department, 1986. Xerox available from Natural Energy Works, P.O. Box 1148, Ashland, Oregon 97520. Book version under preparation, 1997.

2

A SHORT HISTORY OF THE INSTITUTIONALIZATION OF INVOLUNTARY SEXUAL MUTILATION IN THE UNITED STATES

Frederick Hodges

For the past 130 years, the American medical industry has been involved in the business of removing part or all of the external sexual organs of male and female children. While the origin of sexual mutilation among prehistoric primitive peoples is a matter for theory and speculation, the origin and spread of sexual mutilation in American medical practice can be precisely documented. Seen in the proper context of the entire scope of Western history, the modern American enigma of institutionalized sexual mutilation is an historic aberration of profound significance and degree, one that could never have been predicted, and one that perhaps could not have been avoided.

1. MODERNIZATION

The introduction and spread of institutionalized secular sexual mutilation was a response to the tremendous social and cultural anxieties engendered by the effects of the rapid modernization and industrialization of the early decades of the Nineteenth Century. As the traditional rural agrarian-based economy was transformed into an urbanized capitalist economy, parallel changes occurred in social structure, governmental and nongovernmental institutions, demographics, and technology. One significant result of these changes was the ascendancy of the middle class to positions of economic and political power. The emergent middle class was now in a position to reinterpret social mores and redefine the individual for all of society.

As an outgrowth of the middle class, the medical establishment reflected and validated these social changes and offered treatment for the anxieties they inevitably produced, thereby laying the foundations of the modern Therapeutic State — defined by Thomas Szasz as the political order in which social controls are legitimized by the ideology of health.[1] For instance, in traditional agrarian society, adulthood was considered to begin at puberty. Industrialized, middle-class society extended the boundaries of childhood by more than a decade so that middle-class males could receive the specialized pro-

Sexual Mutilations: A Human Tragedy, edited by Denniston and Milos
Plenum Press, New York, 1997

fessional and academic training required by a modern industrialized society. The formidable anxieties produced by these social changes found expression in an intensified focus on childhood sexuality. In conformity with middle-class social mores, physicians theorized that childhood should be a period of complete asexuality, and, consequently, that children should be kept ignorant of sexual and reproductive information until delayed marriage. The functional significance of this change was that young people, who in previous generations had been expected to marry and commence sexual activity in early adolescence, were now expected to delay commencement of sexual activity until they were in their twenties. Young people who were unable to suppress their sexual drive were subjected not only to societal censure but to medical intervention as well.

2.1. Degenerative Theory of Disease and the Reflex Neurosis Theory of Disease

For reasons unrelated to the rise of the American middle-class, two French physicians in the 1820s, Xavier Bichat (1771–1802)[2] and François Broussais (1771–1838),[3] developed a new model of disease — the *Degenerative Theory of Disease*. This model postulated that the human body was allotted a finite amount of vital energy which could either be conserved through correct living or permanently lost through wrong living. Energy depletion led to degeneration, which in turn led to the production of disease. Middle-class American physicians readily adopted this theory, but they expanded it to imply that manifestations of sexuality necessarily represented life-threatening losses of vital energy. Non-procreative use of the sexual organs, even within marriage, was viewed as dangerous. The result was the formulation of the *Reflex Neurosis Theory of Disease*, which postulated that the sexual organs and the erotic sensations they produced were the cause of all human disease. To validate this theory, American physicians redefined normal human sexual behavior, reproductive anatomy, and sexual function in terms of pathology.

2.1.1. Pathologization of Sexual Behavior. The pathologization of normal sexual behavior resulted in the masturbation hysteria. The term *masturbation* was frequently used in a generalized way to describe any sexual activity outside the context of heterosexual marital coitus for the purpose of procreation, but, in practice, a diagnosis of masturbation generally followed discovery of a child's either having sexually stimulated himself or having engaged in sexual behavior with another person. Physicians relied on specious logic to support the pathologization of sexual behavior. Clinical interviews with patients suffering from what would today be ascribed to the effects of malnutrition, overwork, venereal disease, bacterial infections, mental disorders, or tobacco and alcohol poisoning, invariably revealed a past history of masturbatory activity. On this basis, it was concluded that masturbation had brought on these pathological conditions. The inhabitants of the United States were at first reluctant to accept the theory that masturbation was harmful. Many resisted interference on the part of physicians in the private lives of their children, but the rising flood of medical journal articles that allegedly proved the harm of masturbation empowered physicians to meet this resistance with determination.

2.1.2. Pathologization of Sexual Anatomy. In order to validate the *Reflex Neurosis Theory of Disease*, physicians were compelled to pathologize the three distinguishing qualities of the immature juvenile foreskin, e.g., generous length, adherence to the glans, and narrowness of the preputial orifice, under the general diagnosis of *phimosis*. Physicians coined the term *congenital phimosis* to specify that the adhesion of the foreskin to the glans in infants was, in fact, a congenital birth defect. They adopted the term *acquired phimosis* to indicate a fictitious condition in which a previously unadhered foreskin became adhered as a result of masturbation. The term *hypertrophic phimosis,* or *redundancy*, indicated a type of phimosis whose sole symptom was a foreskin that was arbitrarily determined to be too long.

Since the foreskin is the most highly innervated part of the penis, and since masturbation in genitally intact boys generally involves manually stimulating and manipulating the foreskin as well as manually sliding the mobile sheath of the penile skin over the shaft (a wide range of motion made possible by the double fold of the foreskin), masturbation was seen as a cause of reflex disease through the medium of the foreskin. In the absence of the *Germ Theory of Disease,* those American physicians who did not see masturbation alone as the primary cause of disease attributed bacterial, viral, and fungal diseases, as well as the pathological symptoms of malnutrition and overwork, to phimosis. Even in the absence of a diagnosis of phimosis, the foreskin itself was inculpated as a cause of disease. Phimosis in females, defined as an adherence of the clitoral prepuce to the clitoris, was viewed in the same light.

2.1.3. Pathologization of Sexual Function. In accordance with the *Reflex Theory of Disease*, erotic sensation was redefined as *irritation,* orgasm was redefined as *convulsion*, and erection of the penis was redefined as *priapism.* Physicians argued that these manifestations of sexual function were both symptoms and causes of disease, and, likewise, that stimulation of the genitals could cause disease in distant parts of the body such as the heart, brain, back, digestive organs, and eye.

The pathologization of normal male sexual function led first to the 'discovery' of *spermatorrhea.* Physicians defined spermatorrhea as a serious venereal disease whose sole symptom was the ejaculation of sperm under any condition other than connubial bliss. The release of sperm due to nocturnal emissions or masturbation was now classified as a venereal disease as dangerous as any other, if not more dangerous because more people suffered from it more often. Hundreds of case reports published in medical journals world-wide proved, to the satisfaction of most physicians, the harm of spermatorrhea. French physicians such as Claude-François Lallemand (1790–1853) and Léopold Deslandes (1797–1852)[4] were the acknowledged world authorities on the treatment of spermatorrhea. They stuck long steel rods, also known as *bougies,* up the urethra, and, using silver nitrate, cauterized the urethra, prostate, and seminal vesicles in order to prevent the production and loss of sperm. In 1836, Lallemand also advised amputation of the foreskin in the most difficult cases of spermatorrhea as a way of preventing masturbation.[5]

In the United States, Lallemand's use of circumcision caught the attention of Edward H. Dixon (1808–1880). In his 1845 book, *A Treatise on Diseases of the Sexual Organs,* Dixon revealed himself to be one of the first North American advocates of both therapeutic foreskin amputation and universal imposition of the ancient Hebrew rite of infant circumcision.[6] Dixon claimed that phimosis, which he defined as an elongation of the foreskin, was the primary cause of most serious diseases. For a time, the American medical establishment ignored Dixon and Lallemand's advocacy of circumcision. Circumcision was forgotten for the next two decades while other surgical treatments for masturbation, phimosis, and spermatorrhea were developed.

2.2. Castration

Since surgical amputation of body parts in general was considered thoroughly modern and advanced, physicians experimented with specific amputations of the sexual organs to treat masturbation. On June 22, 1842, the *Boston Medical and Surgical Journal* reported that Dr. Winslow Lewis of Boston had severed and tied the left spermatic artery of a young man being treated for "excessive masturbation."[7] In 1843, however, one of the first reports of castration for masturbation was published by Dr. Josiah Crosby of Meredith Bridge, New Hampshire.[8] After cathartics and emetics had failed to cure a 22-year-old youth whose health had reportedly been ruined by masturbation, Crosby castrated the boy and pronounced him cured. The American medical profession responded with interest. Two years later, in 1845, Dr. Samuel McMinn published in the pages of the *Boston Medical and Surgical Journal* a revolutionary case report of an insane woman living outside Tuscaloosa, Alabama, who had taken a razor and amputated "the whole of her external organs of generation." McMinn arrived at the scene and fully expected the woman to die from her massive wounds, but she survived. As her wounds healed, her reason miraculously returned. Fascinated by this development, McMinn speculated:

> And the results of this case may suggest a remedy. Whether it was the great loss of blood, the removal of the external organs and the counter-irritation consequent, that cured the patient, is a question for the consideration of the profession.[9]

The title he gave to his report, however, betrayed his and, presumably, the journal editor's opinion on the source of the cure. The report was dramatically entitled "Insanity Cured by Excision of the External Organs of Generation."

Ten years later, in 1855, Dr. William T. Taylor published a similar report involving a cigar-maker from Philadelphia who had gone insane and then hacked off his penis and testicles with a broken bottle.[10] Although he bled profusely, his wounds healed, and, miraculously, his reason was completely restored. No further proof was needed. A revolutionary new medical response to masturbatory insanity had been established just as the innovation of aseptic surgery was developing. Orthodox American medicine now embarked upon the wholesale amputation of the sexual organs as a cure for seemingly unrelated diseases. Insane asylums castrated inmates on a massive scale to prevent their masturbating and, ostensibly, to cure their insanity. Until the beginning of the Twentieth Century, boys who had been caught masturbating were frequently committed to insane asylums, circumcised, castrated, and shackled in their cells.[11-12] Females were likewise subjected to "female castration," a surgery involving removal of the ovaries, with the intent of curing them of hysteria, epilepsy, or nymphomania.

2.3. Spermectomy, Neurectomy, and Other Treatments

Various other surgeries for masturbation were developed in order to destroy sexual desire. The operation of spermectomy was developed as a less drastic alternative to castration, and consisted of the surgical removal of the spermatic ducts rather than the testicles.[13] Neurectomy also had a certain vogue in the 1890s. In this operation, commonly performed on boys who had been caught masturbating, the physician severed the dorsal nerves of the penis in order to destroy penile sensation and function completely and permanently.[14-15] American physicians also resorted to relatively less drastic measures such as slitting open the urethra,[16] cauterizing the prostate,[17] inflicting corporal punishment,[18] blistering the penis raw with caustic acids,[19] flaying the penile skin with razor blades,[20] sewing the prepuce shut with metal wire,[21] encasing the genitals in plaster[22] or in lockable metal cages,[23] or fitting the penis with penile rings studded with sharp metallic teeth to discourage erections.[24]

For females, the preferred method of treatment for epilepsy and masturbation was clitoridectomy. One of the very first reports of therapeutic clitoridectomy was published in the *San Francisco Medical Press* in 1862. An abstract of the report read:

> Dr. E. S. Cooper, Editor of the *San Francisco Medical Press*, relates two cases of removal by the scalpel of the clitoris in young girls who were inveterately addicted to the habit of masturbation, and for whom there was apparently no other alternative but hopeless insanity or an early grave. The result was a perfect cure in one case, and in the other the practice was broken up, and all the mental faculties improved except the memory, which is not restored.[25]

In the late 1860s, the British physician Isaac Baker Brown developed and promoted clitoridectomy as a cure for epilepsy. His claims of miracle cures through clitoridectomy led to the universal adoption of clitoridectomy in the English-speaking world as a cure for epilepsy, hysteria, and masturbation. In 1867, Dr. Baker Brown's conduct was called into question, and the London Obstetrical Society ordered him to cease performing the surgery. Although few doubted the proven value of clitoridectomy, Baker Brown was charged with failing to provide informed consent to his female patients. It was his method to chloroform and clitoridectomize all females who came into his clinic regardless of their ailment. The British medical press was unanimously in favor of banning Baker Brown from performing surgery, but he was vigorously defended in the American medical press. The editor of the New York-based journal, the *Medical Record*, strongly criticized the anti-clitoridectomy crusade in England, demanding to know, "What now will be the chance of recovery for the poor epileptic female with a clitoris?"[26]

3. CIRCUMCISION AS THERAPY

On December 1, 1855, English physician Jonathan Hutchinson (1828–1913) published his famous paper, "On the Influence of Circumcision in Preventing Syphilis."[27] During the 1850s, London experienced a massive immigration of Jews from the ghettos of Eastern Europe. Hutchinson reported that, at the Metropolitan Free Hospital located in London's immigrant Jewish slum, fewer Jews than Englishmen sought treatment for syphilis. Being innocent of any understanding of the principles of statistical analysis, epidemiology, the *Germ Theory of Disease,* or the quarantine effect of the ghetto, Hutchinson speciously argued that only circumcision could account for the difference in disease rates. Hutchinson's paper was widely reprinted in foreign medical journals. Two years later, it was used as evidence in a religious tribunal. In 1857, a certain Dr. Levit, a Viennese Jew, under the influence of his Western education and, perhaps, the anti-circumcision movement within Reform Judaism, refused to allow his newborn son to be circumcised. The local Rabbinate, under the direction of Dr. Joseph Hirschfeld, held up Hutchinson's paper as evidence of the medical indications for circumcision and as sufficient justification for the Rabbinate to seize custody of Levit's son and forcibly circumcise the child. Levit was left without legal recourse to protect his own son.[28]

On the strength of Hutchinson's paper, the concept of circumcision as a therapeutic intervention now made a cautious reappearance in orthodox American medicine. At the

August 12, 1861, meeting of the Boston Society for Medical Improvement, a Dr. White presented a paper in which he mentioned that circumcision could prevent masturbation.[29] Seven years later, in 1868, Dr. Charles Bliss of Syracuse, New York, published an account of his successes in curing masturbation by partial amputation of the prepuce.[30] In 1869, a learned article appeared by the Baltimore physician, A. B. Arnold, describing the history of circumcision in the religious and tribal context of Jews, Muslims, and African animists.[31] This new surgery was now legitimized by placing it in the context of a long history, albeit an Asiatic, non-Western history.

3.1. The American Medical Association

Hailed in his lifetime as the father of orthopedics and indeed as one of "the most distinguished benefactors whom the American medical profession has produced for the glory of medicine and the good of mankind,"[32] Dr. Lewis A. Sayre (1820–1900) was certainly among the most distinguished believers in the therapeutic powers of circumcision. Sayre served as vice-president of the American Medical Association in 1870 and eventually as president in 1880. At the 1870 meeting of the American Medical Association, Vice-President Sayre delivered a remarkable paper, "Partial Paralysis from Reflex Irritation, Caused by Congenital Phimosis and Adherent Prepuce."[33] Supporting his claims with numerous case studies, and, using the most scientific methodology available at the time, Sayre proved to the satisfaction of his audience that a long, adherent foreskin was not only the cause of paralysis, but also hip-joint disease (tuberculosis of the hip joint), hernia, bad digestion, inflammation of the bladder, and clumsiness. In each case, Sayre reported that amputation of the foreskin had cured the disease. Throughout his career, Sayre urged physicians to examine the penis in all cases of childhood diseases. When phimosis, as defined by reflex theory, was found, Sayre advised immediate preputial amputation. Because of Sayre's professional reputation and impeccable credentials, major American medical schools readily adopted his theories of reflex disease and phimosis into their curricula.

During the late 1860s and throughout the next decade, epilepsy increasingly became the focus of national attention, as indicated by the dramatic increase in the number of scientific publications on epilepsy. Capitalizing on the epilepsy hysteria, Sayre reported to the New York Pathological Society, in 1870, that phimosis was the cause of epilepsy.[34] A few English physicians had been experimenting with circumcision to treat epilepsy since 1865,[35] but they connected the foreskin to masturbation and cited the prevention of masturbation as playing a role in the cure of epilepsy. Sayre maintained that a long foreskin, all by itself, had the power to induce violent epileptic convulsions, and that circumcision had cured every case of epilepsy. As with paralysis, hundreds of case reports were published over the next 75 years, validating Sayre's advocacy of circumcision to cure epilepsy.

At the 1875 meeting of the American Medical Association, Sayre delivered another important lecture on phimosis. He informed his audience that he had discovered that a long, adherent foreskin could cut off circulation to the spinal column and thereby cause lameness, curvature of the spine, paralysis of the bladder, and club-feet.[36] Miraculously, he reported, circumcision brought immediate cure to all patients, including the patient with club-feet. In the same lecture, he also presented several cases in which clitoridectomy brought instantaneous cure to paralytic girls.

3.2. The Masturbation Hysteria and Circumcision

The masturbation hysteria continued unabated throughout the last decades of the Nineteenth Century. From 1800 to the early 1870s, there was an astounding 750% increase in the number of medical journal articles on masturbation. From the 1870s to the 1880s, the number of articles on masturbation increased by 25% and, from the 1880s until 1900, the rate of increase was augmented to 30%. Among the more influential physicians who noticed this dramatic increased focus on masturbation and contributed to it were Abraham Jacobi and M. J. Moses. Jacobi (1830–1919) was the President and founder of the American Pediatric Society, the first Chairman of the Section on Diseases of Children of the American Medical Association, President of the New York State Medical Society, President of the New York Academy of Medicine, and President of the Association of American Physicians. Both Jacobi and Moses claimed that Jews were immune to masturbation solely because they were circumcised, and that non-Jews were especially prone to masturbation and to the horrible diseases that resulted from masturbation solely because they had a foreskin. Moses' and Jacobi's authoritative studies, alleging that the foreskin caused epilepsy, paralysis, malnutrition, hysteria, and other nervous disorders, were cited by medical writers for the next few decades.[37]

In 1871, Moses published an exceedingly influential, and widely-cited article, "The Value of Circumcision as a Hygienic and Therapeutic Measure," in the *New York Medical Journal*. Moses stated, in part:

> As an Israelite, I desire to ventilate the subject, and, as a physician, have chosen the medium of a medical journal, that I may not be trammelled in my expressions, as I necessarily would be were I confined to the pages of an ordinary paper....I refer to masturbation as one of the effects of a long prepuce; not that this vice is entirely absent in those who have undergone circumcision, though I never saw an instance in a Jewish child of very tender years, except as the result of association with children whose covered glans have naturally impelled them to the habit.[38]

It is quite clear from the context that the title word "Hygienic" has a different meaning than it does today. At that time, circumcisers used words such as hygiene to denote moral hygiene, not personal hygiene. Moses' paper made a big impact on American physicians who now argued that castration should be abandoned in favor of circumcision since circumcision cured all the same diseases as castration but did not affect procreation, as demonstrated by the example of the Jews. An article that appeared in the *Medical Record* in 1895 explained the anti-masturbation theory of circumcision thus:

> In all cases [of masturbation],....circumcision is undoubtedly the physicians' closest friend and ally....To obtain the best results one must cut away enough skin and mucous membrane to rather put it on the stretch when erections come later. There must be no play in the skin after the wound has thoroughly healed, but it must fit tightly over the penis, for should there be any play the patient will be found to readily resume his practice, not begrudging the time and extra energy required to produce the orgasm. It is true, however, that the longer it takes to have an orgasm, the less frequently it will be attempted, consequently the greater the benefit gained.[39]

3.3. More Miracle Cures

The list of previously incurable diseases that orthodox physicians now claimed to have cured through circumcision continued to grow. An 1895 textbook declared:

Only within recent years, since the physiology of nervous reflexes has become better understood, has [circumcision] become a generally accepted operation with thinking surgeons. Not alone for local conditions is the operation demanded. In all cases in which male children are suffering nerve tension, confirmed derangement of the digestive organs, restlessness, irritability, and other disturbances of the nervous system, even to chorea, convulsions, and paralysis, or where through nerve waste the nutritive facilities of the general system are below par and structural diseases are occurring it should be considered as among the lines of treatment to be pursued.[40]

Thousands of such reports were published in reputable American medical journals. In 1890, Dr. William D. Gentry (1836–1922) published a typical report, "Nervous Derangements Produced by Sexual Irregularities in Boys," which detailed the frightening and varied consequences of phimosis as well as the miracle cure to be found in circumcision.

Whilst I was physician to the Children's home at Kansas City, in 1884–5, there was brought to the Home from some similar institution in Chicago, a child two years and a half old, who was blind, deaf and dumb. It was nervous, fretful, and caused the matron a great deal of trouble. It was dwarfed and presented the peculiar general appearance which nearly every boy will present who is afflicted with sexual derangement. As soon as I saw the child the thought came into my mind that his trouble had some connection with such derangement, and on making an examination found that he had phimosis. With the consent of the father of the boy, I operated, and removed the derangement. In two months the child could see and make sounds as if trying to speak. In six months he could hear, see and speak.[41]

3.4. Anti-Sexual Nature of Circumcision

The early promoters of circumcision fully acknowledged the sexual functions of the foreskin and advocated circumcision as an intentional destruction of those functions. One of many such acknowledgments was published in the November 3, 1900, issue of *Medical News*:

Finally, circumcision probably tends to increase the power of sexual control. The only physiological advantage which the prepuce can be supposed to confer is that of maintaining the penis in a condition susceptible to more acute sensation than would otherwise exist. It may increase the pleasure of coition and the impulse to it: but these are advantages which in the present state of society can well be spared. If in their loss increase in sexual control should result, one should be thankful.[42]

In 1902, an editorial in *Medical News*, made clear the anti-sexual motivation behind the doctrine of circumcision as a hygienic measure.

Another advantage of circumcision...is the lessened liability to masturbation. A long foreskin is irritating per se, as it necessitates more manipulation of the parts in bathing....This leads the child to handle the parts, and as a rule, pleasurable sensations are elicited from the extremely sensitive mucous membrane, with resultant manipulation and masturbation. The exposure of the glans penis following circumcision...lessens the sensitiveness of the organ....It therefore lies with the physicians, the family adviser in affairs hygienic and medical, to urge its acceptance.[43]

4. EARLY TWENTIETH CENTURY

After the *Germ Theory of Disease* had become widely accepted and vitamins had been identified, most microbial diseases, such as tuberculosis, were silently removed from the list of diseases caused by phimosis. Still, the majority of American physicians tenaciously clung to the belief that phimosis was the cause of diseases, such as epilepsy, that were not yet properly understood. Year by year, the list of diseases caused by phimosis continued to grow. Physicians even attributed death to phimosis.[44]

4.1. Abraham L. Wolbarst and the Cancer Scare

In the January 19, 1914, issue of the *Journal of the American Medical Association*, Dr. Abraham L. Wolbarst (1872–1952), a urologist practicing, among other places, at Beth Israel Hospital and the Jewish Memorial Hospital in New York, published the first of a series of papers indicting the foreskin as a cause of disease. This marked the start of a nearly forty-year crusade for mass involuntary circumcision. Wolbarst was a prominent and influential member of both the American Medical Association and the notorious American Society of Sanitary and Moral Prophylaxis, a reform organization committed to the abolition of extra-marital and childhood sexuality. His views on sexuality were characteristically extreme. For example, in the 1930s, Wolbarst argued that adult masturbators should be sterilized and forbidden to marry.[45] In his 1914 paper, "Universal Circumcision as a Sanitary Measure," Wolbarst stated:

> [I]t is generally accepted that irritation derived from a tight prepuce may be followed by nervous phenomena, among these being convulsions and outbreaks resembling epilepsy. It is therefore not at all improbable that in many infants who die in convulsions, the real cause of death is a long or tight prepuce.[46]

Wolbarst also added that:

> It is the moral duty of every physician to encourage circumcision in the young....[47]

From the context of his paper, it is clear that the title word "Sanitary" denotes morality rather than the absence of germs or dirt. It is important to note that, until this time, circumcision was primarily used as therapy for children and adults, but not as prophylaxis for infants. As a result of Wolbarst's ceaseless lobbying, the radical notion of universal, non-therapeutic, involuntary neonatal circumcision slowly gained acceptance among American physicians. Medical textbooks were rewritten to instruct obstetricians and pediatricians to examine the penis of every newborn boy to determine if the foreskin was retractable. If not, it was advised that it be immediately amputated.

By the mid-1930s, when most physicians had converted to the theory that epilepsy was a problem of the brain, Wolbarst continued to insist that epilepsy and convulsions were caused by a tight foreskin.[48] While never abandoning this theory, Wolbarst must have sensed the need to reformulate his arguments to appeal to the changing interests of the public. In the early decades of the Twentieth Century, the number of popular magazine articles on epilepsy had steadily dwindled. The number of articles on cancer, however, had risen dramatically, reflecting a shift in national focus. The *Reader's Guide to Periodical Literature* listed thirteen articles in popular magazines under the "cancer" entry between 1900 and 1904. By 1909, the number had doubled, and by 1928, the number of popular articles on cancer had increased by 569% since 1900. At a peak in this surge of national concern over cancer, Wolbarst published the definitive paper on circumcision as preventive of penile cancer in 1932. Based on his contention that Jews were immune to penile cancer, Wolbarst theorized that penile cancer was caused by "the accumulation of pathogenic products in the preputial cavity."[49] No scientific validation was offered in support of this idea, yet based on this paper, the theory that smegma was a carcinogen became widely accepted as fact in the United States.

4.2. Advances in Foreskin Anatomy and Development

In 1932, a research team at the University of Pennsylvania, led by Dr. H. C. Bazett, published a detailed anatomical description of the innervation of the foreskin. They noted that the foreskin was richly innervated and capable of detecting very fine distinctions of touch and temperature.[50] In the following year, Dr. Glenn A. Deibert, of the Daniel Baugh Institute of Anatomy at Jefferson Medical College, made a careful investigation of the development of the foreskin in utero and the process of separation of the foreskin from the glans after birth.[51] Deibert demonstrated that the adherence of the foreskin to the glans was not phimosis or a birth defect, but a normal stage of penile development. In 1935, the British anatomist, Richard H. Hunter, of the Department of Anatomy at Queen's University in Belfast, similarly published a detailed description of the embryological development of the foreskin. Perhaps because their findings did not support the current view of the foreskin as a useless, pathogenic defect, all three studies were ignored by the American medical establishment.[52]

4.3. Invention of the Gomco Clamp

The profit margin for circumcision rose with the mass-manufacture and widespread distribution of the now ubiquitous Gomco Clamp, first invented in 1934 by Aaron Goldstein and Dr. Hiram S. Yellen. Gomco is an acronym for the *GO*ldstein *M*anufacturing *CO*mpany, which later changed its name to the Gomco Surgical Manufacturing Corporation of Buffalo, New York. This steel device is still widely used today to crush the male baby's foreskin prior to its amputation. The standardization of surgical technique made possible the more rapid institutionalization of circumcision.

4.4. Popular Perceptions

The September 1941 issue of *Parents' Magazine* contained the first article on routine circumcision that had ever appeared in a popular magazine of such wide distribution. The author, Dr. Alan F. Guttmacher, an obstetrician at Johns Hopkins University Medical School, presented the public with many of the same myths and scare tactics that had been in use since the Nineteenth Century. For instance, Guttmacher admitted that "circumcision causes blunting of male-sexual sensitivity,"[53] but argued that this was an advantage. In addition to mentioning Wolbarst's relatively new myth regarding penile cancer, Guttmacher presented the public with a myth of his own invention, one that had never appeared in the medical literature, and one that directly contradicted the scientific findings of Deibert and Hunter. With the authority of his professional title and institutional affiliations, he stated to the American people, as fact, that:

Present-day hygiene requires that the prepuce, the hoodlike fold of skin which covers the end of the penis (glans) be drawn back daily and the uncovered glans thoroughly washed. Trouble occurs if this is neglected, for the secretion from the multiple glands lining the inside of the hood becomes caked, and within a few days the material may set up an inflammation. Such inflammation may lead to the growth of slender, strandlike bands of tissue between the inside of the prepuce and the glans, gluing the two together, thus forming an adherent foreskin.[54]

To avert this frightening scenario, Guttmacher advised the public to let their children be circumcised at birth because it "makes care of the infant's genitals easier for the mother," and because it "does not necessitate handling of the penis by the infant's mother, or the child himself in later years, and therefore does not focus the male's attention on his own genitals. Masturbation is considered less likely."[55] Guttmacher's article sought to validate the perceived associations between the foreskin, difficult hygiene, inevitable masturbation, genital defects, and taboo handling of the boy's penis. It also served to legitimize, for the benefit of the public, the increasingly common practice of large urban hospitals instituting programs of involuntary circumcision of the newborn.

4.5. Abraham Ravich and Cancer of the Prostate and Cervix

In 1942, expanding upon Wolbarst's theory of smegma as a carcinogen, and repeating the myth of Jewish immunity to disease, Abraham Ravich (1889–1984), a urologist at Israel Zion Hospital in Brooklyn and one of the Twentieth Century's most active crusaders for mass involuntary circumcision, postulated a causal link between the foreskin and prostate cancer. He also restated the obscure theory (proposed without scientific documentation in 1926[56]) that cervical cancer of the female was caused by male smegma.[57] The popular news magazine, *Newsweek*, reported Ravich's claim and quoted his demand that there "be an even more universal practice of circumcising male infants."[58] Amended to the long list of achievements he prepared for his entry in *Who's Who in America*, Ravich proudly credited himself with being the first to report on circumcision of newborn males to prevent genital cancers.[59]

5. WORLD WAR II

During World War II, certain military medical doctors instituted a campaign of mass circumcision of soldiers in all branches of the armed forces. Even at the height of the war, Navy physician Lieutenant Marvin L. Gerber confidently stated in the pages of the *United States Naval Medical Bulletin* that circumcision was one of the most commonly performed surgical operations in the Navy, even more commonly performed than trauma surgery.[60] Military medical records alleged that an epidemic of phimosis and paraphimosis among soldiers had justified the mass circumcision campaign. Soldiers were subjected to unannounced inspections of their penises, called "short arm inspections." Soldiers with intact penises were declared "phimotic" and sent off to be circumcised, sometimes under threat of court martial.

5.1. Sexually Transmitted Diseases and the Scapegoating of Blacks

Military documents reveal that Blacks were blamed for spreading venereal disease in the military and were thus especially targeted for involuntary circumcision. Military physicians such as Eugene A. Hand (1909- circa 1972), a dermatologist who practiced during the war at the Naval Hospital at St. Albans, New York, were responsible for the military adopting this view of Blacks as dangerous disease carriers. Another physician, Captain Leonard L. Heimoff, an officer in the Medical Corps of the United States Army, declared that "Negro troops were causing 70 percent of all new cases of venereal disease." Heimoff organized covert military units to monitor the sexual activities of civilian Black communities.[61] Heimoff's report, like that of Hand and others, concluded that Blacks could not be taught to practice personal hygiene and that they could not be trusted to avoid contracting venereal diseases.

The war coincided with an increased national focus on venereal disease. From 1930 to 1940, there was a dramatic 192% increase in the number of popular magazine articles on venereal disease. Following a surge between the years 1941 and 1943, the number of popular articles on venereal disease increased at a rate of 17% from 1940 to 1947, but dropped precipitously thereafter. At the height of the popular hysteria over venereal disease, Hand delivered a paper, entitled "Circumcision and Venereal Disease," at the annual meeting of the American Medical Association, held in Atlantic City on June 12, 1947. Comparing the rates of venereal disease between Jews, Gentiles and Blacks, Hand theorized that circumcision could prevent venereal disease. He wrote:

> Circumcision is not common among Negroes....Many Negroes are promiscuous. In Negroes there is little circumcision, little knowledge or fear of venereal disease and promiscuity in almost a hornet's nest of infection. Thus the venereal rate in Negroes has remained high. Between these two extremes there is the gentile, with a venereal disease rate higher than that of Jews but much lower than that of Negroes.[62]

In the same study, he also found that cancer of the tongue was more common among those with foreskins than among Jews. *Newsweek* reported Hand's sensational findings in detail, thereby increasing the popular perception that a policy of mass involuntary circumcision was both scientifically based and of critical importance for the security of the nation.[63]

5.2. Fate of the Foreskin

In December 1949, the *British Medical Journal* published the landmark study, "The Fate of the Foreskin," by a bright young Cambridge physician, Douglas M. T. Gairdner (1910–1992).[64] Drawing on the embryological and histological research of Deibert and Hunter, and presenting his own meticulous research on preputial adhesion and retractability in children, Gairdner successfully debunked the phimosis myth. Demonstrating that non-retractability, adherence, and length were normal conditions of the juvenile foreskin, Gairdner also confidently debunked all the alleged benefits of circumcision. His paper generated enormous interest among physicians and attracted the interest of the British government. On the basis of Gairdner's findings, the new British National Health Service elected not to pay for neonatal circumcision, causing the rate of neonatal circumcision in Britain to plummet.

6. CORPORATE INSTITUTIONALIZATION OF CIRCUMCISION IN THE COLD WAR ERA

In the United States, however, Gairdner's paper was largely ignored, and the phimosis hysteria continued unabated. Medical textbooks continued to advise obstetricians to examine every newborn boy for a foreskin that was either too long or adherent, and to perform an immediate foreskin amputation if these symptoms of "phimosis" were detected, as they almost always were. In 1953, two obstetricians, Richard L. Miller and Donald C. Snyder, published an influential paper in the *American Journal of Obstetrics and Gynecology*, calling for the immediate circumcision of all newborn males after birth.[65] Ignoring Gairdner and relying heavily upon the writings of Wolbarst, Miller and Snyder argued that 'phimosis' required immediate surgical correction, and that "circumcision will reduce the incidence of onanism [masturbation]," "increase the male libido," and "increase longevity and immunity to nearly all physical and mental illness." They also argued that immediate circumcision following birth was convenient for the doctor and economically in the best interest of the hospital. The leading obstetrical textbooks were rewritten to include Miller and Snyder's arguments.[66]

6.1. New Cancer Scare

The 1950's saw a dramatic increase in the national focus on cancer. While the focus on cancer had abated considerably during the war, the number of articles on cancer appearing in popular magazines increased 182% from 1943 to 1951. From 1951 to 1955, the number of articles increased by 32%, and from 1955 to 1957, the rate increased by another 72%. In timing with this renewed and dramatically increased popular focus, Ravich published another paper in 1951, "Prophylaxis of Cancer of the Prostate, Penis, and Cervix by Circumcision," alleging that 25 thousand cancer deaths each year were caused by the foreskin and that 3 to 8 million American men then living had contracted prostate cancer as a result of having a foreskin. Ravich concluded that a program of mass involuntary circumcision was necessary as an "important public health measure."[67] Dr. Ernest L. Wynder of Manhattan's Memorial Center for Cancer and Allied Diseases took up Ravich's theory of cervical cancer. In 1954, he published a lengthy paper that purported to show that universal male neonatal circumcision could prevent cervical cancer in women.[68] The popular news magazine, *Time*, published a detailed article of Wynder's study, thereby reinforcing popular support and acquiescence to the activities of the burgeoning circumcision industry.[69]

Meanwhile, there were repeated calls for routine female circumcision at birth. In the 1950s, American physicians stepped up their efforts to make adult female circumcision more widely practiced. In 1959, Dr. W. G. Rathmann of Ingelwood, California, published an important article promoting wide-scale female circumcision as a cure for psychosomatic illness and marital problems. He also took the occasion to tout his newly patented female circumcision clamp.[70]

6.2. Kaiser, Gomco, and Europe

Increasing numbers of corporation-run American hospitals and private insurance companies in large urban centers entered into the profitable routine neonatal circumcision business. Private hospitals instituted policies of immediate and automatic circumcision of all male neonates in the delivery room. For instance, in 1950, at Kaiser Foundation Hospital in Oakland, California (flagship of Kaiser Foundation, one of the oldest and largest health management organizations in the United States), out of 889 live male births, 812 (92.1%) were circumcised immediately after birth.[71] Likewise, many urban hospitals adopted policies of circumcising all genitally intact boys during other operative procedures such as tonsillectomy.

In the late 1950s, the American circumcision industry began efforts to spread circumcision to Europe. Of all European countries, East and West Germany were most often targeted for circumcision propaganda from the United States. Around 1957, the Gomco Surgical Manufacturing Corporation established a European distribution network headquartered in the West German city of Ulm.[72] In the same year, Kaiser Foundation Hospital representatives worked with Otto Dietz, a minor communist official in the East Berlin Secret Police, to promote the mass circumcision of German babies.[73] In 1959, 150 German babies born in a state-run clinic in the West German city of Darmstadt were experimentally circumcised without anesthesia as a promotion for the Gomco Clamp.[74] In 1963, Dr. H. Koester arranged for the maternity clinic at the University of Gießen to adopt a policy of mass circumcision by Gomco clamp of all German boys born there.[75] By 1968, arrangements were made for 2,832 East German babies to be circumcised as a promotion for the Gomco clamp.[76]

In the early 1970s, however, circumcision met with increasing disfavor among medical officials in both East and West Germany, and the circumcision experiments came to an end. Meanwhile, Gomco promoters had moved into Denmark and arranged for 18 Danish newborns to be circumcised in 1973.[77] Along with publicity photographs of the Gomco clamp, the results were published in glowing terms in the Danish medical press. The Danish people, however, strenuously resisted the idea of allowing their children's sexual organs to be surgically altered for any reason, and the circumcision campaign faded.

6.3. Professional Opposition to Mass Circumcision

American opposition to involuntary circumcision did exist. In 1956 and 1959, respectively, Dr. Richard K. Winkelmann, a Fellow in Dermatology at the Mayo Clinic in Rochester, Minnesota, published two anatomical studies documenting the intense erogenous innervation of the foreskin and identifying the foreskin as a specific erogenous zone.[78-79] In an era that was growing increasingly hostile to sexuality, however, Winkelmann's studies were ignored. In 1954, Ravich's theory that the foreskin caused prostate cancer was disproven,[80] and as early as 1962, the myth that the male foreskin caused cervical cancer in women was also scientifically disproven.[81] In 1963, another scientific study disproved Wolbarst's theory that penile smegma was a carcinogen.[82] In 1965, the *Journal of the American Medical Association* published a revolutionary article by Dr. William Keith C. Morgan, "The Rape of the Phallus."[83] Morgan's paper carefully debunked all the then-current arguments hospitals used to justify involuntary circumcision and thereby generated enormous controversy in the American medical community.

The year 1968 saw the publication of yet another ground-breaking study on the nature of the juvenile foreskin. The respected British pediatric journal, *Archives of Disease in Childhood,* published the exhaustive research of Danish pediatrician Jakob Øster, who had examined the incidence of preputial adhesion in 9,545 Danish schoolboys aged 6–17 years.[84] Like Gairdner nineteen years earlier, Øster debunked the phimosis myth and demonstrated that balanopreputial adhesion was not a birth defect but a normal stage of penile development. Øster further demonstrated that preputial separation was a normal biological process that, in many cases, required at least a decade to complete. His research revealed that no intervention was indicated and, more importantly, that inappropriate attempts to hasten development of the preputial space could damage the immature foreskin. Øster's study was widely read by European physicians and it significantly advanced the scientific understanding of the penis. In America, Øster seems to have been ignored. In 1970, the

Journal of the American Medical Association published an important study, "Whither the Foreskin?," by Dr. E. Noel Preston, which thoroughly debunked all the circumcision myths.[85] Preston's review of the literature influenced the American Academy of Pediatrics (AAP) Committee on Fetus and Newborn in 1971 to publish the 5th edition of its *Standards and Recommendations for Hospital Care of Newborn Infants* with the following statement on circumcision:

> There are no valid medical indications for circumcision in the neonatal period.[86]

In the late 1970s, as Americans were growing increasingly aware of the abuses of power rampant throughout the nation's social institutions, influential grass-roots movements protesting the forced circumcision of American children sprang up nationwide. In the face of ridicule and pressure from health-care professionals, many American parents actively refused to permit their newborn sons to be circumcised. At the same time, the sweeping reforms gained by the informed-consent movement now required doctors to explain the probable outcome of any surgery, state the known risks, offer alternative treatments, and obtain written consent from the patient. Circumcision, too, now required a consent form, but since the person being operated on was developmentally incompetent to give consent, spokesmen for the circumcision industry claimed that parents could give consent by proxy. By deceptively presenting involuntary circumcision of the newborn as the "parents' choice," circumcision advocates hoped to obfuscate the crucial fact that the person who faced the risks and permanent consequences of surgical alteration of his sexual organs was still not allowed a choice. Critics countered that doctors had no legal power to concede control of the baby's genitals to the parents because doctors had no de jure legal power over the genitals of babies in the first place.

6.4. Backlash from the Circumcision Industry

The 1970s saw the high-water mark of involuntary circumcision in the United States. With and without parental consent, some hospitals raised the rate of neonatal circumcision to over 90% during the late 1970s and early 1980s. Circumcision advocates from large urban areas accepted positions in small rural hospitals in America's heartland and instituted programs of mass involuntary circumcision of the newborn in parts of the country where routine circumcision was previously unknown.

As part of this backlash, babycare books, popular medical magazines, and popular health books circulated myths to the effect that a boy not circumcised in infancy would be psychologically damaged if he ever realized that his father's circumcised penis differed from his own.[87–89] Another myth that was especially effective in controlling middle-class parents played upon their anxieties concerning conformity and social status by alleging that an intact boy would be made to feel inferior to his circumcised classmates in a high-school locker room.[90]

Anatomical and physiological information on the foreskin was omitted from American anatomy textbooks and replaced with pro-circumcision arguments.[91–92] Even anatomical representations of the penis in standard urology textbooks silently omitted the foreskin and presented the penis as being circumcised, as if it were so by nature.[93] Those few anatomical drawings of the natural human penis that could be found generally represented the anatomy of the foreskin incorrectly. The natural human penis became unfamiliar to the new generation of Americans — physicians and laymen alike — many of whom had never seen one. As an example of the type of information disseminated to American medical stu-

dents in the 1970s, the third edition of *Campbell's Urology*, the standard and most respected American urological textbook, declared:

> Phimotic stenosis causes extreme difficulty of urination with straining and crying; hernia or
> rectal prolapse may be secondary end results. Urinary infection is a frequent complication,
> and is often directly predisposed to by the preputial obstruction. Malnutrition, epistaxis, con-
> vulsions, night terrors, chorea, and epilepsy have all been reflexly attributed to phimosis.[94]

The same textbook also declared:

> Parents readily recognize the importance of local cleanliness and genital hygiene in their chil-
> dren and are usually ready to adopt measures which may avert masturbation. Circumcision is
> usually advised on these grounds.[95]

The masturbation hysteria, though well over 100-years-old, was obviously not over.
In October 1972, the American Academy of Pediatrics Section of Urology appointed a
committee to meet with a committee from the Fetus and Newborn Section and a representative from general pediatrics to discuss the question of circumcision in the newborn in
order to provide guidance to health insurance carriers who had been asking the AAP
whether routine neonatal circumcision should be covered in their insurance programs. The
results were never officially published as such, but were unofficially presented by Dr.
Thomas H. Guthrie, the chairman of the committee, in a paper delivered to the Urology
Section of the American Medical Association Convention in New York City in June of
1973, and later published in *Pediatrics*.[96] Guthrie argued for the adoption of more widespread routine neonatal circumcision and continuation of insurance coverage.

Female circumcision had not entirely disappeared from American medical practice
and, in 1973, Dr. Leo Wollman, a gynecological surgeon at Maimonides Hospital in
Brooklyn, published an article advocating female circumcision as a cure for frigidity.[97]
Wollman's appeal was geared to the ethos of the sexual revolution of the 1970s. Surgical
reduction of male and female genitalia, it was argued, would improve and increase the
pleasure of orgasm. This was the exact opposite of the message given a hundred years earlier, and the sudden reversal of strategy convinced critics that American circumcisionists
were willing to say anything to push genital amputation on a gullible but increasingly rebellious public. The search for new excuses to justify routine circumcision is revealing.

To make matters worse for the advocates of circumcision, a newly formed American
Academy of Pediatrics ad hoc Task Force Committee on Circumcision issued an even
stronger policy statement on circumcision in 1975. The statement concluded:

> There is no absolute medical indication for routine circumcision of the newborn....A program
> of education leading to continuing good personal hygiene would offer all the advantages of
> routine circumcision without the attendant surgical risk. Therefore, circumcision of the male
> neonate cannot be considered an essential component of adequate total health care.[98]

6.5. Legal Action for Children's Rights

In the early 1980s, the medical press reported that several lawsuits had been filed in
California against doctors and hospitals, charging that they had violated the constitutional
rights of the plaintiffs by circumcising them without their permission soon after birth.[99–100]
These cases were filed in order to establish in a court of law that parents have no right to
consent to a medically unnecessary surgery on their child based on the 1975 AAP policy

statement that circumcision was medically unnecessary. The acknowledged lack of medical justification for circumcision put circumcisers at risk for litigation, but more importantly, the Constitutional challenge to the practice of subjecting children to involuntary circumcision threatened to dismantle the lucrative circumcision industry, which, in 1986, was estimated to generate more than $200 million annually.[101] If the practice of involuntary circumcision of the newborn were to survive, a new medical excuse would have to be found.

6.6. The Urinary Tract Infection Scare

In the mid-1980s, urinary tract infections (UTI) emerged as that new excuse. While no articles on this rare disorder had yet appeared in popular magazines, the medical literature reflected a surge of scientific interest in UTI. For the period from 1966 to 1974, a MEDLINE database keyword search uncovered only 4 published studies on UTI, yet from 1975–1979, 65 studies were published. From 1980 to 1984, the number had nearly tripled, and from 1985 to 1989, 350 studies were published. While the national rate of UTI had not changed from 1966 to 1989, the astounding 8,650% increase in the number of published studies reflected a definite surge in scientific interest. As part of this increased interest, Dr. Charles M. Ginsburg and Dr. George H. McCracken, Jr. of Dallas, Texas, in 1982, quietly published a study of 100 infants with acute UTI. Because only 3 of the 62 male infants were circumcised, the authors briefly speculated that non-circumcised males might have an increased susceptibility to UTI, but admitted that "perineal hygiene was inadequate in many patients."[102] In 1985, evidently intrigued by the possibilities of this speculation, Dr. Thomas E. Wiswell (1951-), then a neonatologist at Brooke Army Medical Center in Texas, sought to verify it by publishing in *Pediatrics* the first of many studies promoting the theory that circumcision might reduce the rate of UTI.[103] Wiswell's first nonrandomized, retrospective review of hospital charts suggested a UTI rate of 1.4% for intact boys and 0.14% for circumcised boys. Although the difference in rates was only 1.2 percentage points, it was made to appear significant by being stated in terms of a 10% increase. Proponents greeted the publication of Wiswell's study as the long-awaited indication for the practice.

Significantly, one of the published letters to the editor of *Pediatrics* regarding Wiswell's study directly addressed the California lawsuits. The author, Dr. Aaron J. Fink (1926—1994), a urologist from Mountain View, California, like Wolbarst and Ravich before him, actively lobbied for mass involuntary circumcision. Fink's publications reveal that he was among those most disturbed by the prospect of legal action against circumcisers. In his letter, Fink ridiculed the contention that circumcision required the consent of the patient.[104] In his published reply, Wiswell assented that the alleged medical indication he had discovered obviated any requirement to obtain patient consent before operating.[105] McCracken, however, later stated that "because the long-term outcome of UTI in uncircumcised male infants is unknown, it is inappropriate at this time to recommend circumcision as a routine medically indicated procedure."[106]

Nevertheless, popular medical books and babycare books were updated to include the UTI myth.[107–109] National news magazines, such as *Newsweek*[110] and *U.S. News and World Report*,[111] ran feature stories on Wiswell and the new UTI excuse for subjecting infants to involuntary circumcision. Most males have never experienced a UTI, and the UTI myth had little power to influence fathers, but sociological research had shown that it was mothers, far more than fathers, who signed the circumcision consent form.[112–114] Unpleasant and painful bouts of UTI are significantly more common among females,[115–116] and the new UTI scare tactic proved to be especially efficient in frightening young mothers into agreeing to the circumcision of their sons. Unlike the unsubstantiated or disproven excuses for neonatal circumcision, such as the prevention of geriatric genital cancers and sexually transmitted diseases, UTI could afflict infants. Wiswell alleged that the foreskin posed a serious threat to the individual's life in the first few weeks after birth and its presence could increase the risks of the potential complications of UTI, such as kidney failure, meningitis, or death.[117-118]

An article in the September 1986 issue of *Pediatric News* uncovered the fact that Wiswell and Dr. Terry D. Allen were petitioning the AAP to form another ad hoc Task Force Committee on Circumcision in order that it might issue a policy statement supporting routine circumcision. Reacting to the trend of insurance companies ceasing payment for neonatal circumcision on the basis of the 1975 AAP policy statement on circumcision, Wiswell warned, "If 10 years from now there are uncircumcised children on dialysis with kidney damage associated with UTI, insurers who wouldn't pay for circumcision might be held liable."[119] Oddly, Wiswell presented himself to reporters as an opponent of routine circumcision, saying, "I tell them [parents] that I personally don't like the procedure and don't recommend it, but if they want if performed, I will do it." Under the leadership of Dr. George W. Kaplan, the chairman of the AAP Urology Section, the AAP resisted this pressure for three years.

In 1989, a new AAP Task Force Committee on Circumcision was formed and chaired by Dr. Edgar J. Schoen (1925-), a pediatrician practicing at Kaiser Foundation Hospital in Oakland since 1954. After intense debate, the Task Force was able to issue a new statement that took into account Wiswell's UTI hypothesis. The statement tenuously concluded:

> Newborn circumcision has potential medical benefits and advantages as well as disadvantages and risks. When circumcision is being considered, the benefits and risks should be explained to the parents and informed consent obtained.[120]

By closing the legal loophole created by the 1975 statement, the 1989 statement effectively protected circumcisers from any further lawsuits while avoiding making any overtly unscientific claims. Sensitive to the embarrassing fact that European countries had traditionally rejected American attempts to export involuntary or even voluntary circumcision, Schoen, from his office at the renamed Kaiser Permanente Medical Center in Oakland, tried in 1991 to persuade Northern European countries to adopt programs of routine infant circumcision.[121] The terse reply to Schoen's overtures, written by two of Sweden's most eminent physicians and published in a leading Swedish medical journal, invoked the critical issues of fairness, human rights, and medical ethics. Indicating that it was a violation of human rights to be subjected to such a procedure, the authors asserted that it was only fair to postpone a decision until the young male could make a choice of his own. Moreover, the authors patiently explained, since an Ethics Committee on Experimental Animals would never accept a procedure such as unanesthetized circumcision on laboratory animals, Europe could hardly justify subjecting its own children to such a procedure.[122]

6.7. The HIV Scare

In the early 1980s, the emergence of the human immunodeficiency virus (HIV) and acquired immune deficiency syndrome (AIDS) attracted the attention of both the American people and the medical establishment. As an indicator of this surge in national focus on AIDS, the number of popular magazine articles on AIDS rose from 9 in 1982 to 68 in 1983. From 1983 to 1987, the number of popular articles increased by 657%. Capitalizing on this surge in national focus, Dr. Aaron J. Fink published his newly-invented theory that circumcision could prevent AIDS. In an unexpected departure from its fastidiously high scientific standards, the *New England Journal of Medicine* actually published Fink's theory in 1986, without demanding any scientific substantiation.[123]

During 1987 and 1988, Fink tirelessly lobbied the California Medical Association (CMA) to adopt a resolution endorsing a program of routine infant circumcision as "an effective public health measure" (Resolution 305–88). Fink's resolution had been rejected by the Scientific Committee of the CMA in 1987, but in 1988 he managed to get it passed by a voice vote of the CMA's House of Delegates without the recommendation of the Scientific Committee. Unlike his success with the AIDS theory, his other invented excuses for circumcision, such as the prevention of group ß-streptococcal disease[124] and "sand balanitis"[125] never succeeded in getting national attention.

Fink's theory that circumcision prevents AIDS has recently been taken up with great vigor by several North American circumcisionists, such as Francis A. Plummer, J. Neil Simonsen, Stephen Moses, Allan R. Ronald, and Joan K. Kreiss. Plummer, especially, has achieved a large measure of popular fame because of his ceaseless advocacy of a campaign of mass involuntary circumcision of the newborn to prevent AIDS.

6.8. The Future of Involuntary Circumcision

Since the 1980s, private hospitals have been involved in the business of supplying discarded foreskins to private bio-research laboratories and pharmaceutical companies who require human flesh as raw research material. They also supply foreskins to transnational corporations such as Advanced Tissue Sciences of San Diego, California,[126] Organogenesis,[127] and BioSurface Technology,[128] who have recently emerged to reap new corporate profits from the sale of marketable products made from harvested human foreskins. In 1996 alone, Advanced Tissue Sciences could boast of a healthy $663.9 million market capitalization performance.[129]

Despite these market incentives to maintain the practice of involuntary circumcision of the newborn, the circumcision rates in the United States have continued to fall, largely due to the educational outreach of popular and professional anti-circumcision groups. According to the National Center for Health Statistics of the United States Department of Health and Human Services, the rate of neonatal circumcision in the Western United States fell from 64% in 1979 to 34.2% in 1994. As the result of an increase in the circumcision rate in the Midwest, the cumulative national rate, however, only fell from 64.5% to 62.1% during the same time period for all hospitals reporting.

In February 1996, a research team at the University of Manitoba, led by Dr. John R. Taylor, published in the *British Journal of Urology* the most significant anatomical investigation of the foreskin since Winkelmann.[130] Their paper, "The Prepuce: Specialized Mucosa of the Penis and its Loss to Circumcision," described the structural and functional components of the foreskin and established its rich erogenous innervation and vascularization. Since involuntary circumcision had been initially instituted to ablate these very features, it is not surprising that the medical establishment in the United States has not yet assessed the obvious implications of Taylor's work, even though other organizations have. After extensive review of the medical literature on circumcision — including Taylor's study — both the Australian College of Paediatrics and the Canadian Paediatric Society published policy statements on neonatal circumcision in 1996.[131–132] Both organizations recommended that circumcision of newborns should not be routinely performed, and both statements acknowledged that involuntary circumcision may contravene human rights.

Prominent voices in the world medical community have recently condemned the American practice of involuntary neonatal circumcision as a human rights violation.[133–138] The consensus among critics is that, regardless of the alleged validity of the arguments used to justify involuntary circumcision of the newborn, involuntary circumcision ipso facto represents an intrusion into the personal lives of individuals and an unwarranted deprivation of personal property. Ultimately, the constitutional conflict between human rights and the American medical establishment's program of involuntary circumcision may be settled by the courts.

7. CONCLUSIONS

The historical record makes it clear that American physicians in the late Nineteenth Century institutionalized the sexual mutilation of children as a means of attempting to eradicate childhood sexuality. Physicians performed circumcision on boys to denude, desensitize, and disable the penis to such an extent as to make masturbation theoretically impossible. The clitoridectomy of girls was introduced on the same grounds. While the medical establishment's use of the fear of masturbation to justify mass circumcision has remained fairly constant since the Nineteenth Century, the supplementary and subsequent medical excuses offered to justify the surgical reduction of the genitals of children follow an established pattern: whatever incurable disease happens to be the focus of national attention in any given time period will be the disease that circumcision advocates will use as an excuse for circumcision. In the 1870s, when epilepsy was the focus of national attention, circumcision advocates claimed that circumcision could cure and prevent epilepsy. In the 1940s, when sexually transmitted diseases were the focus of national attention, circumcision advocates claimed that circumcision could cure and prevent the spread of sexually transmitted diseases. In the 1950s, when cancer was the focus of national attention, circumcision advocates claimed that circumcision could cure and prevent cancer of all sorts — from cancer of the penis, cancer of the tongue, cancer of the prostate, to cancer of the female cervix. Since the late 1980s, when HIV and AIDS have become the focus of national attention, predictably, circumcision advocates have claimed that circumcision can prevent HIV infection.

Ironically, the United States today has both the highest percentage of sexually-active circumcised males in the Western world and the highest rates of genital cancers and sexually transmitted diseases. The paradox implicit in this history is that, even though the program of mass involuntary circumcision has been ineffective as a public health measure to prevent or reduce the ever-increasing rates of genital cancers and sexually transmitted diseases, the American medical establishment has failed to abandon involuntary circumcision in favor of more conservative and more effective public health measures. It has, instead, tried to invent new justifications for circumcision. This unscientific allegiance to a perpetually ineffective, radical, and prejudicial surgical procedure corroborates the hypothesis that there is a deeper, non-rational, psychosexual dynamic behind circumcision advocacy.[139]

The history of the institutionalization of involuntary circumcision of the newborn in the United States demonstrates that society has not always hesitated to pursue what it perceived to be scientific measures at the expense of personal liberties. It is tempting to dismiss circumcision as merely a quaint example of medical quackery pursued by a small handful of zealous physicians. It would be better to remember that, in the name of science, hundreds of millions of American citizens have been subjected to involuntary sexual mutilation. In the face of increasing international condemnation and Constitutional challenges, it is uncertain how much longer the American medical establishment will be able to continue to indulge in the kind of flawed thinking and disregard for human rights that support this activity.

8. REFERENCES

1. Szasz TS. Law, Liberty, and Psychiatry. Syracuse: Syracuse University Press. 1989:212.
2. Bichat X. General anatomy, applied to physiology and medicine. 2 vols. Boston: Richardson and Lord. 1822.
3. Broussais F JV. A treatise on physiology applied to psychology. Philadelphia: H.C. Carey and I. Lea. 1826.
4. Deslandes L. De l'onanisme et des autres abus vénériens considérés dans leurs rapports avec la santé. Paris: A. Lelarge. 1835.
5. Lallemand C-F. Des pertes séminales involontaires. Paris: Béchet Jeune, 1836:465–6.
6. Dixon E H. A treatise on diseases of the sexual organs. New York: Burgess, Stringer, 1845:158–165.
7. Editor. Tying the spermatic artery. Boston Medical and Surgical Journal 1842;26:321.
8. Crosby J. Seminal weakness - castration. Boston Medical and Surgical Journal 1843;29:10–1.
9. McMinn SN. Insanity cured by excision of the external organs of generation. Boston Medical and Surgical Journal 1845;32:131–2.
10. Taylor WT. Castration: recovery, followed by phthisis pulmonalis. American Journal of the Medical Sciences 1855;30:85–6.
11. Editor. Castration for masturbation. Medical Record 1894;46:534.
12. Gilbert J A. An unusual case of masturbation. Medical Record 1915;88:608–10.
13. Haynes T. Surgical treatment of hopeless cases of masturbation and nocturnal emissions. Boston Medical and Surgical Journal 1883;109:130.
14. Clark AC, Clark HE. Neurectomy: a preventive of masturbation. Lancet 1899;2:838.
15. M'Cassey JH. Adolescent insanity and masturbation: with exsection of certain nerves supplying the sexual organs as the remedy. Cincinnati Lancet-Clinic 1896;37:341–3.
16. Edson B. Concerning a case for circumcision. Medical World 1902;20:476–7.
17. Ford. Cauterization by injection for spermatorrhœa. Transactions of the American Medical Association 1851;4:264.
18. Garwood A. Onanism in a boy seven years old. American Journal of the Medical Sciences 1854;27:553–4.
19. Keating JM. Masturbation. In: Cyclopædia of the Diseases of Children, Medical and Surgical. Vol. III. Philadelphia: J.B. Lippincott, 1890:710.
20. Warren CE. Genocatachresia. St. Louis Medical and Surgical Journal 1892;63:201–15.
21. Kellogg JH. Plain facts for old and young. Burlington, Iowa: I.F. Segner, 1888:295–6.
22. Flood E. An appliance to prevent masturbation. Boston Medical and Surgical Journal 1888;119:34.
23. Editor. Masturbation harness. Medical World 1910;28:133.
24. Editor. Treatment of spermatorrhœa. Boston Medical and Surgical Journal 1861;48:121.
25. Cooper ES. Excision of the clitoris as a cure for masturbation. Boston Medical and Surgical Journal 1862;66:164.
26. Editor. Clitoridectomy. Medical Record 1867;2:71.
27. Hutchinson J. On the influence of circumcision in preventing syphillis. Medical Times and Gazette 1855;2;542.
28. Hirschfeld J. The jewish circumcision before a medical tribunal. American Medical Monthly 1858;9:272–5.
29. White. Phimosis in new-born children. Boston Medical and Surgical Journal 1861;65:121.
30. Bliss C. Spermatorrhœa - a new method of treatment. Boston Medical and Surgical Journal 1868;77:536–8.
31. Arnold AB. Circumcision. New York Medical Journal 1869;9:514–24.
32. Fishbein M (ed). A History of the American Medical Association, 1847–1847, Philadelphia: W.B. Saunders Co, 1947:636–7.

33. Sayre LA. Partial paralysis from reflex irritation, caused by congenital phimosis and adherent prepuce. Transactions of the American Medical Association 1870;21:205–11.
34. Sayre LA. Circumcision Versus Epilepsy, Etc. Medical Record 1870;5:233–4.
35. Heckford N. Circumcision as a remedial measure in certain cases of epilepsy, chorea, &c. Clinical Lectures and Reports by the Medical and Surgical Staff of the London Hospital 1865;2:58–64.
36. Sayre L A. Spinal anæmia with partial paralysis and want of coordination, from irritation of the genital organs. Transactions of the American Medical Association 1875;26:255–74.
37. Jacobi A. On masturbation and hysteria in young children. American Journal of Obstetrics 1876;8:595–606.
38. Moses MJ. The value of circumcision as a hygienic and therapeutic measure. New York Medical Journal 1871;14:368–74.
39. Spratling EJ. Masturbation in the adult. Medical Record 1895;45:442–3.
40. Fisher CE. Circumcision. In: A hand-book on the diseases of children and their homeopathic treatment. Chicago: Medical Century Co, 1895:875.
41. Gentry WD. Nervous derangements produced by sexual irregularities in boys. Medical Current 1890;6:268–74.
42. Editor. The advantages of circumcision. Medical News 1900;77:707–8.
43. Mark EG. Circumcision. American Practitioner and News 1901;31:122–6.
44. Taylor AS. Case of congenital phimosis leading to death at the age of 83. Lancet 1891;1:1040.
45. Wolbarst AL. Persistent masturbation. Journal of the American Medical Association 1932;90:154–5.
46. Wolbarst AL. Universal circumcision as a sanitary measure. Journal of the American Medical Association 1914;62:92–7.
47. Wolbarst AL. Universal circumcision as a sanitary measure. Journal of the American Medical Association 1914;62:92–7.
48. Wolbarst A L. Does circumcision in infancy protect against disease? Virginia Medical Monthly 1934;60:723–8.
49. Wolbarst AL. Circumcision and penile cancer. Lancet 1932;1:150–3.
50. Bazett HC, McGlone B, Williams RG, Lufkin HM. Sensation: I. depth, distribution and probable identification in the prepuce of sensory end-organs concerned in sensations of temperature and touch; thermometric conductivity. Archives of Neurology and Psychiatry 1932;27:489–517.
51. Diebert GA. The separation of the prepuce in the human penis. Anatomical Record 1933;57:387–99.
52. Hunter RH. Notes on the development of the prepuce. Journal of Anatomy 1935;70:68–75.
53. Guttmacher AF. Should the baby be circumcised? Parents' Magazine 1941;16(9): 26, 76–78.
54. Guttmacher AF. Should the baby be circumcised? Parents' Magazine 1941;16(9): 26, 76–78.
55. Guttmacher AF. Should the baby be circumcised? Parents' Magazine 1941;16(9): 26, 76–78.
56. Ewing J. The causal and formal genesis of cancer. In: Cancer Control. Chicago: The Surgical Publishing Company of Chicago, 1927:168.
57. Ravich A. The relationship of circumcision to cancer of the prostate. Journal of Urology 1942;48:298–9.
58. Editor. Circumcision vs. cancer. Newsweek 1943;21:110–1.
59. Who's Who in America. 42nd edition. 1982–1983. volume 2. Chicago: Marquis Who's Who, 1982/83:2752.
60. Gerber ML. Some practical aspects of circumcision. United States Navy Medical Bulletin 1944;42:1147–9.
61. Heimoff LL. Venereal disease control program. Bulletin of the United States Army Medical Department 1945;3:93–100.
62. Hand EA. Circumcision and venereal disease. Archives of Dermatatology and Syphilography 1949;60:341–6.
63. Editor. Circumcision and VD. Newsweek 1947;30:49.
64. Gairdner D. The fate of the foreskin: a study of circumcision British Medical Journal 1949;2: 1433–7.
65. Miller RL, Snyder DC. Immediate circumcision of the newborn male. American Journal of Obstetrics and Gynecology 1953;65:1–11.
66. vide: Obstetrics. ed. J.P. Greenhill. 13 edition. Philadelphia: W.B. Saunders, 1960:1049. and: Eatman NJ, Hellman LM, eds. Williams Obstetrics. 12th edition. New York: Appleton-Century-Crofts, 1961:1101.
67. Ravich A, Ravich RA. Prophylaxis of cancer of the prostate, penis, and cervix by circumcision. New York State Journal of Medicine 1951;51:1519–20.
68. Wynder EL, Cornfield J, Schroff PD, Doraiswami KR. A study of environmental factors in carcinoma of the cervix. American Journal of Obstetrics and Gynecology 1954;68:1016–52.
69. Editor. Circumcision and Cancer. Time 1954;63:96–7.
70. Rathmann WG. Female circumcision, indications and a new technique. GP 1959;20:115–20.

71. Dietz O, Dougherty EC. Vergleichende Studie zur Frage der Beschneidung in Deutschland und in den Vereinigten Staaten. Deutsche Gesundheitswesen 1957;12:193–6.
72. Kelâmi A. Die sogenannte Gomecotomie als Methode der Wahl für Circumcision. Der Chirurg 1966;37:512–3.
73. Dietz O, Dougherty EC. Vergleichende Studie zur Frage der Beschneidung in Deutschland und in den Vereinigten Staaten. Deutsche Gesundheitswesen 1957;12:193–6.
74. Hofmeister KB. Über erste Erfahrungen mit der routinemäßigen Beschneidung des Neugeborenen in Deutschland und Gedanken zur krebsprophylaxe. Geburtshilfe und Frauenheilkunde 1959;19:20–31.
75. Koester H. Zur Frage der Zirkumzision neugeborener Knaben. Geburtshilfe und Frauenheilkunde 1963;23:934–43.
76. Dietz O. Erfahrungsbericht über 2800 Zirkumzisionen. Dermatologische Monatsschrift 1970;156:1029–34.
77. Bock JE, Rebbe H. Neonatal Circumcisio. Ugeskrift for Laeger 1973;135:1890–2.
78. Winkelmann RK. The cutaneous innervation of human newborn prepuce. Journal of Investigative Dermatology 1956;26:53–67.
79. Winkelmann RK. The erogenous zones: their nerve supply and its significance. Proceedings of the Staff Meetings of the Mayo Clinic 1959;34:39–47.
80. Gibson EC. Carcinoma of the prostate in jews and circumcised gentiles. British Journal of Urology 1954;26:227–9.
81. Stern E, Neely PM. Cancer of the cervix in reference to circumcision and marital history. Journal of the American Medical Women's Association 1962;17:739–40.
82. Govinda Reddy D, Baruah IJSM. Carcinogenic action of human smegma. Archives of Pathology 1963;75:414–20.
83. Morgan WKC. The rape of the Phallus. Journal of the American Medical Association 1965;193:223–4.
84. Øster J. Further fate of the foreskin: incidence of preputial adhesions, phimosis, and smegma among danish schoolboys. Archives of Disease in Childhood 1968;43:200–3.
85. Preston EN. Whither the foreskin? a consideration of routine neonatal circumcision. Journal of the American Medical Association 1970;213:1853–8.
86. Committee on Fetus and Newborn. Circumcision. In: Hospital Care of Newborn Infants. 5th edition. Evanston, Ill: American Academy of Pediatrics, 1971:110.
87. The Boston Children's Medical Center. Pregnancy, Birth and the Newborn Baby. Boston: Delacorte Press, 1971:285.
88. Pomeranz VE, Schultz D. The Mothers' and Fathers' Medical Encyclopedia. Boston: Little, Brown and Company, 1977:109.
89. Livermore B. Like father, like son. Health 1987;19:15.
90. Barton S. Your Child's Health. New York: Bantam Books, 1991:113–8.
91. Masters WH, Johnson VE, Kolodny RC. Human Sexuality. 4th edition. New York: HarperCollins, 1992:58–9.
92. Miller MA, Drakonitides AB, Leavell LC (eds). Kimber-Gray-Stackpole's Anatomy and Physiology 17th edition. New York: Macmillan, 1977:577.
93. Snell RS. Atlas of Clinical Anatomy. Boston: Little, Brown and Company. 1978:136.
94. Campbell MF. The male genital tract and the female urethra. In: Campbell MF, Harrison JH, eds. Urology. vol. 2. Third edition. Philadelphia: W.B. Saunders, 1970:1836.
95. Campbell MF. The male genital tract and the female urethra. In: Campbell MF, Harrison JH, eds. Urology. vol. 2. Third edition. Philadelphia: W.B. Saunders, 1970:1836.
96. Burger R, Guthrie TH. Why Circumcision? Pediatrics. 1974;54:362–4.
97. Wollman L. Female Circumcision. Journal of the American Society of Psychosomatic Dentistry and Medicine 1973;20:130–1.
98. Committee on Fetus and Newborn. Report of the Ad Hoc Task Force on Circumcision. Pediatrics 1975;56:610–1.
99. Editor. Two suits charge circumcision malpractice. Contemporary Ob/Gyn 1986;28(4):150.
100. Editor. Calif. suit raises liability questions in circumcision. Ob.Gyn. News 1986;21(22):1,18 passim.
101. Editor. Two suits charge circumcision malpractice. Contemporary Ob/Gyn 1986;28(4):150.
102. Ginsburg CM, McCracken GH, Jr. Urinary tract infections in young infants. Pediatrics 1982;69:409–12.
103. Wiswell TE, Bass JW. Decreased incidence of urinary tract infections in circumcised male infants. Pediatrics 1985;75:901–3.
104. Fink AJ. In defense of circumcision. Pediatrics 1986;77:265–6.
105. Wiswell TE. Reply to: In defense of circumcision. Pediatrics 1986;77:266–7.
106. McCracken GH Jr. Options in antimicrobial management of urinary tract infections in infants and children. Pediatric Infectious Disease Journal 1989;8:552–5.

107. Burch FW. Baby Sense. New York: St. Martin's Press, 1991:226.
108. Santesteban A. Child Care for the '90s. Bedford: ABC & I Press, 1993:18.
109. Dollemore D, Holman M, Kaufman BP, et al. Symptoms: Their Causes & Cures. Emmaus: Rodale Press, 1994:199.
110. Monmaney R, Raine G. Doubts about circumcision: fewer boys are now cut. Newsweek 1987;109:74.
111. Silberner J, Carey J. Circumcision. U.S. News and World Report 1988;104:68.
112. Rand CS, Emmons CA, Johnson JWC. The effect of an educational intervention on the rate of neonatal circumcision. Obstetrics and Gynecology 1983;62:64–7.
113. Bean GO, Egelhoff C. Neonatal circumcision: when is the decision made? Journal of Family Practice 1984;18:883–7.
114. Lovell JE, Cox J. Maternal attitudes toward circumcision. Journal of Family Practice 1979;9:811–3.
115. Eriksen NH, Poulsen PN, Friis HM, Vejlsgaard R. Urinary tract infectionsm etiology, diagnosis and treatment with effective antibiotics. Nordisk Medicin 1989;104(2):35–8.
116. Shabad AL, Minakov NK, Mkrtchan GG, et al. The pathogenesis and prevention of urinary tract infection in women. Urologiia I Nefrologiia 1995;(4):8–12.
117. Wiswell TE, Geschke DW. Risks from circumcision during the first month of life compared with those for uncircumcised boys. Pediatrics 1989;83:1011–15.
118. Wiswell TE. Routine neonatal circumcision: a reappraisal. American Family Physician 1990;41:859–63.
119. Ahmann S. Academy holds fast to position on circumcision. Pediatric News 1986;20:38–9.
120. Task Force on Circumcision. Report of the task force on circumcision. Pediatrics 1989;84:388–91.
121. Schoen EJ. Is it time for Europe to reconsider newborn circumcision? Acta Paediatrica Scandinavica 1991;80:573–4.
122. Bollgren I, Winberg J. Reply to: Is it time for Europe to reconsider newborn circumcision? Acta Paediatrica Scandinavica 1991;80:575–7.
123. Fink AJ. A possible explanation for heterosexual male infection with AIDS. New England Journal of Medicine 1986;315:1167.
124. Fink AJ. Is hygiene enough? Circumcision as a possible strategy to prevent neonatal group B streptococcal disease. American Journal of Obstetrics and Gynecology 1988;159:534.
125. Fink AJ. Circumcision and sand. Journal of the Royal Society of Medicine 1991;84:696.
126. Manson B. Forget pork bellies, now it's foreskins. San Diego Reader (May 4, 1995):12, 14 passim.
127. Brewer S. New skin twin life- and look-save. Longevity (September 1992):18.
128. Rosenberg R. Companies see $1.5b market in replacement skin products. Boston Globe (October 19, 1992): 22–23.
129. Hall CT. Biotech's Big Discovery. San Francisco Chronicle. October 25, 1996:E1, E4.
130. Taylor JR, Lockwood AP, Taylor AJ. The prepuce: specialized mucosa of the penis and its loss to circumcision. British Journal of Urology 1996;77:291–5.
131. Australian College of Paediatrics. Position statement: routine circumcision of normal male infants and boys. Australian College of Paediatrics. 27/05/96.
132. Fetus and Newborn Committee, Canadian Paediatric Society. Clinical practice guidelines: Neonatal circumcision revisited. Canadian Medical Association Journal 1996;154:769–80.
133. Menage J. Male Genital Mutilation. British Medical Journal 1993;307:686.
134. Sorger L. To ACOG: stop circumcisions. OB.GYN.News 1994;(November 1):8.
135. Fleiss PM. Female circumcision. New England Journal of Medicine 1995;322:189.
136. Mullick S. Circumcision. British Medical Journal 1995;310:259.
137. Warren JP, Smith PD, Dalton JD, et al. Circumcision of children. British Medical Journal 1996;312:377.
138. Fleiss PM. More on circumcision. Clinical Pediatrics 1995;34:623–4.
139. Bigelow J. The Joy of Uncircumcising! 2nd edition. Aptos: Hourglass, 1995:89–112.

3

JEHOVAH, HIS COUSIN ALLAH, AND SEXUAL MUTILATIONS

Sami A. Aldeeb Abu-Sahlieh

Female sexual mutilation is practiced in about twenty-eight countries. Many of these countries are Arab or Muslim. Among those practicing female sexual mutilation under religious pretext, we must mention here Sudan, Somalia, Eritrea and Egypt. In Egypt, about 3,600 girls are excised daily.[1] Other Arab and Muslim countries do not practice female sexual mutilation, such as several North African Countries, Syria, Iraq, Jordan, Saudi Arabia (with some exceptions) and Iran.

Male sexual mutilation is practiced by approximately one billion Muslims, 300 million Christians and about 16 million Jews. From this fact, we can consider Muslims to be the major religious group in the world practicing male and female circumcision for religious reasons. It is, then, important to understand the arguments which are behind these two practices in order to determine the most effective way to work against them.

1. GENERAL REMARKS ON MALE AND FEMALE SEXUAL MUTILATION

1.1. Male Sexual Mutilation

According to Islamic law, male circumcision involves the cutting of the foreskin, preferably the whole foreskin. If the child is born without a foreskin, some Islamic writers are of the opinion he should be left as such, while for others, the knife should be passed over the emplacement of the foreskin to fulfil the Commandment. If the circumcision is incomplete, it should be completed.[2]

Sexual Mutilations: A Human Tragedy, edited by Denniston and Milos
Plenum Press, New York, 1997

1.2. Female Sexual Mutilation

There are many different kinds of female sexual mutilation. *Sunnah* circumcision, which means circumcision according to the tradition of Mohammed, is limited to cutting the clitoral hood or a part of the clitoris. *Clitoridectomy*, or excision, consists of the ablation of the clitoris and for some also the labia minora. It is the operation of choice in Egypt. *Infibulation*, or *pharaonic* circumcision, involves the complete ablation of the clitoris, labia minora and part of labia majora. The two sides of the vulva are then sewn together in order to close the vulva, except for a very small opening for the passage of urine and menstrual flow. In some tribes, the woman is sewn up each time her husband goes travelling and is opened again each time he returns. In case of divorce, the woman is sewn up to forbid any possibility of intercourse.

1.3. Circumcision of the Hermaphrodite

The opinions of classical authors differ with regard to the circumcision of hermaphrodites — persons with ambiguous genitalia, or both penis and vulva. Some authors state that both sets of genitalia must be circumcised, while others hold that only the organ passing urine should be cut. Another group suggests that circumcision must be delayed until it is possible to tell which one of the two organs is predominant. Cautiously, Al-Sukkari, a modern author, chooses the first opinion, the circumcision of both sexes, to minimize the chance of mistake.[3]

1.4. Age for Male and Female Circumcision

For the Jews, the age at which male sexual mutilation occurs is determined by the passage in the Bible that states: "Every male among you shall be circumcised when he is eight days old" (see below).

Muslim jurists are not unanimous regarding the age at which male and female sexual mutilation should be carried out. Different opinions can be found: at any time; at puberty; before 10 years of age; at about 7 years.[4]

Jurists have asked themselves if males who died without having been circumcised should be circumcised post mortem. The majority reject such an idea. Other jurists are of the opinion that circumcision of the deceased is necessary, and that his foreskin should be placed in the shroud. They support this with reference to a saying of Mohammed, according to which one must do to the dead what is done to those getting married.[5] The same controversy exists concerning uncircumcised Jews who die in Israel.

1.5. Practice of Male and Female Sexual Mutilation

Often male and female sexual mutilations are performed without anesthesia in a barbaric manner by persons without any medical training, such as barbers or midwives, using rudimentary instruments that cause complications sometimes leading to death.

2. RELIGIOUS ARGUMENTS

Before giving the religious arguments about circumcision found in Islamic sources, it is important to mention briefly those arguments found in the holy books of Jews and Christians, to which Islamic sources very often refer.

2.1. The Bible Is the Major Basis for Male Sexual Mutilation

The Bible does not contain any statements concerning female circumcision, but it constitutes the major basis for male circumcision, not only for Jews, but also for Muslims.

The most important text in the Bible concerning male circumcision is in Chapter 17 of *Genesis*, which reports that God appeared to Abraham at the age of 99 years and established a covenant with him and his descendants. When Abram was 99 years old, the Lord appeared to Abram, and said to him:

I am God Almighty... No longer shall your name be Abram, but your name shall be Abraham... I will establish my covenant between me and you, and your offspring after you throughout their generations, for an everlasting covenant, to be God to you and to your offspring after you. And I will give to you, and to your offspring after you, the land where you are now an alien, all the land of Canaan, for a perpetual holding; and I will be their God. God said to Abraham, "As for you, you shall keep my covenant, you, and your offspring after you throughout their generations. This is my covenant, which you shall keep between me and you and your offspring after you: Every male among you shall be circumcised. You shall circumcise the flesh of your foreskin; and it shall be a sign of the covenant between me and you. Throughout your generations every male among you shall be circumcised when he is eight days old, including the slave born in your house and the one bought with your money from any foreigner who is not of your offspring. Both the slave born in your house and the one bought with your money must be circumcised. So shall my covenant be in your flesh an everlasting covenant. Any uncircumcised male who is not circumcised in the flesh of his foreskin shall be cut off from his people; he has broken my covenant.[6]

We find many references to circumcision in the Bible, which uses the term "uncircumcised" as a synonym of "unclean." For this reason, the uncircumcised are not permitted to enter the Sanctuary, or even Jerusalem:

Thus says the Lord God: No foreigner, uncircumcised in his heart and uncircumcised in his flesh, shall enter into my sanctuary, nor any strangers who are among the children of Israel.[7]

Awake, Awake, O Zion; put on your beautiful garments, O Jerusalem, the holy city; for henceforth there shall no more come into you the uncircumcised and the unclean.[8]

We find a gradual shift in the conception of circumcision in the Bible. Circumcision of the skin gradually is replaced by the circumcision of the heart. Let us quote just this text of Jeremiah:

Circumcise yourselves to the Lord, and take away the foreskins of your heart, you men of Judah and inhabitants of Jerusalem.[9]

Nevertheless, with few exceptions, male circumcision is still considered by Jews as a religious obligation, even though they have abandoned forever many other Biblical laws such as the *lex talionis*: "Life shall be for life, eye for eye, tooth for tooth, hand for hand, foot for foot,"[10] or the stoning of those who have committed adultery:

If there is a damsel who is a virgin and who is betrothed to a man, and another man find her in the city and lie with her; then you shall bring them both out to the gate of that city, and you shall stone them with stones, that they die.[11]

2.2. Christians Abandon the Obligation of Male Sexual Mutilation

Jesus Christ attacked the *lex talionis*[12] as well as the law concerning the stoning of adulterous women.[13] We do not find any concrete position of Jesus Christ concerning male circumcision in any of the four Gospels. The Gospel of St. Luke merely reports that Jesus had been circumcised "when eight days were fulfilled."[14] We find one more reference to male circumcision in the Gospel of St. John:

> Jesus answered them [the Jews], I performed one work, and all of you are astonished. Moses gave you circumcision (it is, of course, not from Moses, but from the forefathers; and you circumcise a man on the Sabbath. If a man receives circumcision on the Sabbath in order that the law of Moses may not be broken, are you angry with me because I healed a man's whole body on the Sabbath. Do not judge by appearance, but judge with right judgment.[15]

Notice here that Jesus does not say that circumcision is from God, but from the forefathers. Since the first Christians were Jewish converts, male circumcision was not questioned because these converts were already circumcised. When non-Jews became Christians, however, there was a heated debate concerning male circumcision because the Jews considered uncircumcised persons to be unclean. There are many verses in the book of the *Acts of the Apostles*[16] and in the *Epistles* of St. Paul concerning this question.

The *Acts of the Apostles* tell us that certain individuals came down from Judea and were teaching the brethren: "Unless you are circumcised according to the custom of Moses, you cannot be saved."[17] Most of the apostles, especially St. Paul, were against imposing circumcision onto the Pagans. Peter is reported to have received in his dream a message from God, saying: "What God has made clean, you must not call unclean."[18] St. Paul wrote:

> Was anyone at the time of his call already circumcised? Let him not seek to remove the marks of circumcision. Was anyone at the time of his call uncircumcised? Let him not seek circumcision. Circumcision is nothing, and uncircumcision is nothing, but obeying the commandments of God is everything. Let each of you remain in the condition in which you were called.[19]

> And have clothed yourselves with the new self, which is being renewed in knowledge according to the image of its creator. In that renewal there is no longer Greek and Jew, circumcised and uncircumcised, barbarian, Scythian, slave and free, but Christ is all and in all.[20]

These texts from the New Testament do not forbid circumcision in itself, but destroy its mandatory character. We should also notice that we do not find any reference in these texts or in any other text in the Old Testament or in the New Testament relating to the question of the inviolability of physical integrity of a non-consenting person. There is also no reference to medical justification of circumcision. Today, these are the main arguments used when discussing male and female sexual mutilation. It is important for scholars to study why these arguments are missing in the writings of the holy books of Jews and Christians. One has the impression that Paul's intention was to find a way to let the pagans enter the new community without angering the Jews who had converted to Christianity. His arguments have more to do with stratagems than with human rights.

2.3. Male Circumcision in Islamic Sources

Jews and Muslims believe that only God can indicate what is good or bad. For this reason, he sent many prophets to whom he revealed a message indicating the right path for humanity.

Jews consider that only the Old Testament prophets received direct revelation from God. For Christians, divine revelation is extended to include the writings in the New Testament.

Muslims add Jesus to the list of Jewish prophets to have received revelation. They also consider Mohammed to be the last prophet to have received direct revelation from God. The revelation of Mohammed is included in the Koran. The Koran requires Muslims to accept all of the laws revealed to the previous prophets, unless these laws contradict the laws of the Koran.

In addition to the Koran, whose revelations are considered to be the primary basis for Islamic law, Muslims give great importance to the *Sunnah* (tradition), Mohammed's commentaries on the Koran. The Sunnah is considered as the second source of Islamic law. For Muslims, Mohammed is an infallible prophet; whatever he said or did must be applied. Many years after his death, the apocryphal sayings and deeds of Mohammed were collected and preserved in various books. The authenticity of these books is questioned even by Muslim scholars who, nevertheless, refer to these books to interpret or to complete the Koran. Muslims make a clear distinction between the Koran, whose author, according to them, is God himself, and the Sunnah, whose author is Mohammed. Male and female sexual mutilation is justified through these two sources.

2.4. Male and Female Circumcision in the Koran

The Koran, the first source of Islamic law, mentions neither male nor female circumcision. Muslims nevertheless find a justification for male circumcision in verse 2:124:

> When Abraham was put to the test by his Lord, through certain commandments, he carried them out. God then said: "I am appointing you a guide for the people."

Using some apocryphal sayings of Mohammed, the words "test" and "commandments" are interpreted by classical and modern Muslim authors as referring to the circumcision of Abraham as mentioned in Genesis (Chapter 17). As Abraham is a model for Muslims (Koran 16:123), they must do as he did. This interpretation is rejected by Mohammed 'Abdou who considers it as an invention of the Jews to ridicule the Islamic religion.[21] It is also rejected by Imam Mahmud Shaltut who considers it excessive (israf fil-istidlal).[22] These two religious authorities do not question male circumcision in itself. They consider it to be based on the Sunnah of Mohammed (see below). The above-mentioned Koranic justification of circumcision can easily be destroyed by a more accurate reading.

The only explicit reference to circumcision in the Koran can be found in two verses (2:88 and 4:155), which use the term "uncircumcised" in association with "hearts" (*qulubuna ghulafun*), in reference to the Jews. This expression, which clearly comes from Biblical terminology, is wrongly translated by Muslims into English by "our hearts are sealed" or "our hearts are hardened." Muslims never refer to these two verses when discussing circumcision.

One would have expected the term "uncircumcised" in verse 9:28, which limits access to holy places to foreigners (see above): "O you who believe, assuredly the idolaters are unclean, so let them not approach the Sacred Mosque after this year of theirs" (9:28). The Bible explicitly forbids uncircumcised persons from entering holy places. Contrary to the Bible, the Koran does not specifically name these persons as "uncircumcised."

This quasi-silence of the Koran is in contrast with the large debate about male circumcision in the Old and the New Testaments. This would indicate that the Koran ignores this practice, or at least considers it to be unimportant. One can even say that male (as well as female) circumcision is contrary to the philosophy of the Koran as indicated in the following verses:

> Our Lord! You have not created these in futility. Glory be to You: guard us then against the torment of the fire (3:191).

> Everything with Him is by measure (13:8).

> He has created everything and meted it out in perfection (25:2).

> No change is there in God's creation (30:30).

> Who has perfected everything He created (32:7).

> He created not the heavens and the earth, and what is between them for futility (38:27).

> He shaped you, and perfected your forms (40:64).

> Indeed everything we have created in measure (54:49).

> He fashioned you, and perfected your shapes (64:3).

> Truly We created man in the best shape (95:4).

> [Satan said]: "I will surely take of Your servants an appointed portion. And I will surely lead them to perversity, and I will stir whims in them, and I will enjoin them and they will cut off the cattle's ears; and I will enjoin them and they shall alter God's creation. But whoever takes Satan for patron, apart from God, shall surely suffer a plain perdition" (4:119).

One can easily deduce from the first ten verses that the foreskin is an integral part of the human body created by God, and that one should not imagine that, by cutting it off, one is perfecting the work of God. The third verse considers the alteration of God's creation as obedience to the Devil.

It is very important to notice here that the argument of the perfect shape in which God created man is used by those Muslims who condemn female circumcision. Doctor Nawal El-Saadawi, an Egyptian woman, herself circumcised, writes:

> If religion comes from God, how can it order man to cut off an organ created by Him as long as that organ is not diseased or deformed? God does not create the organs of the body haphazardly without a plan. It is not possible that He should have created the clitoris in a woman's body only in order that it be cut off at an early stage in life. This is a contradiction into which neither true religion nor the Creator could possibly fall....[23]

Aziza Kamel, adversary of female circumcision, refers to verse 32:7, and adds: "Circumcision is a distortion of what God created because God is satisfied with His creation."[24]

The only Muslim author to have cast doubts on male circumcision by using a new interpretation of the Koran has had legal action brought against him and might be sentenced to death for apostasy. I am speaking of (retired) Judge Mustafa Kamal Al-Mahdawi, who is today under a ferocious attack led by Libyan religious circles in the mosques as well in the press.

This Libyan judge insists that male circumcision is a Jewish custom; the Jews believe that God cannot recognize them unless they create distinctive marks such as circumcision or blood-stained doors. He refers here to God's command given to the Jews that the blood from sacrificed lambs be put on jambs and lintels of houses at the time of Passover because God intended to kill all firstborn in Egypt.[25] The Libyan judge adds that the Koran does not mention this "peculiar logic." For him, God does not devote Himself to such banter no more than He created the foreskin as a superfluous object destined only to be cut off. He quotes verse 3:191, which states: "Our Lord, You did not create all this in vain."[26]

2.5. Male and Female Circumcision in the Sunnah

As we said above, Muslims consider the Sunnah (tradition) of Mohammed as the second source of Islamic law. Classical and modern jurists generally quote the apocryphal sayings of Mohammed to justify male and female circumcision. I will try here to glean them from the works of contemporary Arab authors.

The most frequently cited myth reports a debate between Mohammed and Um Habibah (or Um 'Atiyyah). This woman, known as a circumciser of female slaves, was one of a group of women who had immigrated with Mohammed. Having seen her, Mohammed asked her if she kept practicing her profession. She answered affirmatively adding: "Unless it is forbidden and you order me to stop doing it." Mohammed replied: "Yes, it is allowed. Come closer so I can teach you: if you cut, do not overdo it (la tanhaki), because it brings more radiance to the face (ashraq) and it is more pleasant (ahza) for the husband."[27] The Shi'is cite Al-Sadiq as the reporter of this narration.[28] I shall hereinafter refer to this tale as the Circumciser's Tale.

Mohammed said: "Circumcision is a sunnah for the men and makrumah for the women."[29] The term sunnah here means that it conforms to the tradition of Mohammed himself, or was simply a custom at the time of Mohammed. The term makrumah is far from clear, but it can be translated by a meritorious action, which means that it is better to do it, even though it is not obligatory from a religious standpoint. The Shi'is quote Imam Al-Sadiq who states: "Female circumcision is a makrumah, and is there anything better than a makrumah?"[30]

Mohammed said: "Let him who becomes a Muslim be circumcised, even if he is old."[31]

Someone asked Mohammed if an uncircumcised man could go on a pilgrimage. He answered: "Not as long as he is not circumcised."[32]

Mohammed said: "Five laws define fitrah: shaving of the pubis, circumcision, moustache trimming, armpit depilation and nail clipping."[33] The laws of fitrah are believed to be those taught by God to His creation. The man in pursuit of perfection must conform to these laws. They are not compulsory, but simply advisable.[34]

Mohammed stipulated: "If both circumcised parts (*khitanan*) meet or if they touch each other, it is necessary to wash before prayer."[35] From this, it may be deduced that men and women were circumcised in Mohammed's time.

Mohammed said: "The earth becomes defiled forty days from the urine of an uncircumcised person."[36] This saying comes from a classical Shi'a book. We have not found it quoted by modern Muslim authors.

It must also be mentioned that classical Muslim authors report a tale in which the Biblical character Sarah, during a jealous quarrelling with Hagar, swore that she would sexually mutilate her. Abraham protested, to which Sarah answered that she had sworn before God that she would do it and would not be made a liar in God's eyes. Abraham relented and indicated to Sarah that she could go ahead and circumcise Hagar. In this way, female circumcision became a custom for women.[37] This strange story represents an attempt to attach female circumcision to the foremother Hagar in the same way that male circumcision was attached to the forefather Abraham.

The supporters of male and female sexual mutilation acknowledge that the sayings attributed to Mohammed concerning male and female circumcision have little credibility.[38] Mahmud Shaltut states that these texts are neither clear nor authentic.[39]

As for male sexual mutilation, some classical authors acknowledge that many people of different races converted to Islam; nobody searched under their clothes to determine if they were circumcised or not.[40] Furthermore, these authors have no unanimous opinion on whether Mohammed himself was circumcised. Some say that he was born circumcised, others think that he was circumcised by an angel or, according to others, he was circumcised by his grandfather.[41]

Whatever the authenticity of the sayings attributed to Mohammed, one has to recognize that there is a contradiction between these sayings and the Koran. This contradiction needs an explanation.

Mohammed 'Abdou, as mentioned above, thinks that the extensive interpretation of the Koranic verse 2:124 was a Jewish invention. We acknowledge here that many Jews converted to Islam. They were very influential in the new community. This Jewish influence is now receiving increasing criticism. Some modern Muslim authors are even demanding that all classical Islamic books be reprinted after first expurgating the interpolations of Jewish origin (*isra'iliyyat*).[42] What about the tales concerning male circumcision? Were they forged by Jews to maintain this Biblical law, the same as they tried to do when they converted to Christianity? This hypothesis must be studied by Muslim scholars if they wish to find a solution to the contradiction between the Koran and the narrations attributed to Mohammed.

2.6. The Gospel of Barnabas

In addition to the Bible, modern Muslim authors refer to the Gospel of Barnabas, a forged book of an unknown author probably from the Thirteenth Century. According to this Gospel, Jesus says to his disciples: "Verily, I say unto you that a dog is better than an uncircumcised man."[43] He also explains why circumcision was ordered by God:

Adam the first man having eaten, by fraud of Satan, the food forbidden by God in Paradise, his flesh rebelled against the spirit; whereupon he swore, saying: "By God, I will cut thee!" And having broken a piece of rock, he seized his flesh to cut it with the sharp edge of the stone: whereupon he was rebuked by the angel Gabriel. And he answered: "I have sworn by God to cut it; I will never be a liar!" Then the angel showed him the superfluity of his flesh, and that he cut off. And hence, just as every man taketh flesh from the flesh of Adam, so is he bound to observe all that Adam promised with an oath. This did Adam observe in his sons, and from generation to generation came down the obligation of circumcision. But in the time of Abraham there were but few circumcised upon the earth because that idolatry was multiplied upon the earth. Whereupon God told to Abraham the fact concerning circumcision, and made this covenant, saying: "The soul that shall not have his flesh circumcised, I will scatter him from among my people forever." The disciples trembled with fear at these words of Jesus, for with vehemence of spirit he spoke. Then said Jesus: "Leave fear to him that hath not circumcised his foreskin, for he is deprived of paradise."[44]

Muslim authors conclude from this text that "each of Adam's descendant is bound to observe all that Adam promised with an oath."[45]

Khalil Saadeh, the translator of this Gospel from English into Arabic, says that the harsh words comparing an uncircumcised man to a dog could not have been originally written by a Christian. He remarks that Muslims in Andalusia imposed circumcision on Christians, and this was one of the reasons for the revolt of Spanish Christians against Islamic authority. He deduces from this observation, among others, that this Gospel was probably forged by a Spanish Jew who first converted to Christianity before converting to Islam.[46] Conservative Muslim scholars, however, maintain that this book is the only authentic Gospel because it acknowledges the prophecy of Mohammed, whereas the four Canonical Gospels do not, and are thus considered forgeries.[47]

2.7. Qualification of Circumcision in Muslim Law

Some adversaries of sexual mutilation regard it as forbidden when it concerns girls. On the other hand, they do not oppose male circumcision and even consider it mandatory. As for the supporters of male and female circumcision, they are divided on the qualification that should be attached to it. Modern authors say that circumcision is compulsory for boys and *makrumah* (meritorious but not obligatory action) for girls.

Al-Sukkari states that male circumcision is mandatory because of what he calls "the repugnant smell of the greasy secretions retained under the foreskin. This uncleanness renders prayer invalid." Since purity is necessary for prayer, circumcision becomes compulsory according to the legal ruling which states: "What is necessary to fulfil an obligation becomes in turn mandatory." On the other hand, female circumcision is only advisable "because the female has no foreskin and therefore no source of impurity down there." Two reasons underlie the recommendation of female sexual mutilation: to fulfil *makrumah* granted by Mohammed; and to avoid violating a taboo.[48]

According to Professor Zakariyya Al-Birri, it is better to carry out female circumcision. Anyone who does not perform it does not sin if he is convinced, in the light of religious texts and doctor's advice, that he is under no obligation to perform it.[49] Al-Qaradawi leaves the choice to parents according to their beliefs, in spite of the fact that he favors female circumcision because it protects girls' morality, "especially nowadays."[50]

A *fatwa* (religious decision) of 1949 from the *Egyptian Fatwa Committee* has declared that abandoning female circumcision does not constitute a sin.[51] Another *fatwa* of 1951 from the same body is contradictory and more rigid. Not only does this *fatwa* not recognize the abandonment of female circumcision as an option, but it is further of the opinion that it is advisable to carry it out because it curbs "nature."[52] A third and much more detailed *fatwa* of 1981 from the same institution is adamantly opposed to giving up female circumcision. The author of this *fatwa* is the present Great Sheikh of Al-Azhar, of the most famous University of the Islamic World in Cairo. He insists that it is impossible to abandon the lessons of Mohammed in favor of the teaching of others, even if they are doctors, because medical science evolves and does not remain constant. The responsibility of female circumcision lies with the parents and with those in charge of the girl's welfare. Those who do not abide by it do not do their duty.[53] The great Sheikh of Al-Azhar, Gad-al-Haq, who signed the last *fatwa*, reiterated in October 1994 his position for the continuation of female sexual mutilation.[54]

This view is strongly disputed by the present Great Mufti, Sheikh Mohammed Al-Tantawi, who issued another *fatwa*, which states that the Koran contains nothing on female circumcision and that the sayings of the Prophet Mohammed are weak on this subject. He adds that one should defer to the opinion of doctors.[55]

Jurists have asked themselves if public authority can force a Muslim to submit to circumcision, especially if he is getting on in years. *Zaydis* and the *Shafi'is* answer affirmatively.[56] In his two above-mentioned *fatwas*, Gad-al-Haq quotes the *Hanafi* School, which says that, if a group rejects male circumcision, the Head of State must declare war against this group![57]

Hanbalis say that male and female sexual mutilation is an Islamic ritual; the man can force his wife to be circumcised as well as to force her to pray. *Ibadis* consider the marriage of a non-circumcised Muslim male invalid even if it has been consummated. The wife of a genitally intact Muslim may ask for legal separation. Even if the husband is circumcised after the consummation of the marriage, the marriage remains invalid; he must go through another wedding ceremony in order to get his wife back. For the Hanbalites, the non-circumcision of the husband is a breach of contract, giving the woman the choice of asking for divorce or continuing the marriage. For some, the non-circumcised man has no right of guardianship of another Muslim and no right to give his consent to the marriage of a Muslim relative. In this case, the marriage is dissolved, unless it was consummated.[58]

Al-Sukkari, a modern author, grants the woman the right to dissolve the marriage if the husband is not circumcised because his foreskin can be a cause of disease. It can also be a source of repulsion, thus preventing the realization of the objectives of marriage, which are love and understanding between partners. The woman has a right to be married to someone handsome and clean, since Islam is supposed to be the religion of cleanliness and purity.[59]

Ahmad Amin emphasizes the importance of circumcision in the Egyptian mind by recounting an anecdote in which a Sudanese tribe wanted to join Islam. The chief wrote to a scholar of the Al-Azhar to ask him what had to be done in order to join. The scholar sent him a list of demands, placing circumcision at the top of the list. The tribe then refused to become Muslim.[60]

According to the Saudi religious authorities, a man who converts to Islam must be circumcised, but if he refuses to join Islam for fear of the procedure, this demand may be postponed until the faith is stronger in his heart.[61]

The non-circumcision of a female has serious consequences. In some countries, non-circumcised girls cannot get married and are regarded by people as if they were guilty of misbehavior, or possessed by the devil. In the Egyptian countryside, the matron who performs circumcision on the local females issues a certificate, which is used as a marriage license.[62] El-Masry reports the statement of an Egyptian midwife who had circumcised more than 1,000 girls. In her opinion, "One should lynch the fathers who were opposed to the circumcision of their daughters, because these fathers were in fact willing to see their girls become whores."[63]

3. REASON SUPPORTING RELIGION: ADVANTAGES AND DISADVANTAGES

The Koran says: "No one questions Him about anything He does, but men are questioned" (21:23). God does not have to justify his laws even if Muslim jurists are of the opinion that divine laws are intended to bring good to man. Today, however, there is a tendency among Muslims as well as Jews to try to justify religious laws *a posteriori*, that is, to pretend that the original intent of the ancient laws commanding sexual mutilation was to confer real or fictitious medical benefits.

3.1. Male Circumcision

3.1.1. Advantages of Male Circumcision. Muslim authors skim over male circumcision. They only see advantages. In fact, they simply repeat what circumcision advocates in the West say in favor of male circumcision. According to Al-Hadidi, non-circumcision of the male can cause penile infections arising from urine droplets. It can develop into cancer, requiring the penis to be amputated entirely. Doctor Al-Fangari is of the opinion that circumcision prevents cancer in the circumcised man's sexual partner. He also believes that it helps to extend the length of copulation, thanks to the liberation of the glans.[64] Jewish authors make the same type of argument.[65]

Imam Shaltut does not find any basis for male or female circumcision in either the Koran or in the Sunnah of Mohammed. Therefore, the practice must be judged according to the general Islamic consensus which forbids hurting anyone, unless the advantages outweigh the disadvantages. For boys, he states that circumcision is beneficial because it cuts off the foreskin which harbors filth and promotes cancer and other diseases. As such, it is a protective and preventive measure; thus its mandatory quality in Muslim law.[66]

3.1.2. Disadvantages of Male Circumcision. Muslim authors completely ignore the criticism of increasing numbers of Western writers against male circumcision.

3.2. Female Circumcision

3.2.1. Advantages of Female Circumcision in Compliance with the Sunnah. Certain Muslim religious scholars are opposed to female circumcision only when it is not in compliance with the Sunnah. They outline the advantages of female circumcision as follows: it maintains cleanliness; it prevents diseases; and it is believed that there is less promiscuity among circumcised women. This prevents the transmission of deadly diseases to the husband.[67] Female circumcision prevents vaginal cancer,[68] it also prevents swelling of the clitoris, which could drive the woman to masturbation or homosexual relations.[69] Female circumcision brings calm and gives radiance to the face. Female circumcision shields the girl from nervousness at an early age and prevents her from acquiring a yellow face. This statement is based on a narration by Mohammed: "Circumcision is *makrumah* for women" and "gives them a glowing face."[70]

Female circumcision is also believed to keep married couples together and prevents drug use. Doctor Hamid Al-Ghawabi admits that female circumcision does reduce the sexual instinct in women, but he sees this as a positive effect. With age, male sexual instinct lessens. His circumcised wife will then be at the same level as he. If she were not, her husband would be unable to satisfy her, which then would lead him to drug-use in order to succeed.[71]

It prevents her falling into what is forbidden. Gad-al-Haq, Great Sheikh of Al-Azhar, says that modern times call for female circumcision "because of mixing of the sexes at public gatherings. If the girl is not circumcised, she subjects herself to multiple causes of excitation leading her to vice and perdition in a depraved society."[72]

3.2.2. Disastrous Consequences of Any Kind of Female Sexual Mutilation. Opponents of female sexual mutilation reject it because of the seriousness of the complications, which depend on the method used.

3.2.3. Physical and Mental Damage. Many complications may occur after female circumcision. Doctor Mahran classifies them as follows:[73]

Immediate complications: post-operative shock, pain, hemorrhage, infection, urinary complications and accidental injuries to surrounding organs. Later physical complications: painful scars, keloid formation, labial adherences, clitoridal cysts, vulva mutilation, kidney stones, sterility.

3.2.4. Psychosexual and Social Complications. For the female, the psychosexual complications of circumcision may be a sense of loss of her femininity, lack of libido, less frequent coitus, absence of orgasm, depression and psychosis, and high rate of divorce. For the husband of the circumcised female, the complications included: premature ejaculation, polygamy (lacking pleasure with his circumcised wife, he takes another woman).[74]

The Muslim supporters of female circumcision do not deny these complications, but state that they arise out of the manner in which the surgery is performed, mostly because of lack of attention to the conditions laid down by Muslim law. Al-Sukkari, however, writes: "If one goes to a barber for an appendectomy, must we conclude that this form of surgery has never been provided for in an Islamic book and thus should be banned because the way it is performed is wrong?"[75]

3.2.3. Drug Use. It was noted earlier that the enthusiasts for the type of female sexual mutilation called *sunnah* favor it because it allegedly prevents the use of drugs. The opponents use the reverse argument.[76] The link between female circumcision and the hashish plague in Egypt has been widely exposed by El-Masry. He states that female circumcision distorts sexual relations: "Very few healthy males can fully succeed in bringing a circumcised woman to orgasm. She has lost her capacity for pleasure. The man will soon have to admit that he alone cannot do it. There is only one solution: hashish." Doctor Hanna states: "The man will resort to narcotics to satisfy his wife sexually. Circumcision is responsible for her lack of arousal and the husband has to take drugs to be able to hold his erection as long as necessary." The women are the ones to request that their husbands use drugs before sex: "They know from experience that it is their only chance to reach orgasm, for hashish is the only cure for their mutilated clitoris."[77] The same link is observed between female circumcision and narcotics in Yemen where the plague of qat is widespread.[78]

3.2.4. Ineffectiveness in Preventing Diseases. For Doctor Al-Hadidi, there is no medical value in female circumcision, as opposed to male circumcision, since the woman does not have a foreskin to retain germs.[79] Doctor Nawal El-Saadawi also denies that female circumcision will reduce the incidence of genital cancer.[80]

3.2.5. Maintaining Man's Domination. Nawal El-Saadawi, a victim of excision, explains why female circumcision still goes on in Arab society under the iron will of males:

> The importance given to virginity and an intact hymen in these societies is the reason why female circumcision still remains a very widespread practice despite a growing tendency, especially in urban Egypt, to do away with it as something outdated and harmful. Behind circumcision lies the belief that, by removing parts of girls' external genital organs, sexual desire is minimized. This permits a female who has reached the dangerous age of puberty and adolescence to protect her virginity, and therefore her honor, with greater ease. Chastity was imposed on male attendants in the female harem by castration which turned them into inoffensive eunuchs. Similarly female circumcision is meant to preserve the chastity of young girls by reducing their desire for sexual intercourse.[81]

She adds that female circumcision is a means of dominating women in a patriarchal society where a man can have more than one wife. The society uses various means to sexually bind her to one man and to control who is the father of her children.[82]

In fact, classical Muslim authors understood female circumcision to be a means of reducing the sexuality of the woman, because a non-circumcised woman has an increased sexual attraction for men.[83] Al-Qarrafi recommends that a man circumcise a female slave if he buys her and intends on keeping her in his home. Only if he is willing to sell her is he not obliged to circumcise her.[84]

3.3. Religious Circles Confronted with Reason

As for female sexual mutilation, as stated earlier, Muslim religious circles are opposed to it, if it does not conform to the Sunnah, mostly because of the *Circumciser's Tale*. As far as *sunnah* circumcision itself is concerned, those circles refuse to condemn it on principle and the criteria mentioned above, even if differences of opinion can be noticed among them. The opinions range from unquestioning acceptance to proscription of the practice.

3.3.1. To Apply the Law for the Law's Sake. Hamrush, Chairman of the *fatwa* Committee at Al-Azhar, rejects the idea that female circumcision prevents diseases or keeps girls healthy since, "Contrary to boys, they do not have a foreskin to harbor filth." He also rejects the idea that it is a protection of the woman's honor and morality. If that were the case, then one would assume that circumcision is an obligation, and not just a *makrumah*. The Sheikh, however, holds the opinion that female circumcision should be performed to fulfil the teaching of Mohammed.[85]

3.3.2. The Law Has Benefits Unknown to Reason. The Egyptian *fatwa* of 1951 states:

> Medical theories relative to diseases and to their cure are not constant; they are subjected to changes with time and research. Therefore, it is impossible to use them as grounds to criticize female circumcision. The Lawmaker, wise, expert and knowledgeable, uses his wisdom to rectify the human creation. Experience has taught us that, given time, the true meaning of the Lawmaker's wisdom, which was hidden, is unveiled to us.[86]

3.3.3. Neither Misdeed nor Interdiction. Al-Sukkari states that Mohammed never indicated that he had any reservations about the harmfulness of female circumcision. Given this fact, how can any ordinary man forbid it under the pretense of harmfulness? Can we imagine the Prophet keeping silent about something hurtful to the girl? Man has no power to allow or to forbid, only God does, and his wishes are set out in the Koran or by His Prophet.[87]

3.3.4. To Maintain the Custom in the Absence of Misdeeds. Imam Shaltut does not see any justification for male or female circumcision, either in the Koran or in the Sunnah of Mohammed. To him, female circumcision has no medical value, the girl having no foreskin to "hold filth." He considers that both those in favor of and against female circumcision go too far. He comes to the conclusion that female circumcision could be a *makrumah* for men who are not used to feeling the clitoris protruding; for the girl, it is the same as taking care of her beauty, dabbing perfume or removing axillary hair.[88] Elsewhere, Imam Shaltut is in favor of keeping the tradition of female circumcision until it is proven harmful.[89]

3.3.5. Permitted But Soon to Be Forbidden Because of Adverse Consequences. Doctor 'Abd-al-Wahid presents a strange reasoning. After stating that female circumcision is forbidden the same way as it is forbidden to chop off one's finger, he admits that the Lawmaker (God) gave permission for the *sunnah*, any excess being forbidden. He adds, however, that this form of circumcision is allowed but not mandatory and suggests that it be forbidden due to its medical and psychological consequences, which he recounts in detail.[90]

3.3.6. It Must Be Forbidden. The most daring and most coherent opinion coming from a religious leader against female circumcision is that of Sheikh Abu-Sabib, a Sudanese. He spoke at the Seminar on Traditional Practices (Dakar, 1984). The sayings of Mohammed about female circumcision are not reliable. They and the Koran do not require anyone to suffer, when science proves the harm done by this mutilation.[91] The Egyptian Mohammed Salim Al-'Awwah holds a similar opinion.[92]

4. LEGAL PROHIBITION OF MALE AND FEMALE CIRCUMCISION

4.1. Prohibition of Male Circumcision

Male circumcision is considered to be obligatory by all Muslims. Contrary to female circumcision, it is unimaginable, till today, that this practice could be prohibited in Muslim countries. This situation will continue as long as international organizations and Western countries refuse to take a position against male circumcision in spite of the obligation to do so according to article 24, paragraph 3 of the *Convention on the Rights of the Child*, which states:

> States Parties shall take all effective and appropriate measures with a view to abolishing traditional practices prejudicial to the health of children.

In fact, international organizations have generally refused to involve themselves in the issue of male circumcision. It is likely, they are afraid of being considered anti-Semitic. This is notably the case with the World Health Organization, the United Nations

Fund For Population Activities, UNICEF, and Amnesty International. These organizations, responsible for overseeing the protection of human rights, are always ready to criticize — and correctly so — female sexual mutilation but have become accomplices in the violation of the fundamental human right of male infants to an intact body. The fear of anti-Semitism paralyses them.

During the United Nations Seminar in Ouagadougou (Burkina Faso), the majority of participants agreed that the justifications for female circumcision, which are based on cosmogony and on religion, "must be assimilated to superstition and denounced as such," since "neither the Bible, nor the Koran recommend that women be excised." They recommend ensuring that, in the minds of people, male circumcision and female circumcision be dissociated, the former as a procedure for hygienic purposes, the latter, excision, as a serious form of assault on the women's physical integrity.[93]

This reasoning is specious and extremely dangerous. Using the Bible or the Koran as the basis for modern legal interpretations is absurd. If humanity were obliged to obey all the laws and customs in the Bible and the Koran, we would then have to legitimize the practice of many barbaric laws such as the law of retaliation or other similarly inhuman laws. If female circumcision were specifically commanded in the Bible or the Koran, would it then be allowed no matter what?

In Muslim societies, the only measures that are taken concerning male circumcision are against non-physicians who fail to practice the surgery correctly. The Egyptian courts have convicted a barber for circumcising a boy who died as a consequence. Contrary to the physician, the judgment states, the barber is not protected by law if the result of his action is death or disability. The judge refused to consider laudable or charitable intentions or the absence of criminal intent. In this case, the Court applied Article 200 of the Penal Code, which makes provision for three to seven years of forced labor or imprisonment in cases of voluntary injury without intention to kill, but in fact causing death.[94]

In another judgment, the Court of Cassation stated that a midwife does not have the right to practice circumcision. The right to perform surgery is reserved for physicians only, in pursuance of the first article of law 415/1954. The Court added that any attack on physical integrity, except in cases of necessity authorized by law, is punishable, unless the acts are performed by a physician. The midwife had circumcised a boy and mistakenly amputated his glans penis, causing permanent disability that the Court estimated at twenty-five percent. The midwife was sentenced to six months forced labor, suspended on condition of good behavior after three years.[95]

4.2. Prohibition of Female Sexual Mutilation

Western countries and international organizations that keep silent on the issue of male circumcision condemn female circumcision because it is not practiced by the Jews (if we ignore the Fallachah of Ethiopia).

On July 10, 1958, the *Economic and Social Committee of the United Nations* invited the World Health Organization "to undertake a study on the persistence of customs involving ritual practices on girls and on the measures in effect or planned to put an end to those practices." The answer was clear: "[The World Health Organization] believes that the ritual practices in question, resulting from social and cultural conceptions, are not within the World Health Organization's jurisdiction."[96]

In 1984, the Inter-African Committee stipulated that "for understandable psychological reasons, it is the black women who should have the say in the matter." This committee asked for restraint, in order that the project might be successful, claiming that "the wave of uncontrollable and violent denunciations of those mutilations on the part of Western countries" was doing more harm than good.[97] On the subject of legal prohibition, this same committee warned against "untimely haste which would result in rash legal measures that would never be enforced."[98]

The World Health Organization abandoned its above-mentioned reservations of 1959. In 1977, it became involved in the creation of the first workshop on female circumcision. In February 1979, its Eastern Mediterranean Regional Office organized the first *International Seminar on Traditional Practices Affecting Women's and Children's Health* in Khartoum. This seminar recommended that specific national policies be adopted in order to abolish female circumcision. In 1989, the Regional Committee of the World Health Organization for Africa passed a resolution urging the participating governments "to adopt appropriate policies and strategies in order to eradicate female circumcision; and to forbid medicalization of female circumcision and to discourage health professionals from performing such surgery."[99]

A turnaround was also made by the Inter-African Committee. Whereas in 1984, it had warned against promulgating laws against female circumcision, it requested such laws in 1987, because "neither the efforts nor the research nor the campaigns ever had any real impact."[100] Three years later, it reinforced its position, requesting promulgation of specific laws "forbidding the practice of female genital mutilations and other sexual abuses and making provision for sentencing anyone guilty of such practices." This law should provide "an especially severe punishment for health professionals."[101]

This firm opposition to all forms of female circumcision is not supported by Muslim law, which makes a distinction between the permitted female circumcision, called *sunnah*, while other forms, though widely practiced, are condemned by religious circles. This distinction seems also to apply in Muslim countries.

In Sudan, a law from 1946 classified infibulation as an infraction punishable by a fine and imprisonment. It was abrogated under public pressure and replaced by an authorization for professional midwives to practice *sunnah*.

On an undated flyer, written in Arabic, the *Sudanese Association of Struggle against Traditional Practices* stated:

> Female circumcision (*khafd*) is an attack on the physical integrity and an alteration of the human being created by God in the very best way and in the very best form.

> Female circumcision is a savage butchery that divine religions do not allow.

> Female circumcision is neither a duty nor a *sunnah*, but a practice of the pre-Islamic era (*al-gahiliyyah*: the era of ignorance) against which the Prophet warned us in his narration: "Cut lightly and do not overdo it as it is more pleasant for the woman and better for the husband."

> Female circumcision does not protect chastity which is better guarded by education promoting good morality and healthy teaching of Islam.

> Female circumcision preceded religions and is practiced by many peoples of different religions and beliefs of which only the Sudan, Egypt and Somalia are Muslim.

> Therefore, stop circumcising girls.

This organization, while rejecting female circumcision in general, seems, in the third paragraph, to propose the *sunnah* instead of the *pharaonic* circumcision now prevalent in Sudan.

A similar attitude has been adopted in Egypt. This country has promoted a governmental decree (No. 74–1959) regarding female circumcision. The text is far from clear. It states:

> 1. It is forbidden for physicians to perform the surgical procedure of female circumcision. If one wishes it, then only partial circumcision may be carried, but not total circumcision.

> 2. Female circumcisions are forbidden in the clinics of the Ministry of Health.

> 3. Certified midwives have no right to perform any surgical procedure whatsoever including female circumcision.[102]

On September 7, 1994, during the International Conference on Population and Development held in Cairo, the Cable News Network (CNN) broadcast footage of a screaming 10-year-old girl having her genitals cut by a Cairo barber. The Egyptian authorities arrested the girl's father, the free-lance producer, and the two men who performed the procedure. The father told the police that, as a Muslim, he believes he acted properly.[103] In reaction, the Egyptian Minister of Health, on 29 October 1994, issued a decree that seeks to medicalize female sexual mutilation by designating a number of selected hospitals to perform the operation for a fee of LE 10 (approximately US $3.00).[104]

On October 17, 1995, the Egyptian Minister of Health rescinded the directive of October 19, 1994. He forbade state hospitals to perform female genital mutilations. This change seems to be the result of pressure from women's and human rights groups, as well as fear of economic sanctions from the United States government.

5. STRATEGIES TO STOP CIRCUMCISION

5.1. Scientific Information and Religious Arguments

In the struggle against male and female circumcision, one must examine the reasons used to legitimize these two practices. Many actors are involved here: physicians, nurses, insurance companies, religious authorities, and parents. One argument may work with one group, but not with another. It is necessary, therefore, to develop arguments that will appeal to each of these groups. It is equally important to understand what kind of society one is dealing with.

Western Society can be more receptive to scientific arguments than Jewish and Muslim societies, where circumcision is based on religious argument. In those societies, we first need to reverse these arguments. In September 1994, Professor Shimon Glick, Director of the Centre for Medical Education in Ben-Gurion University, sent me an article showing that circumcised people have a lower risk for AIDS. To this, he attached a note that read: "If God commands an action it cannot be harmful." This proves that even among "intellectuals," scientific arguments are secondary; religion comes first.

5.2. Humor and Sarcasm

With religious leaders, exegeses can be helpful, but there is little chance that these leaders will change their minds. With common people, we have to find a way to help them escape the authority of religious leaders and texts. Rudimentary scientific data will help in this regard, but humor or even sarcastic arguments should not be overlooked. Humor and sarcasm oblige a person to forget his taboos, to revert to reason, to be more human, and to accept the possibility of questioning revelation.

We need more Voltairian than scientific arguments in our struggle against male and female circumcision. Before reaching the nut, one must break the shell. Humor and sarcasm are certainly the best way to break the religious shell which forbids reason to function. Here are a few examples of sarcastic arguments I have found to be effective:

> Is God so stupid and limited that he cannot distinguish between believers and non-believers unless their genitals have been marked? Imagine a man cutting the penis of his horses and donkeys to distinguish them from those of his neighbors! Why do we practice on our children what we would find disgusting if it were practiced on animals?

> If we agree that God could not be so stupid as to ask his believers to cut their penis as a distinguishing mark, we must question whether Abraham — if he ever existed — was really a normal man when he pretended that God ordered him to cut his penis at the age of 99 years, as is related in the Bible (Muslims pretend that he was circumcised when he was 80 or 120 years old). Was he not senile? After telling a Kuwaiti Muslim how old Abraham was when he cut his penis, he was so surprised that he immediately said, "I understand now why in our region we call an idiot, 'Abraham'." When we consider that Abraham is said to have come from that region, we see that the local population has maintained a bad impression of him. Another Kuwaiti said: "Why did he cut his penis at that age? Did he want to anger his wife?" He told me that, in Kuwait, people say: "A person who wants to anger his wife should cut his penis."

> Now, imagine old Abraham, sitting under his tent. He was bored. He had nothing to do. In Arabic, we say that a person who does not have too much to do "plays with his testicles" (meaning his penis). While playing with his penis, Abraham accidentally cut it. Instead of saying that poor old Abraham became senile, his tribe pretended that he received an order from God to do it. Then the tribe performed this mutilation on all the males.

Certainly, such explanations will be shocking to religious leaders. For normal people, however, this way of thinking will open new perspectives. Abraham, this holy personage for Jews, Christians and Muslims, is transformed in this way into a normal man who can become senile when old. If he was senile, why, then, should we follow him?

I spoke about Voltaire who made great contributions to the Enlightenment. Voltaire, however, as a Western thinker, cannot be easily accepted by Muslims and Jews. For this reason, one must find Oriental thinkers who can play the same role in breaking the religious shell, in order to arrive at reason.

Mohammed Ibn Zakariyya Al-Razi (in Latin: Rhazes) (circa 854–925 or 935) is certainly one of the most important Muslim thinkers who may be able to help in this respect. Al-Razi was the director of the hospital of Baghdad. His medical books were used in European universities until the Sixteenth Century. He wrote many philosophical books but, unfortunately, very few were published. We should encourage scholars to publish his manuscripts, if they still exist. From the few available documents, it is clear that this philosopher was the most liberal Muslim thinker who ever existed. He believes in God but rejects the validity of revelation.[105] By weakening the importance of revelation, we can help people to think in a rational way and to reject the barbaric practice of circumcision, which is based on revelation.

6. CONCLUSION: SOME FUNDAMENTAL POINTS

6.1. Circumcision of the Male and Female Is a Question of Principle

You cannot simultaneously be against female circumcision and in favor of male circumcision unless you are willing to convince us that:

- your culture is better than others' cultures
- your religion is better than others' religions
- your holy book is better than others' holy books
- girls have to be protected but not boys.

There is one principle that must be either accepted or totally rejected: the right to physical integrity. If you accept this principle, you must apply it to any person, regardless of his religion, race, color, gender, or culture.

Because I accept the above-mentioned principle, I consider both male circumcision and female circumcision to be crimes that should be punished when they are perpetrated against non-consenting individuals without valid, serious, and immediate medical reason. For this reason, I consider any Western or Eastern legislation that condemns female circumcision but accepts male circumcision to be immoral.

Remember here that male circumcision is the most frequently committed crime on earth that goes without punishment and with the benediction of Jehovah, Allah, legislators, and charlatan physicians all over the world, in "civilized" countries as well as in jungles.

6.2. Differences between Male and Female Circumcision

One can agree that there is a difference between male and female circumcision, and that female circumcision (especially pharaonic circumcision) is more harmful than male circumcision. Likewise, one can agree that to cut off a hand or a foot is different than cutting off a finger. Cutting off a hand or a foot is more harmful than cutting off a finger, but this difference does not give anyone the right to cut off someone else's finger without his consent and without a serious, valid, medical reason.

6.3. Medical Benefits

One may agree that male circumcision, as well as surgical amputation of the hand or foot could be, in very rare instances, practiced for medical reasons, but it seems to me that the alleged medical benefits used to justify male circumcision are *a posteriori* reasons to justify a barbaric act. It seems very pretentious to suppose that Nature made a mistake so serious as to require surgical intervention on such a large scale.

6.4. God's Orders and the Respect of Others' Will

When Abraham pretended to have received the order from God to be circumcised, he was 99 years old, according to the Bible (and 80 or 120 years old according to Islamic sources). In my view, a God who demands that his believers be mutilated and branded on their genitals like cattle is a God of questionable ethics, unless, of course, we suppose that Abraham was not quite sane at such an advanced age, and that God never gave such an order to poor old Abraham. In either case, we can forget Abraham and his strange story.

Those who do not accept this liberal way of interpreting the Bible, must, nevertheless, admit that Abraham circumcised himself when he was 99 years old. He made this decision himself. Why then should we impose our decisions on others? If we respect our children, we must leave them intact until they reach the age of eighteen at the very least, at which time, they can decide for themselves whether they would like to have their penis mutilated. They can even have their ears cut if this is their will.

7. REFERENCES

1. Al-Gumhuriyyah, as quoted by Al-Nahar, August 31, 1996:24.
2. Al-Sukkari, 'Abd-al-Salam 'Abd-al-Rahim: Khitan al-dhakar wa-khifad al-untha min manzur islami. Heliopolis: Dar al-manar, 1988:65–67.
3. Al-Sukkari: Khitan, op. cit., pp. 87–89.
4. Al-Sukkari: Khitan, op. cit., pp. 86 and 90–95.
5. Al-Sukkari: Khitan, op. cit., pp. 78–81.
6. Genesis 17: 1–14.
7. Ezekiel 44:9.
8. Isaiah 52:1.
9. Jeremiah 4:4.
10. Deuteronomy 19:21.
11. Deuteronomy 22:24.
12. St. Matthew 5:38–39.
13. St. John 8:3–11.
14. St. Luke 2:21.
15. John 7:21–24.
16. See Acts of the Apostles Chapters 10, 11 and 15.
17. Acts of the Apostles 15:1.
18. Acts of the Apostles 10:9.
19. 1 Corinthians 7: 18–20.
20. Collosians 3:10–11.
21. Tafsir al-Qur'an al-karim (Tafsir al-manar). 2nd ed., Beirut: Dar al-ma'rifah, 1980;1:373–4.
22. Shaltut, Mahmud: Al-fatawi. 10th ed. Cairo & Beirut: Dar al-shuruq, 1980:332.
23. El-Saadawi, Nawal. The hidden face of Eve, Women in the Arab World. translated and edited by Sherif Hetata. London: Zed Press, 1980:42.
24. Rapport sur les pratiques traditionnelles, Addis Ababa, 1987:83.
25. Exodus 12:7–13.
26. Al-Mahdawi Mustafa Kamal: Al-Bayan bil-Qur'an, Al-dar al-gamahiriyyah, Misratah and Dar al-afaq al-gadidah, Casablanca, 1990;1:348–50.
27. Quoted by Gad-al-Haq, Gad-al-Haq 'Ali: Khitan al-banat, in Al-fatawi al-islamiyyah min dar al-ifta' al-masriyyah, Wazarat al-awqaf, Cairo. 1983;9:3121. and by Al-Sukkari: Khitan, op. cit., pp. 83–84.
28. Al-Gamri, 'Abd-al-Amir Mansur: Al-mar'ah fi zil al-islam. 4th ed. Beirut: Dar al-hilal, 1986:170–1.
29. Quoted by Al-Sukkari: Khitan, op. cit., p. 59.
30. Al-Gamri: Al-mar'ah fi zil al-islam, op. cit., pp. 170–171.
31. Quoted by Al-Sukkari: Khitan, op. cit., p. 50.
32. Quoted by 'Abd-al-Raziq, Abu-Bakr: Al-khitan, ra'y al-din wal-'ilm fi khitan al-awlad wal-banat. Cairo: Dar Al-i'tissam, 1989:71.
33. Quoted by Al-Sukkari: Khitan, op. cit., p. 55.
34. Al-Sukkari: Khitan, op. cit., pp. 55–56.
35. Quoted by Al-Sukkari: Khitan, op. cit., p. 51.
36. Al-Tubrussi: Makarim al-akhlaq. Beirut: Mu'assasat al-A'lami, 1994:220.

37. Ibn ʿAbd Al-Hakim: The history of the conquest of Egypt, North Africa and Spain, known as the Futuh Misr, ed. by Charles C. Torrey. New Haven: Yale University Press, 1922:11–12. See also Al-Tabari: Tarikh Al-Tabari, 3rd ed. Beirut: ʿIz-ad-Din, 1992;1:130.

38. Al-Sukkari: Khitan, op. cit., pp. 103–107.

39. Shaltut, Mahmud: Al-fatawi. 10th ed. Cairo & Beirut: Dar al-shuruq, 1980:331.

40. Ibn-Qudamah: Al-Mughni. Riyad: Maktabat al-Riyad al-hadithah, 1981;1:85.

41. Al-Asbahani: Kitab dalaʾil al-nubuwwah. Riyad: ʿAlam al-kutub, 1988:99–105. See also Al-Sukkari: Khitan, op. cit., pp. 67–68.

42. Al-Nimr, ʿAbd-al-Munʾim: ʿIlm al-tafsir. Cairo & Beirut: Dar al-kitab al-Masri, Dar al-kutub al-islamiyyah & Dar al-kitab al-lubnani, 1985:159–60.

43. The Gospel of Barnabas. Edited and translated by Lonsdale and Laura Ragg. Oxford: Clarendon Press, 1907. reprint Chapter 22 in: Lahore: Al-Kitab, 1981:45.

44. The Gospel of Barnabas, op. cit., chap. 23, pp. 47–49.

45. ʿAbd-al-Raziq: Al-khitan, op. cit., p. 16.

46. Saadah, Khaleel: Mugaddimat Ingil Barnaba. Cairo: Magallat al-Manar, 1908: introduction, page "j."

47. See the foreword written by Qazi Muhammad Hafizullah to the reprinted English edition of the Gospel of Barnabas, op. cit.

48. Al-Sukkari: Khitan, op. cit., pp. 46, 62–63.

49. Al-Birri, Zakariyya: Ma hukm khitan al-bint wa-hal huwa daruri, in ʿAbd-al-Raziq: Al-Khitan, op. cit., pp. 95–96.

50. Al-Qaradawi, Youssef: Huda al-islam, fatawi muʾassirah. 3rd ed. Kuwait: Dar al-qalam, 1987:443.

51. Makhluf, Hassanayn Muhammad: Hukm al-khitan, in: Al-fatawi al-islamiyyah min dar al-iftaʾ al-masriyyah. Cairo: Wazarat al-awqaf, 1981;2:449.

52. Nassar, ʿAllam: Khitan al-banat, in Al-fatawi al-islamiyyah min dar al-iftaʾ al-masriyyah. Cairo: Wazarat al-awqaf, 1982;6:1986.

53. Gad-al-Haq: Khitan al-banat, op. cit., pp. 3119–3125.

54. Gad-al-Haq, ʿAli Gad-al-Haq: Al-khitan, annex to the periodical Al-Azhar, October 1994.

55. Al-Ahram, October 9, 1994:8.

56. Al-Sukkari: Khitan, op. cit., pp. 75–77.

57. Gad-al-Haq: Khitan al-banat, op. cit., p. 3120.

58. Al-Sukkari: Khitan, op. cit., pp. 73–75.

59. Al-Sukkari: Khitan, op. cit., pp. 75–77.

60. Amin, Ahmad: Qamus al-ʿadat wal-taqalid wal-taʾabir al-masriyyah. Cairo: Maktabat al-nahdah al-masriyyah, 1992:187.

61. See the two Saudi fatwas in Magallat al-buhuth al-islamiyyah, Riyad: 1987;(20):161. and 1989;(25):62.

62. Zenie Ziegler, Wedad: La face voilée des femmes d'Egypte,. Paris: Mercure de France, 1985:66–7.

63. El-Masry, Youssef: Le drame sexuel de la femme dans l'Orient arabe, Paris: Laffont, 1962:3.

64. Al-Fangari, Ahmad Shawqi: Al-tib al-wiqaʾi fil-islam. Cairo: Al-hayʾah al-masriyyah al-ʿammah lil-kitab, 1980:143.

65. See these arguments in Bigelow, Jim: The Joy of Uncircumcising, Aptos: Hourglass, 1992:29–45.

66. Shaltut: Al-fatawi, op. cit., pp. 333–334.

67. Al-Ghawabi, Hamid: Khitan al-banat bayn al-tib wal-islam, in ʿAbd-al-Raziq: Al-Khitan, op. cit., p. 57.

68. Al-Salih, Muhammad Ibn-Ahmad: Al-tifil fil-shariʾah al-islamiyyah. Cairo: Matbaʾat nahdat Masr. 1980:85.

69. Al-Ghawabi: Khitan, op. cit., p. 62.

70. Al-Ghawabi: Khitan, op. cit., p. 51.

71. Al-Ghawabi: Khitan, op. cit., p. 57.

72. Gad-al-Haq: Khitan al-banat, op. cit., p. 3124.

73. Mahran, Maher: Les risques médicaux de l'excision (circoncision médicale), reprint of a paper published in Bulletin Médical de l'IPPF 1981;15(2):1–2.

74. For more about those complications, see Rapport sur les pratiques traditionnelles, Addis Ababa: 1990:56–7.

75. Al-Sukkari: Khitan, op. cit., p. 106.

76. For the link between drugs and female circumcision, see Amin: Qamus al-ʿadat, op. cit. p. 188; Al-Hadidi, Muhammad Saʾid: Khitan al-awlad bayn al-tib wal-islam, in ʿAbd-al-Raziq: Al-khitan, op. cit., pp. 67–70.

77. El-Masry: Le drame sexuel, op. cit., pp. 56–69.

78. El-Masry: Le drame sexuel, op. cit., pp. 61–62.

79. Al-Hadidi: Khitan al-awlad, op. cit., pp. 67–70.

80. El-Saadawi: The hidden, op. cit., p. 38.

81. El-Saadawi: The hidden, op. cit., p. 33.

82. El-Saadawi: The hidden, op. cit., pp. 40–41.
83. Ibn-Taymiyyah: Fatawi al-nissa.' Beirut: Dar al-qalam, 1987:17.
84. Al-Qarrafi: Al-dhakhirah. Beirut: Dar al-gharb al-islami, 1994;13:278–9.
85. Hamrush, Ibrahim: Khitan al-banat, in 'Abd-al-Raziq: Al-khitan, op. cit., p. 75.
86. Nassar: Khitan al-banat, op. cit., p. 1986.
87. Al-Sukkari: Khitan, op. cit., pp. 33–37, 39–40.
88. Shaltut: Al-fatawi, op. cit., pp. 333–334.
89. Shaltut: Khitan al-banat, op. cit., pp. 89–90.
90. 'Abd-al-Wahid, Nigm 'Abd-Allah: Nazrat al-islam hawl tabi'at al-gins wal-tanassul. Kuwait: Matabi' al-manar, 1986:109–16.
91. Unabridged Arab text on the issue in Report on Traditional Practices, Dakar: 1984:247–250; basic French translation, pp. 72–73.
92. Text in Al-Sabbagh, Muhammad Ibn-Lutfi: Al-hukm al-shar'i fi khitan al-dhukur wal-inath. Alexandria: Munazzamat al-sihhah al-'alamiyyah, 1995:26–34.
93. Report of the United Nations Seminar related to Traditional Practices affecting the Health of Women and Children, Ouagadougou, Burkina Faso, April 29-May 3, 1991, E/CN.4/Sub.2/1991/48, Jun.12, 1991:9.
94. Magmu'at al-qawa'id al-qanuniyyah 1931–1955, Penal Division, March 28, 1938 Session, vol. 2, p. 824.
95. Qararat Mahkamat al-naqd, Penal Division, March 11, 1974 Session, Judicial Year 25, p. 263.
96. WHO, 12th World Health Assembly, 11th Plenary Meeting, May 28, 1959.
97. Rapport sur les pratiques traditionnelles, Dakar, 1984, p. 67.
98. Ibid., p. 71.
99. WHO, Resolution of the Regional Committee for Africa, Thirty-ninth session, AFR/RC39/R9, Sep. 13, 1989.
100. Report on Traditional Practices, Addis Ababa, p. 77.
101. Ibid., pp. 8–9.
102. Arabic text in: Al-halqah al-dirassiyyah 'an al-intihak al-badani li-sighar al-inath, Cairo: 1979:54–6.
103. Time magazine, September 26, 1994, p. 65; Middle East Times, September 18–24, 1994:1, 16 passim.
104. Equality now, Women's action 8.1, March 1995; Akhbar al-Yom, October 29, 1994:13.
105. See on this philosopher, Encyclopédie de l'Islam, new edition, Leiden: Brill. 1995;8:490–3.

4

THE SKOPTZY

The Russian Sect of the Castrated

Didier Diers and Xavier Valla

Editors' note: Some Christian sects practiced sexual mutilation, including partial or complete amputation of the testicles and penis. A sect in Russia, which began this practice in 1757, and which continues to the present day, is described. Proselytizing among unsuspecting peasants, the leaders of this sect promised converts that redemption would follow mutilation. The underlying motivation for castration was that sexuality led to damnation. Circumcision may follow similar reasoning.

Partial or complete amputation of the external sexual organs is an ancient practice that is not limited to Judaism or Islam. Although Christian dogma is officially opposed to sexual mutilations such as castration and circumcision, a variety of Christian religious sects have arisen down through the ages whose members have imitated the act of self-mutilation performed by Origen, an early father of the Christian Church. The fact that there are seventy-two eunuchs to be found in the list of Christian saints indicates the special place castration has earned in traditional Christianity.

In the Eleventh Century, Valesius founded the first Christian community of castrates, in accordance with the Christian idea that the more the body suffers, the happier the soul. Christian castration expanded rapidly during the Byzantine Empire. Even in Italy, up until the end of the Eighteenth Century, about four thousand boys were emasculated each year — with the pope's benediction — to supply the choirs of Europe with castratos. Today, in some Sicilian villages, it is still possible to find antique shops selling old signs reading, "Boys castrated here for a modest price." Despite this seemingly universal Christian tendency towards castration, there is no other Christian country where castration was more wide-spread than Russia.

During the Eighteenth Century, a deep mystical movement swept through the Russian Empire. In 1757, André Ivanov, a rebellious member of the sect of flagellants, reacted against the perceived licentiousness of the Klysty, and founded the sect of the Skoptzy, or Castrates. He launched the new sect by castrating himself and then thirteen of his disciples. Soon thereafter, Ivanov was arrested by the authorities and deported to Siberia, where he eventually died.

Rather than forsaking the new religion, the martyrdom of Ivanov served to strengthen the commitment of the remaining Skoptzy disciples and proselytes. The sect declared that Kondrati Sselivanoff, one of the original disciples, was "the new Christ descended among men" and, under his leadership, the new sect grew in size and power. His followers walked around the Russian Empire and propagated the simple message: "Everyone can be a tsar through this conversion." By 1770, Sselivanoff was finding a wider audience and could even be found preaching his doctrine in St. Petersburg. He eventually became the protégé of the Baroness of Krudener, the mistress of the Tsar. The Baroness reportedly considered Sselivanoff to be a saint.

In the middle of the Nineteenth Century, Russian authorities put the number of castrates living in the Empire at 10,000. Skoptzy converts could be found in every social class, gaining considerable strength among the banking and capitalist classes, but the majority of converts were peasants, whose tendency for religious fanaticism opened them to exploitation by Skoptzy task-masters. The majority of Skoptzy were converts from the Greek Orthodox Church, but a fairly significant minority were Roman Catholics, Lutherans, Muslims, and Jews. Initiated sect members, however, did not break with the Orthodox Church. In order to divert suspicion, they became outwardly more zealous and devout than before. The austere life-style of the Skoptzy, coupled with their doctrinal devotion to money-making, placed many a Skopet castrate into the realm of millionaires. Many of these castrates rose to positions of power and influence throughout the Empire. One such high-placed castrate, a certain Mr. Elensky attained the position of chamberlain to Tsar Alexander I. In 1804, Elensky proposed to the Tsar a plan to convert the entire Russian Empire into a castrate empire. Elensky did not find an enthusiastic audience in the Tsar, and a few years later, Alexander I decreed that any Skopets caught by the police would be sent to the mines.

In 1859, three young men from prominent St. Petersburg families died as a result of their initiatory rites. The public outcry over these deaths led to increased popular opposition to the Skoptzy, forcing many of them to flee to Romania, where the State's policy of fostering complete religious freedom could be relied on to shield the Skoptzy from persecution.

The Skoptzy did, however, reject the fundamental dogmas of the Greek Orthodox Church, including the dogma of the redemption of Christ. The Skoptzy held that Sselivanoff was the true Christ, sent by God to teach the world the principle of sexual mutilation for the redemption of mankind.

In Russia, the Skoptzy, united by their common mutilation, worked to attract new members and influence the power structure of the Empire in their favor through incessant propaganda about their sect and its rites. Members of the sect divided and shared their patrimony communally. Their small communities, called 'Naves,' found new members among the middle class. Workers employed by factories that were owned by members of the castrate sect were required to adhere to a vegetarian diet, abstain from alcohol, work hard, and accept castration. The sexual mutilations imposed on the workers prevented them from leaving the sect.

There were several steps involved in becoming a member of the Skoptzy. After marriage and the birth of a second child, members of the sect were required to submit to the rites of castration. The first stage of the initiation was called "the first purification" or "the little mark." Initially, the first stage was performed by burning off testicles with a red-hot iron, but this technique proved to be too barbaric even for the Skoptzy. Later, the scrotum and testicles were cut off with a knife or razor blade. In Skoptzy theology, the testicles were considered to be the "keys to hell," and their amputation conferred upon the initiate "the right to mount the spotted horse."

The second stage of initiation, called "the great seal," the "imperial seal," or simply, "the second purification," involved the amputation of the penis. This stage was usually delayed for a few years after the removal of the testicles. The penis was amputated with scissors, a razor, a pocketknife, a pruning knife, a chisel, a piece of sheet metal, a bone from a bull, or a hatchet, and was performed without much ceremony, though frequently the rite involved a ritual dance. Hemorrhage was stopped with ice and resin, and the urethra was plugged with a tin or lead tube. In Skoptzy theology, the penis represented the "key to the abyss." Amputation of the penis gave the initiate the right to "mount the white horse of the apocalypse" and saved him from hell. After emasculation, the novice was admitted into the sect. Wearing a long white shirt, the novice recited the following oath:

> I swear to endure torture, exile, fever, whip, block or hatchet rather than give my secret to the enemy.

Following this, the novice received a candle and a net to signal his status as a full-fledged member of the sect.

For the women of the sect, the initial ritual mutilation involved the amputation of the nipples. This mutilation was called "the little seal." The so-called "great seal" involved the total ablation of the breasts, the ablation of labia minora, and sometimes the ablation of labia majora and the clitoris.

Some castrates underwent a third purification, in which part of the breast muscle was cut off and a triangle of flesh was removed from the hip. The third step, involved much whirling or jumping to induce a trance state. In the castrate theology, all these mutilations represented the five wounds of the Christ. At the end of the Eighteenth Century, Skoptzy proselytizers often quoted the German writer Jakob Böhme — then popular among the Russian intelligentsia — who said, "The only difference between men and angels is the lack of sexual organs."

Because of constant persecution from the authorities, castrates who were arrested shielded the sect and its members by never admitting how they had become castrated or revealing the name of the person who had castrated them. Instead, they invented stories about accidents.

The methods of recruitment used by the Skoptzy were simple and effective. Proselytizers distributed pamphlets containing Biblical texts which refer to castration. In many cases, children were forcibly castrated to mark them as members of the Skoptzy community. Capitalist Skopets pressured their workers into conversion through economic slavery, irresistible cash incentives, or by providing free housing for the poor or for orphans in exchange for their castration. Younger members of the sect were used for proselytism because of their ability to attract others of their age.

In the middle of the Nineteenth Century, tsarist authorities began to banish members of the sect to Siberia. Article 197 of the tsarist criminal code allowed for deportation of heretic sects, but did not specifically mention forbidding sexual mutilation. Article 201, passed a few years later, was more explicit. The sentence for self-castration was deportation to Siberia. The sentence for castrating another person was six years of hard labor. After the Revolution of October 1905, the Skoptzy were granted the right to live where they wanted in Russia, but in 1910, 142 castrates were arrested and deported.

After the Bolshevik Revolution, Article 123 of the new penal code replaced the anti-heretical articles of the former regime. This law was formulated during the anti-religious trials of the late 1920s and early 1930s. Sexual mutilation was specifically outlawed under Article 142 of the new legal code. In May of 1929, members of the sect were sentenced before the Leningrad tribunal in what was the biggest anti-Skoptzy trial that had ever taken place. One-hundred-fifty sect members were sentenced and deported.

Soon the State apparatus took emergency actions against the Skoptzy. A number of well-known castrates came under constant police surveillance. Administrative action was taken to isolate fanatics and castrators. Mr. Bontch-Brouevitch, a specialist in the study of mystical sects, wrote in 1928:

> It is time now, in the 20th Century, to stop the propaganda in favor of religious mutilations because circumstances have changed. In their place, there are now pressing goals which call for energy, strength and will. These rituals invented by uneducated people must change.

Eradication of the Skoptzy was not achieved quickly. Even as late as 1931, the newspaper, *Without God*, ran a front-page story with the banner headline: "Rid Moscow of the Castrate Infection."

Presumably, the Soviet authorities were successful in their campaign to rid the country of the Skoptzy, but even as late as the 1970s, there were still about 100 followers of this sect living in the USSR. Today, in St. Petersburg, the house where Sselivanoff lived for 18 years still stands in Kovenski Passage. It is now a youth club.

BIBLIOGRAPHY

Derbes VJ. The keepers of the bed: castration and religion. Journal of the American Medical Association 1970;212:97–100.

Volkov N. La Secte Russe des Castrats. Paris: Les Belles Lettres, 1995.

von Stein F. Die Skopzensekte in Russland, in ihrer Entstehung, Organisation und lehre. Zeitschrift fur Ethnologie 1875;7:37–69.

Volkov NN. Skopchestvo i sterilizatsiia; istoricheskii ocherk. Moskva: Izd-vo Akademii nauk SSSR, 1937.

5

FUNCTIONAL AND EROTIC CONSEQUENCES OF SEXUAL MUTILATIONS

Gérard Zwang

Infant and childhood sexual mutilations carry immediate risks, such as uncontrollable hemorrhage, urinary tract infection, tetanus, gangrene, and septicemia. These complications can often be fatal. The risk of fatality is also an element of the mutilative rites of passage imposed on adolescents in animist societies. It is intolerable that certain occidental enthusiasts for Third World cultures romanticize the mythical benefits of these traditional initiation rites, when these same "civilized" peoples are traumatized by the slightest sore and will do anything to spare their offspring the harsh rigors of their own society's "rites of passage," such as the final examinations of secondary school or university selection examinations.

The long-term consequences for the survivors of sexual mutilation are precisely those desired by the mutilators, who permanently mark the unfortunate children who pass into their hands. The injuries are perhaps less severe for males than for females, but the mutilation of the two sexes are inextricably linked. One cannot eradicate one without eradicating the other.

1. THE COMPLICATIONS OF FEMALE SEXUAL MUTILATION

Many immediate complications of female sexual mutilation are identical with the immediate complications of male sexual mutilation. These include: pain, hemorrhage, and infection.

1.1. Immediate Complications

One complication of clitoridectomy is injury to the urethra, either at its orifice or along the interior canal. The immediate result is urinary retention and reflux, which requires emergency medical attention, although this is not always possible in countries without adequate medical care. Later, the injured urethra generally develops a cicatricial

Sexual Mutilations: A Human Tragedy, edited by Denniston and Milos
Plenum Press, New York, 1997

stenosis. This condition of the urethra results initially in dysuria, making each micturition difficult and painful. Above the stenosis of the urethra, there may develop an ascending distention of the urinary canal, reaching the bladder, the ureters, and the kidneys, bringing grave risk of infection and chronic kidney damage.

1.2. Long-Term Complications

The long-term complications of female sexual mutilation are of three types: obstetric, coital, and erotic.

1.2.1. Obstetric Complications. Once known only in the countries where these mutilations are practiced, obstetric complications were treated by what used to be called "colonial" medicine and surgery. As a result of African immigration to the larger cities of France, these complications are, unfortunately, found today in urban maternity clinics to such an extent that obstetricians now publish two sets of morbidity statistics: one for the normal population, and one for the excised population. This fact was first revealed in 1977 at a press conference on female sexual mutilation held in Geneva.

Obstetrical complications are largely the result of infibulation, but also of clitoridectomy, particularly when it is associated with the excision of the labia. If the excision and cutaneous sutures in the area of the anterior portion of the vulva are only centimeters from the vulvular orifice and body of the clitoris, the mutilator, using backward motions of the razor blade, can extend the cuts around the vaginal orifice. This may happen as a result of clumsiness, haphazard cutting, or cutting too deeply at the intersection of the labia. It may also be a result of the victim struggling and causing the knife to slip.

In every case, the result of mutilation may be an extensive sclerosis of the vulvoperineal cicatrices. This is the classic cause of perineal dystocia, causing the head of the fetus to ram against the cicatricial, sclerotic, and indilatable vagina at the perineal floor.

Sometimes the fetus remains lodged in the vaginal canal. If medical attention is not received immediately, the risk becomes twofold. For the infant, there is the mortal risk of asphyxiation. For the mother, there is the risk of perineal fistulas. The recto-vaginal and especially the vesico-vaginal partitions necrotize around the impacted fetal head. This is the usual cause of the recto-vaginal and vesico-vaginal fistulas that afflict so many African women.

Sometimes the fetus ruptures the perineum. The vaginal orifice may be the only one shredded, but often the rupture lacerates the fibrous nucleus of the perineum, the anal sphincter, the anal canal, and its orifice. This massive rupture cannot properly cicatrize without immediate surgical attention. Such attention is rare, leaving the victims to suffer from fecal or urinary incontinence. Their perineum becomes a cesspool.

Evidently, the ethnic groups that perpetrate sexual mutilation of their females either attach little importance to the physical integrity of the female or are obedient to a blind fatalism by pretending that, without excision, women will not be able to give birth correctly. Despite the obvious obstetrical complications caused by mutilation, this myth continues to be disseminated by tribal chiefs and practitioners of mutilation — those whom ignorant occidentals naively consider to be the "depositaries of ancestral wisdom."

1.2.2. Coital Complications. Excised women may not only suffer from frigidity, but may also suffer from dyspareunia. The first coital experience of infibulated women is usually accompanied by excruciating pain, since the suture of the labia majora must be cut open with a knife. The lucky ones cicatrize fairly well, such that the penile penetration

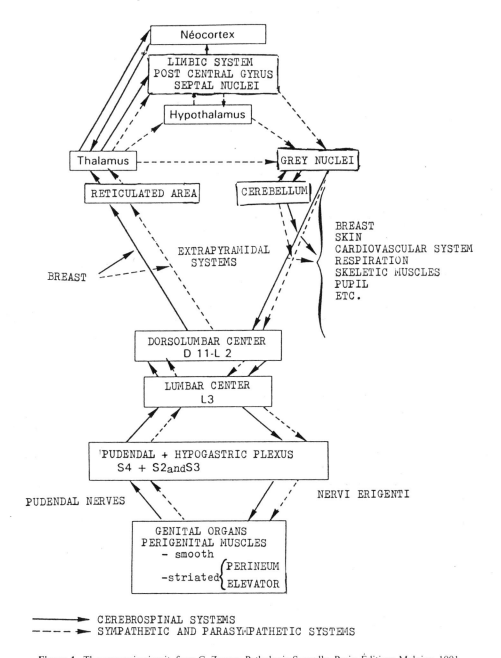

Figure 1. The orgasmic circuit. from G. Zwang. Pathologie Sexuelle. Paris: Éditions Maloine, 1991.

into the vagina becomes painless. A certain number of other women develop indurated, fragile, painful, and bleeding cicatrices. Each act of sexual intercourse causes pain. The pain increases for those who have been subjected to periodic refibulation and defibulation and to women whose perineum has been destroyed by the obstetrical complications described above.

The amputation of the clitoris may also result in chronic, agonizing pain caused by the development of a neuroma on the scar where the dorsal nerve was cut. Beyond the spontaneous pains that can generate phantom clitoral pain (identical to the phantom pain suffered by limb amputees), the least touch in this region can bring about fulgurating pain. For these women, each sexual experience is torturous.

1.2.3. Erotic Complications. Regardless of the justifications proffered to Westerners by the perpetrators of sexual mutilation, the excision of the clitoris has but one precise goal: to prevent women from experiencing orgasm. The great majority of excised females suffer from primary anorgasmia.

Orgasm is a complex systemic reflex. It encompasses numerous pathways and nervous connections of such magnitude that one can speak of a vast orgasmic circuit.

At birth, this circuit only exists in a rudimentary state. Similarly, other nervous circuits, such as that which controls bipedal locomotion and that which regulates spoken language, exist in a rudimentary state at birth. The establishment of these circuits is epigenetic, that is, secondary to birth, and depends on the full development of these connections and the synapses connecting the neurons under the influence of endogenous stimulation.

In young humans, the epigenetic connections of the orgasmic circuit begin to fuse effectively around age 2 or 3. The normal mechanism for activation of this circuit is handling and fondling of the external sexual organs, as inevitably and innocently practiced by children as they explore their body. Little boys, with their projecting penis, have an advantage in this respect. They have even been observed masturbating in the womb. Little girls, however, fondle the clitoris during infancy, and their orgasmic circuit becomes functional around 6 or 7 years of age. Consequently, masturbation in late childhood and adolescence, even when it is not regular, continues to involve the clitoris and trains the functional pathways of the reflex circuit. Certainly, there exist other feminine methods of reaching solitary orgasm. Thigh rubbing exercises the pelvic musculature, the anal elevator muscles, and the perineal muscles. Although thigh rubbing can be considered a "trial run" of the orgasmic physiology of the lower vagina, it is not effective until after the establishment of the orgasmic reflex by clitoral stimulation.

It is only in the second decade of life that human females attain genital development sufficient to engage in copulation. Although they are not exactly of the same type as those of the clitoris, the vagina possesses orgasmogenic erogenous receptors which permit the triggering of the orgasmic reflex after a time of coital practice. This is possible only if the orgasmic circuit has been established and has become functional. For many females, self-induced clitoral orgasm is a necessary preliminary for attaining vaginal orgasm.

It should be acknowledged that the complete branching of the reflex connections of orgasm can only be established during the crucial period of early childhood. Likewise, this is the same crucial period of life for the development of language skills. After that, it is too late. The physiology of the orgasmic reflex must therefore be established in the first years of life, before 6 or 7 years of age. It will later be reactivated by functional stimulation. Otherwise, it will fall into disuse. This is the classic mechanism whereby under-utilized nervous circuits wither and degenerate.

It is, therefore, easy to understand why females who have been subjected to clitoridectomy are anorgasmic. Young girls excised in the first years of life, even at birth, will never establish the functional connection of the synapses. Adolescent girls mutilated between the ages of 10 and 15 are no longer able to receive the necessary stimulation to maintain these reflexes. In either case, they will be unable to connect their vaginal sensations into the potential or transferred nervous circuit. No longer having a clitoris, at adulthood, they cannot trigger orgasm from either of these two primary erogenous zones.

Occasionally, it is claimed, that certain excised females have attained vaginal orgasm. This could be possible if they were mutilated rather late in life, such that their reflex circuit, being well established and well maintained, particularly by thigh rubbing, could be functionally engaged through vaginal stimulation. All doubt would be removed if the actual function of the orgasmic reflex of such women were subjected to objective, controlled, clinical study. As yet, there is no scientific data to prove or refute this claim.

The World Health Organization has already recognized the concept of sexual health, and has issued its recommendations for the abolition of sexual mutilation. Those countries that practice excision, and do nothing to stop it, can no longer turn a deaf ear. They must face the severest condemnation if they continue to create, in an experimental way, women who, because of clitoral mutilation, are unable to satisfy the orgasmic needs that humans of both sexes normally feel. In these countries, men do not deprive themselves of opportunities to satisfy their sexual appetites, and in order to find satisfaction, claim that they require the erotic services of more than one woman. Excision is a destruction of erotic function. Mutilated women can never experience the beauties of this world in all its dimensions or realize all their corporeal abilities. This is precisely the goal of these societies: to transform these women into enslaved beings.

2. THE COMPLICATIONS OF CIRCUMCISION

Ablation of the clitoris, a primary erotic zone, easily earns the contempt of all those who understand the seriousness of this act. The ablation of a "little piece of skin" at the end of the penis of little boys, however, seems, by comparison, to be so much less injurious. Because of this misconception, it is often difficult to raise consciousness against this odious and harmful practice. Circumcision is, however, very damaging, even though this fact is difficult to accept for those people who cling tenaciously to its mythology and who still want to mark their unfortunate offspring in this indelible way. It would be useful here to provide a succinct description of the anatomy and functions of the foreskin.

2.1. Anatomy and Physiology of the Foreskin

The foreskin is part of normal human anatomy. Its development is genetically programmed. It is present in all male newborns regardless of their ethnic make-up. Its physiological characteristics are identical, regardless of its pigmentation, size, length, or shape.

As a folded prolongation of the penile skin sheath, the foreskin consists of a thin epidermal layer without hair follicles or subdermal fat layer. It continues towards its attachment at the coronal sulcus. The posterior zone is advanced, forming a unique fold, called the frenulum, that finds its point of attachment at the urethral meatus. In its normal state, the foreskin rolls freely over the surface of the glans penis. This anterior-posterior, backward and forward motion of eversion and reversion can occur spontaneously or deliberately. The classic comparison is the action of the eyelid over the surface of the eye. The role of the foreskin is both protective and erotic.

2.1.1. Protective Role: The Static Function of the Reverted Foreskin. In childhood, the foreskin is often longer than the glans penis. It protects the integument of the glans from contact with urine. This protective feature is especially important during infancy and prior to the establishment of urinary continence. It prevents infections and irritation. During the uncontrollable micturitions of infancy, urine courses through the nozzle of the foreskin with sufficient force such that little or no urine droplets remain inside the foreskin. In the normal child, urine is sterile. Stagnant urine can ferment in the diapers, especially if it comes in contact with fecal mater. The longer and more adherent the foreskin is to the glans, the more the glans penis and, especially, the urethral meatus, are protected.

In adulthood, a portion of the glans may or may not remain uncovered. This occurs during puberty because the penile shaft develops, in terms of length, faster than the foreskin. The glans (*acorn* in Latin) takes its name not only because of its conical shape, but because of the configuration of the foreskin, which forms an epithelial capsule around it, similar to the acorn. The foreskin protects the most sensitive parts of the glans penis: the zone of insertion for the frenulum; and the corona glandis. The basal zone of the foreskin is rich in sebaceous glands, ensuring proper lubrication of the rolling mechanism.

2.1.2. Erotic Function of the Foreskin. The erotic role of the foreskin is realized in the anterior-posterior rolling movement over the surface of the glans penis. This is usually the result of habitual manual stimulation. During erection, preputial eversion occurs spontaneously in normal men. This liberates the glans penis without the least effort. The elastic quality of the preputial skin permits the foreskin to revert over the glans with great ease and, indeed, great pleasure.

The surface of the glans, with its reduced keratinization and increased complement of corpuscular erogenous nerve receptors, cannot tolerate direct, dry friction without experiencing pain. During coitus, stimulation of the glans occurs naturally by the lubricated vaginal epithelium. Fellatio, due to the salivary lubricant, is also a very effective stimulant. Direct manual stimulation, however, is unpleasant, and has no possibility of triggering the orgasmogenic physiology. Held between the thumb and index finger, the foreskin is in precisely the right place to mediate digital stimulation of the glans penis, with the backward and forward motion that is the standard mechanism of erogenous excitation. This natural mechanism of balanic stimulation generally functions in two areas.

2.1.2.1. Auto-Eroticism. Masturbation is a universal phenomena among boys. As in females, masturbation develops the orgasmic circuit by establishing and reactivating its neural connections. Additionally, masturbation liberates any remaining preputial adherences and prevents the development of most cases of constitutional preputial stenosis (phimosis) by passing the glans penis through the preputial orifice, even if a little bit tight.

2.1.2.2. Heterosexual Intercourse. During sexual activity, penile stimulation is performed by the female partner. If desired, preputial stimulation can lead directly to orgasm. During foreplay, the glans is stroked through the medium of the foreskin. Erection is a phenomenon that should be maintained, at least before copulation. The foreskin allows easy and quick stimulation to maintain erection. It is quickly appreciated and can be done without fuss, in an almost automatic way, especially at the moment where the female partner is experiencing her own subjective reactions to erogenous excitation and hardly has time to think about complicated maneuvers. In this way, the foreskin demonstrates its useful and beneficent role: to serve as a natural intermediary of feminine erotic tenderness. The man who has been subjected to a ritual circumcision has thus been unjustifiably deprived of a useful body part, and this is precisely the object of the mutilation.

2.2. Consequences of Preputial Mutilation

The injurious consequences of preputial mutilation, or "circumcision," are seen in childhood and throughout adulthood. They include immediate operative complications, such as pain, hemorrhage, inflammation, and infection. Long-term complications include erotic, aesthetic, and ethical harm.

2.2.1. Immediate Complications. The immediate operative complications of circumcision affect children and adolescents, but they also affect males mutilated in adulthood.

2.2.1.1. Pain. With or without reasonable justification, it is unpardonable to inflict suffering on infants and young children who are unable to defend themselves. Ritual circumcision is neither a vaccination nor a healthful surgical operation. Of course, a "proper traditional circumcision" is performed without anesthesia. The child mutilated at seven years of age will always remember the gashing of the razor or the cutting of the scissors between his legs.
A certain number of mutilated children will develop a real phobia for pain. They cannot tolerate the least amount of pain, such as that experienced during medical examinations and vaccination, without suffering panic attacks or hysteria. If, during the mutilation of the child, the perpetrators — particularly the mother — are affected by his screams, they do not seem sufficiently affected to rush to the defense of the child and protect him from harm.

2.2.1.2. Hemorrhage. Injury to the frenular artery, which is necessarily severed during circumcision, can cause severe hemorrhage. This is especially dangerous for infants afflicted with hemophilia, a condition that is not obligatorily diagnosed in countries where medical care is rudimentary or nonexistent.

2.2.1.3. Inflammation. Directly exposed to prolonged contact with urine, the urinary meatus can become inflamed and ulcerated. This is the classic cause of dysuria, as well as urinary distention and inflammation of the ascending urethra.

2.2.1.4. Infection. Where asepsis is unknown, the amputation wound is directly exposed to all sorts of infectious agents, from common germs, to tetanus, and to gangrene. Every year, countless children die of the infectious complication of circumcision.

2.2.1.5. Mechanical Complications. In cases of hypospadias, the loss of the foreskin prevents a straight-forward repair surgery and subjects the child to a much more complex and hazardous surgery.

2.2.2. Long-Term Harm. Circumcised males have been subjected to three levels of harm: erotic, aesthetic, and ethical.

2.2.2.1. Erotic Harm of Circumcision. Erotic damage is inflicted in two ways. First, circumcision entails a loss of the physiological mechanism of manual stimulation of the glans. The glans of the circumcised penis can obviously benefit from masturbatory stimulation, but less easily than manual stimulation mediated through the foreskin. Alternative pressure, longitudinal and cautiously-applied friction, necessitate the application of auxiliary artificial lubrication, or, more often than not, saliva. Female sexual partners can be instructed in the particular modalities of manual stimulation of the glans of the circumcised penis, but in a way that is unnatural and less spontaneous. In many countries where circumcision is performed systematically (in Arabo-Muslim countries and in the United States), women must often become accustomed to performing fellatio (the so-called "Berber wake-up call").

2.2.2.1.1 Hypersensitivity of the Glans. Contrary to a tenacious mythology, the thickened glans of the circumcised penis is not always immune to pleasurable surfeit when brought in contact with vaginal mucous membrane. By leaving the glans permanently externalized, circumcision may indeed cause the formation of a protective corneal layer, but it is incorrect to claim that this permits circumcised men to engage in coitus for hours and hours, bringing their partners endless hours of vaginal ecstasy. Among the clients of Masters and Johnson, there were still large numbers of circumcised American premature ejaculators. Furthermore, there are many other circumcised males who have directly incriminated their mutilation for their lack of staying power. The tight, foreshortened, immobilized, often sclerotic skin of the circumcised penis is also more liable to laceration, bleeding, and pain during intercourse. Some circumcised men have identified their mutilation as the cause of the discomfort they suffer when their circumcised penis comes in contact with underclothes, consigning them to a permanently uncomfortable place in a world that requires clothes.

2.2.2.3. Aesthetic Harm. The scar created by ritual circumcision, practiced in a workmanlike manner by non-doctors — be they mohels or barbers — is usually unsightly, tortuous, and irregular, especially if it has suppurated. Western sculpture and painting regularly depict intact men (with foreskin) as the classical aesthetic canon of the human penis. The violation of the standards of Western aesthetics is a cause of legitimate complaint for men whose foreskin has been ablated, whose remnant penis has been scarred, and whose glans is permanently externalized.

2.2.2.4. Ethical Harm. Many men who were subjected to involuntary foreskin amputation in childhood come to regret that they were deprived of a part of their body without anyone having first obtained their consent. This regret is double where ritual circumcision is practiced towards the end of early childhood, when, after the boy has lived contentedly for 7 to 10 years with a foreskin, he is subjected to a brutal foreskin amputation without anesthesia.

3. CONCLUSIONS

All of these recriminations are expressed in the movement to abolish circumcision that has slowly emerged at the end of the Twentieth Century. These recriminations are also made by circumcised men, despite attempts to correct the mutilation. The eradication of this practice in the West has a twofold justification. First, it is necessary for Western countries to preserve the anatomical integrity of their children and not to force involuntary sexual mutilation on individuals who have not given their consent. Second, it is hypocritical for Western countries to condone sexual mutilation of males while condemning the sexual mutilation of females.

When Westerners inquire of non-Westerners the reasons for their aggression against the sexual organs of their offspring, they are often told an old myth: the myth that humans are inherently bisexual and must be subjected to "anatomical correction." Ignoring the hypocrisy of this myth for a moment, this is a perfect example of idiocy. The vast majority of men and women, like other mammals, come into the world completely male or female. The condition of intersexuality is exceedingly rare. According to the myth of the inherent bisexual nature of humans, the foreskin is supposed to be a tube identical to the vagina, and the clitoris an organ identical to the penis. Consequently, a male must have his feminizing foreskin removed in order to become a true male, and a female must have her masculizing clitoris removed in order make her a true female.

It is unfortunate that the myth of the inherent bisexual nature of humans has been enshrined in certain occidental writings. The explanation — indeed, the justification — for sexual mutilation as a "perfection of sexual anatomy" is found in Freudian psychoanalysis, which has adopted this myth. Of course, some people in the Third World take these myths as gospel truth. These Freudian myths have been succeeded today by an intellectual movement, of which E. Badinter is the leading spokesman, that pretends, on the contrary, that the two sexes are the same. This, too, opens the door to all kinds of controverted legitimizations for forcibly modifying the sexual organs of males and females.

Among the victims of ritual circumcision figure numerous Israelites living in the West and "Christian" citizens of the United States, where this mutilation has for a long time been practiced in a routine fashion in maternity wards. These circumcised men are among those medics who are working in the Third World, individually or under cover of international organizations, against childhood sexual mutilations. We have observed that the most dedicated and persuasive occidental missionaries against clitoridectomy are women working closely with third-world mothers. We have practically never seen, on the other hand, occidental men working against ritual male circumcision in Africa or the Middle East. Traditionalist immigrants, such as Israelites, Muslims, and autochthonous Africans, even attempt to prevail upon French hospitals to perform "proper circumcisions" on their children, at the cost of swindling the French Social Security system.

Perhaps these medics or missionaries are circumcised themselves and because "it didn't kill them" they do not have the desire or the will necessary to save little native boys from their cruel fate. Perhaps they may still have an intact penis, but they think in a perfunctory and perfectly controverted way that "circumcision is a proper hygienic measure for little Negro boys," and that it is more convenient to work to preserve the physical integrity of girls.

This resignation in the face of ritual male circumcision is one of the reasons that induces traditionalist Africans not to heed contradictory warnings, which seem to be just more examples of the incomprehensible "ways of white folks." For these groups, to cut boys and to cut girls has the same goal: to correct and perfect human anatomy. It seems inconsistent to them to be obliged to leave girls in their native state, while still being permitted to "correct" boys. We will never be able to completely eradicate clitoridectomy of little girls while we still allow boys to be cut.

The movement against female sexual mutilation must begin with the eradication of ritual or routine male circumcision in our own countries. This is a difficult struggle, one that is contrary to many prejudices, many habits, and, indeed, one that must confront many organized lobbies, such as the circumcision lobby in the United States. This is not, however, a reason to be discouraged.

4. BIBLIOGRAPHY

Zwang G. Pourquoi continuer à circoncire nos petits garçons? Gyn, Obs 1996;350(15 avril).

Zwang G. Quel avenir pour la circoncision? Contraception, Fertilité, Sexualité 1995;23(5):348–54.

Zwang G. Histoire des Peines de Sexe. Paris: Éditions Maloine, 1994.

Zwang G. Pathologie Sexuelle: les Troubles de la Fonction Érotique et du Comportement Sexuel de l'Adulte. Paris: Éditions Maloine, 1990.

Zwang G. Sexologie. 4e édition Paris: Masson, 1990.

Zwang G, Romieu A. Précis de Thérapeutique Sexologique: Traitement des Dysfonctionnements Érotiques de Couple. 4e édition. Paris: Éditions Maloine, 1989.

Zwang G. La Statue de Freud. Paris: R. Laffont, 1985.

Zwang G. La Fonction Érotique. Paris: Éditions Robert Laffont, 1978.

Zwang G. La circoncision, pour quoi faire? Contraception, Fertilité, Sexualité 1977;5:247–53.

Zwang G. Abrégé de Sexologie. Paris: Masson, 1976.

Zwang G. Le Sexe de la Femme. Paris: La Jeune Parque, 1967.

6

THE HUMAN PREPUCE

Mervyn M. Lander

The information prepared in this paper comes as a result of 27 years of clinical experience as a pediatric surgeon in the management of children, and, in this context, of male children, their penises, and their concerned parents; it is a personal reflection that has arisen out of analytical clinical practice.

1. INTRODUCTION

Males are born as they are meant to be and as they were destined to remain, yet a disposable society continues to want to routinely dispose of the human foreskin rather than accepting that, "if the cap fits, wear it!"

2. LANGUAGE

Normal or intact males are often labeled as being "uncircumcised." It is irrational to define the normal as "not operated upon," as if the mutilated variant is the norm. The normal male should be addressed as such, or referred to as "intact."

3. NORMAL PREPUCE

The normalcy of the human foreskin can conveniently be considered under the headings of the "PREPUTIAL P's."

3.1. Possession

It seems unlikely that humanity has been created perfectly, apart from the male prepuce. It is heresy to state, as routine male infant circumcision vividly does, that the creator

Sexual Mutilations: A Human Tragedy, edited by Denniston and Milos
Plenum Press, New York, 1997

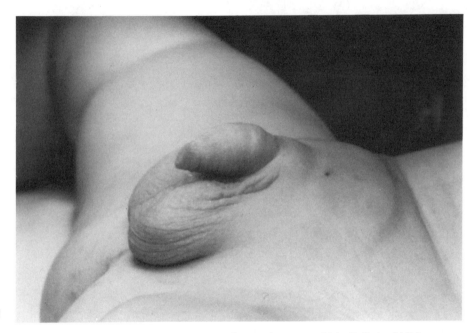

Figure 1. Normal penis of human baby. (Photograph courtesy of John R. Taylor, M.D.)

God erred in His design of the penis of every male, to such an extent that doctors and others have to surgically restore "normalcy." Boys, like girls, are, in general, born in total perfection. The human foreskin is a standard fitting, not an optional extra.

3.2. Protection

The prepuce affords protection:

- to the glans
- to the external urinary meatus
- against injury

3.3. Puberty

For many intact males, the glans remains fully covered at puberty; for some, the glans is partially covered, while, for a significant number of intact men, the foreskin is always retracted behind the glans.

3.4. Play

The intact penis has twice as much integument as the circumcised penis. This provides many innovative possibilities for play, compared to the tight, immobile skin of the circumcised penis.

3.5. Performance

The intact male has adequate skin to maximize his erectile potential. Many circumcised males have suffered radical skin removal at the time of circumcision. As a result, they lose penile length, experience pain, and have hairs and scrotal skin displaced along the shaft of the erect penis.

3.6. Pleasure

The prepuce maximizes a male's erogenous potential from:

- a sensitive, protected glans
- the prepuce itself
- the frenulum (God's gift to man). The frenulum is a male's most sensitive erogenous zone; the frenulum is usually excised in neonatal circumcision.

3.7. Procreation

When the prepuce is fully retracted, traction is exerted upon the frenulum, which deviates the glans ventrally. This occurs normally at ejaculation, placing the ejaculate at the entrance of the cervix.

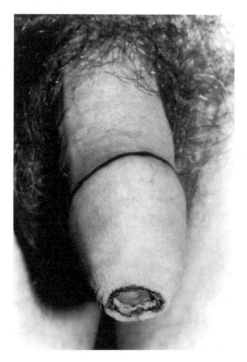

Figure 2. Three Zones of Penile Skin 1. Penis slightly tumescent. The area between the groin and the upper line is (1) the skin covering the shaft. The area between the upper line and the lower line is (2) the foreskin's outside fold. The outside fold is almost as long as the skin covering the shaft. *Well over half of the total penile skin is foreskin!* See also Figures 3–6. (Photograph courtesy of John A. Erickson)

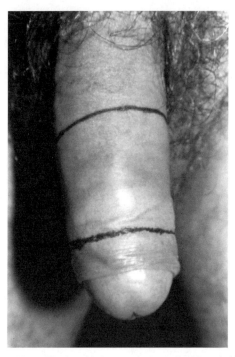

Figure 3. Three Zones of Penile Skin 2. The foreskin retracted (manually) about half an inch. The area between the upper line and the lower line is (2) the foreskin's outside fold. The area below the lower line is first half inch or so of (3) the foreskin's everting inside fold. (Photograph courtesy of John A. Erickson)

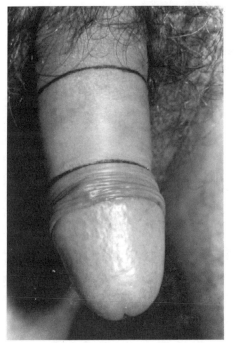

Figure 4. Three Zones of Penile Skin 3. The foreskin everted. The area between the upper line and the lower line is (2) the foreskin's everted outside fold. The area below the lower line is (3) the foreskin's inside fold, now gathered behind the coronal sulcus. (Photograph courtesy of John A. Erickson)

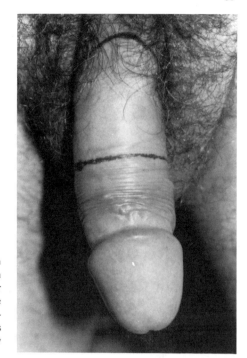

Figure 5. Three Zones of Penile Skin 4. The foreskin everted farther. Almost the entire shaft is now covered with foreskin. The area between the upper line and the lower line is (2) the foreskin's outside fold. The area between the lower line and the glans is (3) the foreskin's retracted inside fold. If the skin were released, it would return to its position in the previous photograph. (Photograph courtesy of John A. Erickson)

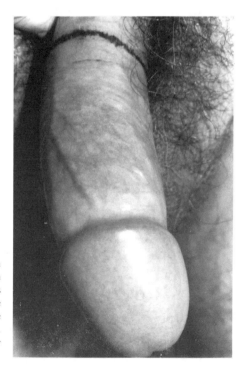

Figure 6. Three Zones of Penile Skin 5. The foreskin everted as far as it will comfortably go. The area between the lower line (the only line now visible) and the glans is (3) the foreskin's fully everted inside fold. The entire penile shaft is now covered with foreskin. Well over half of the penile shaft is covered with the foreskin's inside fold. Veins, arteries, capillaries and smooth glans texture clearly visible. (Photograph courtesy of John A. Erickson)

3.8. Penetration

With intercourse, both intact and circumcised men experience contact with the vaginal wall with penetration and withdrawal. The intact male also slides in and out of his prepuce and places intermittent tension on his frenulum. He experiences a "triple treat" compared to the circumcised man. The action of the intact male is also more gentle to the vagina.

3.9. Perfume

The intact penis has a distinctive "odor," which is normal and should not be regarded as pathological in our deodorized society.

4. RELATIONSHIP OF THE GLANS AND PREPUCE

At birth, the glans and prepuce are attached to each other. Separation occurs on its own, both distally around the meatus (and this is often eccentric), and in areas over the glans, giving rise to yellow smegma collections under the foreskin. These are normal and require no treatment. Full separation may occur normally at any age from birth to marriage.

4.1. Glans Color

The glans of the intact male of European descent is usually purple, compared to the dull pink glans of the circumcised male.

4.2. Advice to Parents Regarding Care of the Intact Penis

LEAVE IT ALONE!
Older males should retract their prepuce fully (if fully separated) or to the level of normal attachment with their daily ablutions. NO SPECIAL CARE IS REQUIRED.

5. PATHOLOGY

As with all body parts, the prepuce may be the site of pathological processes.

5.1. Narrow Preputial Orifice

The narrow preputial orifice may present as:

• infection
• non-retractability
• ballooning with micturition

The treatment of the narrow preputial orifice is:

• gentle eversion of the inner layer
• steroid cream

In the absence of scarring, the phimotic prepuce is salvageable.

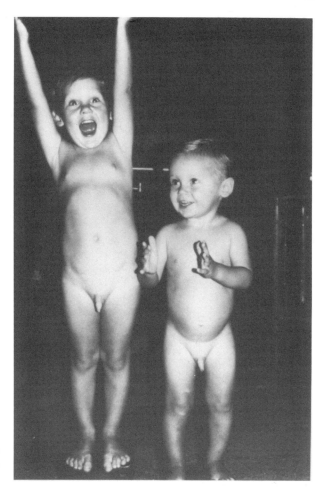

Figure 7. Two intact boys. (Photograph courtesy of John R. Taylor, M.D.)

5.2. Indications for Circumcision

The only surgical indication for circumcision is established balanitis xerotica obliterans. In its early stages, this condition may respond to steroid cream, but at the present state of medicine, if scarring is established, then a circumcision may be indicated.

Such circumcisions should:

- retain as much of the penile skin as possible
- excise all but a rim of the inner layer
- retain the frenulum

6. CONCLUSION

Infant circumcision is not only the unkindest cut of all and a rip-off, it has significant legal and human rights implications. It must remain the right of every man to shape his own end.

7

NORM UK AND THE MEDICAL CASE AGAINST CIRCUMCISION

A British Perspective

John P. Warren

Necessity is the plea for every infringement of human freedom. It is the argument of tyrants; it is the creed of slaves.

William Pitt
British Prime Minister, 1783.

1. NATIONAL ORGANISATION OF RESTORING MEN OF THE UNITED KINGDOM (NORM UK)

NORM UK was set up in 1994 as an organization whose aims are:

- To oppose genital mutilation of children of both sexes in Britain and elsewhere.
- To provide information about the normal genitalia, and the importance of retaining them.
- To provide information about conservative treatment of disorders of the foreskin in boys.
- To provide accurate information and psychological help and support for men who have been circumcised and want to recover their glans and have a more normal looking penis. For this purpose NORM UK operates support groups in Britain (currently one in Hertfordshire and one in Manchester, but more will be established as the need arises).

The history of routine neonatal circumcision in Britain was similar to that of the United States up to 1950, when the newly established National Health Service declined to

Sexual Mutilations: A Human Tragedy, edited by Denniston and Milos
Plenum Press, New York, 1997

pay for the surgery. Consequently, routine neonatal circumcision swiftly disappeared from Britain. Since 1950, the cumulative circumcision rate in boys has dropped from about 30% to about 6 or 7%. Given that other developed Western European nations, such as Denmark, have a cumulative national circumcision rate of 1.6% for boys under 15 years of age[1] — most of whom are Jewish or Moslem immigrants — it is clear that an excessive number of late circumcisions continue to be performed on older boys in Britain. This may be due to a high level of unfamiliarity among older medical personnel with normal prepu-tial anatomy and development. There is also a degree of unfamiliarity with the many exist-ing alternative, conservative, less-invasive, and more rational treatments for actual pathological conditions of the prepuce.

During 1996, NORM UK prepared a report on circumcision for the Law Commis-sion of England as a result of a consultation document published by the Commission, *Con-sent in the Criminal Law*. Amongst many other proposals, this document proposes a change in English law to make religious circumcision of children legal by statute. In the past, the practice has not been clearly illegal, but neither has it been wholly legal.

2. ANATOMY OF THE PREPUCE

The prepuce has been defined, in the past, as merely a fold of skin covering the glans. This is a gross oversimplification. The prepuce is a complex structure analogous to the eyelids or lips.

Taylor, et al., in a study of autopsy material, found that the mean length of the nor-mal adult prepuce was 6.4 centimeters.[2] The mean length of the penile shaft was 6.9 centi-meters, so that the prepuce was long enough to cover 93% of the shaft. They found that,

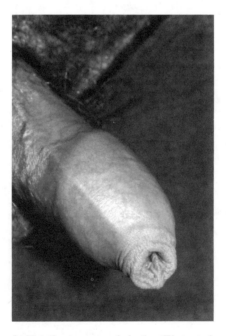

Figure 1. Prepuce of adult male. Note the strong vascularization. (Photograph courtesy of John A. Erickson)

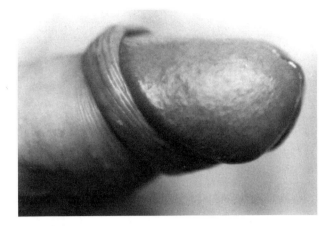

Figure 2. Ridged band, displaced behind corona glandis, of everted prepuce. (Photograph courtesy of John A. Erickson)

when retracted, the inner surface of the prepuce displays two zones, "ridged" and "smooth." The first, a transversely-ridged band of mucosa 10–15 millimeters wide, lies against the true skin edge. When magnified, the "ridged band" has a pebbled or coral-like appearance. Unretracted, the adult ridged band usually lies flat against the glans; retracted, the "ridged band" can be everted on the shaft of the penis. The remainder of the preputial lining between the "ridged band" and the glans is smooth and lax. The "ridged band" was shown to be intensely vascular.

The inner surface of the prepuce is lined by variably keratinized squamous epithelium similar to the frictional mucosa of the mouth, vagina and esophagus. The epithelium is papillated by stromal or "corial" tissue and is rich in nerves, Schwann cells, lymphoid cells and capillaries. Papillae are continuous with a highly vascular, loose-knit tissue layer that resembles the corium of oral mucosa. Preputial mucosa also lacks the dense collagenous zone seen in most areas of true (skin) dermis and, again unlike true skin of the penile shaft and outer surface of the prepuce, the mucosal surface of the prepuce is completely free of hair follicles and sweat glands.

Histological cross-sections of the "ridged band" showed focal, spiky, or more rounded, broader, and flatter ridges interspersed with sulci. Meissner's corpuscles were more plentiful in some subjects than in others, but, perhaps significantly, they were only seen in the crests of the ridges, occasionally in small clumps that expanded the tips of the

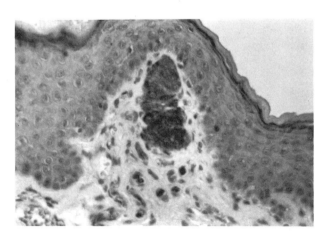

Figure 3. Meissner's corpuscle and myelinated nerve fibers in crest of preputial ridged band. S100 stain. x 100. (Photograph courtesy of John R. Taylor, M.D.)

corial papillae. End-organs were not seen in the sulci between ridges. The "ridged band" was found to be richly innervated and contained additional end-organs and myelinated nerve fibers within papillae. Sections of "smooth mucosa" showed no ridging of the mucosal surface, slightly shallower corial papillae, and few Meissner's corpuscles. Taylor et al. suggest that their findings support the view that the lining of the prepuce is identical to or a prolongation of the common squamous mucosa of the glans and the balano-preputial sulcus.

Meissner's corpuscles of the prepuce may be compared with similar nerve-endings in the finger-tips and lips, which respond in a fraction of a second to contact with light objects that bring about deformation of their capsules. Complex sensation, however, at least in the glans penis, may be mediated by free nerve endings rather than by specialized end-organs. The mode of transmission of stimuli from the prepuce and glans penis has not been fully elucidated.

Taylor, et al., postulate that the "ridged band," with its unique structure, tactile corpuscles, and other nerves, is primarily sensory tissue, and that it cooperates with other components of the prepuce. In this model, the "smooth" mucosa and true skin of the external fold of the prepuce act together to allow the "ridged band" to move from a forward to a "deployed" position on the shaft of the penis. The prepuce, then, should be considered a structural and functional unit made up of more or less specialized parts.

Taylor, et al., suggest that, whereas it is generally thought that the prepuce protects the glans, it is equally likely that the glans shapes and protects the prepuce. In return, the glans and penile shaft gain excellent, if surrogate, sensitivity from the prepuce. Possibly, the "ridged band" helps mediate the afferent limb of the ejaculatory reflex.

On the underside of the glans, the advanced point of preputial attachment forms the frenulum, which, in conjunction with the muscle fibers of the prepuce, helps return the everted prepuce to its forward position. The frenulum contains a high concentration of nerve endings, and is often excised at circumcision. Both the prepuce and the frenulum contain erogenous nerve endings, which, when stimulated, trigger erection and orgasm. Retraction, rolling, and stretching of the prepuce stimulate erogenous stretch receptors, which comprise the bulk of the sexual sensations of the erect penis.[3]

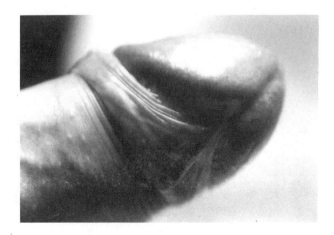

Figure 4. Ventral view of frenulum and contiguous ridged band of everted prepuce. (Photograph courtesy of John A. Erickson)

2.1. Development of the Prepuce

The embryological development of the prepuce has been described by Gairdner,[4] who showed that, at the time of birth, the prepuce is still developing, and that its attachment to the glans at this age contributes to its non-retractability. He found that 4% of newborns have a fully retractable prepuce, that in 54% the prepuce could be retracted sufficiently to reveal the meatus, while, in the remaining 42%, even the tip of the glans could not be uncovered. He found the following rates of non-retractability: at 6 months, 80%; at 1 year, 50%; at 2 years, 20%; at 3 years, 10%.

In a longitudinal study, Øster extended Gairdner's observations for older boys in a Danish population, where circumcision is rarely practiced.[5] He showed that non-retractability is found in 8% of 6–7 year-olds, in 6% between 8 and 11 years, 3% at 12–13, and only 1% at 14–17. He also showed that preputial adhesions decreased with advancing age in the boys in the study, so that these were present in 63% of 6–7 year-olds, but only 3% of 16–17 year-olds. Øster also pointed out that the nature and origin of smegma were not elucidated.

2.2. Functions of the Prepuce

The prepuce plays an important role in the mechanical functioning of the penis during sexual acts, such as penetrative intercourse and masturbation. The penile shaft skin is unique in its laxity and mobility. The reason for this is clearly to allow free movement of the skin over underlying structures during sexual activity. An ample surplus of skin is necessary both to allow for expansion of the organ during erection and to permit comfortable sexual stimulation. During sexual activity with an intact penis, there is a rolling action of the inner prepuce over the glans, and these two layers of specialized erogenous tissue are stimulated simultaneously. After circumcision, the shaft skin is often tightly stretched at erection, and none of these mechanisms can function. After circumcision, the surface of the glans is thickened and it loses sensitivity.[6] Loss of the sensory input from the specialized erogenous tissue of the prepuce is an inevitable consequence of circumcision.

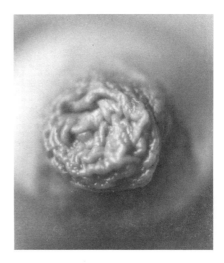

Figure 5. Eversion of the prepuce 1. Preputial orifice slightly dilated. Mucosal fold of inner prepuce exposed, but still closed. (Photograph courtesy of John A. Erickson)

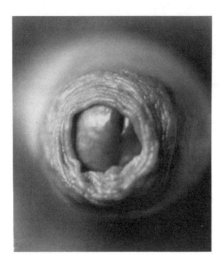

Figure 6. Eversion of the prepuce 2. Preputial orifice more widely dilated. Meatus slightly exposed. (Photograph courtesy of John A. Erickson)

3. CLARIFICATION OF PREPUTIAL CONDITIONS

3.1. Phimosis

The term *phimosis* comes from a Greek word meaning "muzzling." It is properly used to describe a self-limiting condition whereby a formerly retractable prepuce becomes unretractable as the result of scarring or dermatological pathologies. As reported above, the studies of Gairdner and Øster have shown that non-retractability is physiological, normal, and probably protective in children. Pathological phimosis due to disease must, therefore, be distinguished from the normal, physiological non-retractability of the prepuce of children. Unfortunately, many medical practitioners have failed to make this distinction, and unnecessary circumcisions of children have resulted. Topical therapy with corticosteroid has been found to be effective in relieving true, pathological phimosis in a number of studies.[7–9] Alternative, prepuce-saving surgical techniques have also been reported.[10-15]

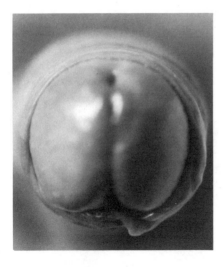

Figure 7. Eversion of the prepuce 3. Preputial orifice dilated, prepuce everted. (Photograph courtesy of John A. Erickson)

Most cases of phimosis go undiagnosed and probably resolve on their own. No treatment, however, should be undertaken before the male is post-pubescent and can weigh the therapeutic options for himself and give informed consent.

3.2. Balanitis Xerotica Obliterans

Gordon and Collin suggest that the 1% of 17-year-olds noted by Øster to have non-retractile prepuces may have had a case of Balanitis Xerotica Obliterans (BXO).[16] The condition also affects other parts of the penis, such as the glans and urethra. Little is known about this extremely rare condition, including its cause. It is characterized by dermal edema, lymphocytic infiltration, basal cell degeneration and atrophy of the stratum malpighii. The treatment of BXO has not been fully investigated. Spontaneous resolution has been reported, as has response to medical and laser treatment.[17] Response to intradermal steroid injection has been reported.[18-19] Much research is yet to be done into this condition.

3.2.1. Inappropriate Circumcision Referrals. In Britain, a cumulative national circumcision rate of 6% by the age of 15 has been reported by Rickwood and Walker.[20] This is clearly in excess of the 1% of adolescent boys who have persistently non-retractile foreskins. The authors point out that 21,000 boys under 15 are circumcised annually under the National Health Service in England, at an estimated cost of £5.2 million at the time they wrote. They found that the majority of referrals for circumcision had developmentally non-retractile prepuces rather than true, pathological phimosis, and no examples of true phimosis were seen in boys under 5 years. Ironically, most circumcisions performed in the Mersey Region were before this age, leading the authors to conclude that two-thirds of the operations were unnecessary.

3.3. Paraphimosis

Paraphimosis is the name given to the condition where the immature prepuce, having been forcibly retracted, becomes trapped in the sulcus behind the glans and cannot be brought forward again. It is extremely rare in boys and is always due to interference with a prepuce that is not ready to be retracted, possibly by the boy himself, or more usually his parents, or a misguided doctor or nurse. It is unusual for the boy to do this by himself, as stretching the immature prepuce sufficiently to produce paraphimosis is painful. Education concerning proper care of the prepuce is the most effective way of preventing paraphimosis from occurring.

When this condition has been induced, the glans soon becomes edematous, making reduction more difficult. Squeezing the glans between thumb and index finger until the volume of the glans is sufficiently reduced will allow the prepuce to slide forward again.

3.4. Balanoposthitis

Balanitis is the name given to inflammation of the glans, while posthitis refers to inflammation of the prepuce, and balanoposthitis implies inflammation of both structures. Balanoposthitis was reported by Escala and Rickwood to affect no more than 4% of boys with intact prepuces, with most boys suffering only a single attack. No link with phimosis was found.[21] It occurs most commonly in preschool children who, at a self-exploratory stage, intermittently touch their anus and penis. In a retrospective study of 272 intact and

273 circumcised boys, Herzog and Alvarez found balanitis more frequently in the intact children (6% versus 3%), but the difference was not statistically significant.[22] There is, therefore, no clear evidence that circumcision prevents balanitis. Balanitis may very well be under-reported in circumcised boys.

4. CIRCUMCISION

Circumcision is the surgical excision of the prepuce with the aim of artificially externalizing the glans penis. The operation may be one of the oldest known to humanity, and its origins are lost in prehistory. We do not know why the operation was performed at that time and can only speculate. For some, circumcision has been a puberty rite. The operation was taken up by the Jews as a religious rite, and has continued for over 3000 years. Circumcision is also practiced by some African animists, Australian Aborigines, and Moslems. It was undoubtedly practiced in early Arabia, but is not mentioned in the Koran. Circumcision does not have a prominent place in Islamic books of law, but great value is attached to it in popular estimation. In many Moslem countries, boys are circumcised between the age of 3 and 7 years with great pomp. The operation is usually performed by a barber, without anesthesia. In other parts of the world, Moslem boys may be circumcised at birth or as old as 15 years.

Medical circumcision became common in the late Nineteenth Century in English-speaking countries. At first, it was alleged to prevent masturbation, as masturbation had been linked causally to many diseases including epilepsy and insanity. It was carried out as a routine surgery soon after birth. At this age, no anesthesia was used. In the early decades, doctors probably used a free-hand technique, using scissors to cut a dorsal slit, and then cutting both layers of the prepuce around the circumference of the penis. Sutures were used to close the wound and achieve hemostasis. Although the original rationale for routine circumcision was discredited or forgotten, the practice continued in a few English-speaking countries, and other reasons for its practice were proposed, such as hygiene and the prevention of cancer. Newer techniques were introduced with clamps, such as the Gomco clamp, which crushed and devitalized the prepuce, obviating the need for sutures.

Nowadays, the practice of routine neonatal circumcision is mainly found in the United States of America, where as many as 60–70% of adult males may have been circumcised, and to some extent in Canada and Australia. It has largely disappeared from the United Kingdom in the last 20 years. Apart from ritual Jewish and Moslem circumcision, the operation is still a traditional practice in other parts of the developing world, particularly in parts of Africa, where it is often found alongside female genital mutilation. It has never been common in mainland Europe. Approximately one-sixth of the world's male population is circumcised, mainly on religious grounds. When circumcision for a medical reason is carried out on older children or adults, some form of anesthesia is used, either local or general.

4.1. Complications of Circumcision

An excellent and comprehensive review of the literature on complications of circumcision has been published recently.[23] Operative complications are hemorrhage, sepsis, removal of insufficient prepuce, removal of excessive amount of skin leading to denudation of the shaft, concealed penis, laceration of the penis and/or scrotum, partial or total

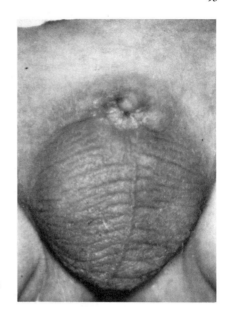

Figure 8. Total amputation of the penis by circumcision. (Photograph by Tom Reichfelder, M.D., courtesy of John Money, M.D.)

amputation of the glans, partial or total amputation of the penis, and formation of urethral fistula.

Bleeding is a common complication because the prepuce is such a vascular structure. It is particularly likely to occur in children with clotting disorders. Death may result from blood loss if appropriate steps are not taken to prevent it. Blood transfusion may be required. Excessively tight circumferential bandaging may obstruct the flow of urine and lead to renal failure.

Infection after circumcision occurs in up to 10% of patients. In the majority of cases, this is mild and manifested only by local inflammatory changes. Occasionally, sepsis may have more serious consequences, and can even lead to death.

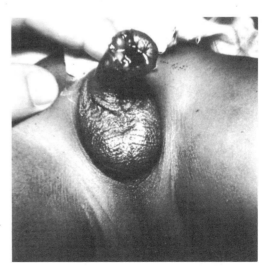

Figure 9. Extensive injury and suppuration of newly circumcised penis. (Photograph by Tom Reichfelder, M.D., courtesy of John Money, M.D.)

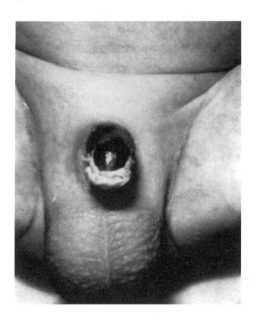

Figure 10. Destruction of penis by electrocautery circumcision. (Photograph by Tom Reichfelder, M.D.,
courtesy of John Money, M.D.)

Gearhart and Rock reported four cases of total loss of the penis in newborn boys following circumcision with use of electrocautery.[24] In all cases, the infants had sex-change
surgery and were raised as girls. There have been other reports of total loss of the penis
following circumcision.

Ulceration of the external urethral meatus occurs in 8–20% of boys following circumcision. It tends to occur 2–3 weeks after the operation. It can lead to permanent narrowing of the meatus, i.e., meatal stenosis. The latter has been advanced as a cause of
recurrent pyelonephritis and obstructive uropathy, for which meatotomy, enlargement of
the meatus, is curative. Meatitis is probably more common than reported. Most circumcised infant boys suffer from an erythematous meatus, which is the result of constant irritation from urine, feces, and friction from rubbing against the diaper (napkin). Many
doctors would consider this finding normal.

In some cases, circumcision results in the formation of a bridge of skin between the
circumcision scar and the surface of the glans. These bridges may cause pain and deformity on erection. When anesthesia is used, risks are incurred. In the case of local anesthetic,

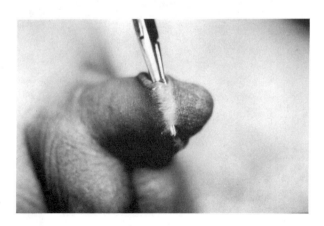

Figure 11. Skin bridge with inserted
probe on circumcised penis. (Photograph
by Tom Reichfelder, M.D., courtesy of
John Money, M.D.)

such as lignocaine, overdosage may result in seizures or cardiac arrhythmias. With general anesthesia, there are the risks of airway obstruction, inhalation of vomit, cardiac arrhythmias, malignant hyperpyrexia, and other drug reactions, for example, to scoline or halothane.

4.1.1. Psychological Complications of Circumcision. Psychological   complications have been explored by some investigators. Alice Miller has pointed out that injured children are likely to grow up into adults who injure children.[25]

Cansever carried out a psychoanalytical study of 12 Turkish boys undergoing circumcision at the age of 4–7 years. She found that intelligence quotient tended to fall and that body image perception showed a tendency to contract after circumcision. She concluded that:

> Circumcision is perceived by the child as an aggressive attack upon his body, which damaged, mutilated, and in some cases totally destroyed him. The feeling of "I am now castrated" seems to prevail in the psychic world of the child. As a result he feels inadequate, helpless and functions less efficiently.[26]

4.1.2. NORM UK Survey. To men who contact NORM UK for information about foreskin restoration, NORM UK sent a postal questionnaire inquiring about their views on the effects of circumcision. Eighty-seven men replied, 48 of whom had undergone neonatal circumcision. There were seven cases of adult circumcision. In most cases of childhood circumcision, dissatisfaction started in childhood, and only in 17 out of 79 cases was it delayed until adult life. Of the complaints listed on the questionnaire, the most frequent reasons for dissatisfaction were the appearance (74%), sense of mutilation (72%), lack of sensitivity (69%), being different from other men (57%), discomfort due to chafing of the glans by clothing (45%), sexual problems (37%), irregular or lumpy scar (30%), variation of skin color (26%), deformity or curvature of penis (15%). Respondents also mentioned many other complaints or gave more detailed information about problems relating to masturbation (12.5%), feelings of inferiority (9%), unspecified psychological effects, feeling exposed, sense of loss and jealousy, feeling assaulted or violated, painful scar, nightmares, being teased, and resentment at not having consented to surgery that altered the sex organ.

This study should alert doctors to the long-term physical and psychological damage that may result from this allegedly trivial operation, and should promote further study of the physiology of the glans and foreskin. In some circumcised men, the glans becomes dysfunctional, with impaired sexual feeling and discomfort on contact with clothing.

4.2. Pain and Circumcision

A recent review of pain control in children pointed out that patients receive less relief from pain than they should, and that this tendency is more pronounced in children than in adults.[27] The authors refer to the myth that very young infants do not have the neurological capacity to experience pain. Neuroanatomical studies, however, have shown that by 29 weeks of gestation, pain pathways and the cortical and subcortical centers involved in the perception of pain are well developed, as are the neurological systems for the transmission and modulation of painful sensations. Behavioral and physiological studies have shown that even very young infants respond to painful stimuli. Premature infants undergoing surgery with minimal anesthesia, which was once standard practice, have significantly higher stress responses (by hormonal and metabolic measures) and significantly higher rates of complications and mortality than those given deeper anesthesia.

A related misunderstanding is the belief that very young children who undergo painful experiences have no lasting memory of the pain, and therefore it has no lasting effect. Recent studies, however, have concluded that pain and distress, such as those associated with circumcision, can endure in memory, resulting, for example, in disturbances of feeding, sleeping, and the stability of the state of arousal.[28] Preliminary data suggest that early experiences of pain may produce permanent structural and functional reorganization of developing nociceptive neural pathways, which in turn may affect future experiences of pain.

In a recent review on stress and pain in infancy and childhood, it was found that the flexor reflex response is present in neonates, and that the threshold for the reflex, which in adults is equivalent to subjective pain sensation, is low in very preterm babies (25–27 weeks gestation).[29] There is spread of the reflex to involve other limbs, receptive field areas are large at birth, and there is long-lasting after-discharge that is more pronounced than the initial response.[30] The threshold increases with gestational age, but at term is still lower than the adult pain threshold. Of additional concern is the fact that repeated stimulation sensitizes the reflex in neonatal rats and in human neonates up to 32 weeks gestation, resulting in a lower threshold and exaggerated response. In neonates of all gestations, repeated heelpricks are associated with increasing severity of distress and heart rate changes.

Memory of pain may be a conscious phenomenon, as in children and adults, or may consist of altered behavior to subsequent stimuli. This is a difficult concept to understand in relation to the neonate and not easily amenable to scientific investigation. Anand and Hickey suggested that the "memory" of pain may disrupt adaptation to the environment, the development of bonding and feeding patterns, and even long-term psychological development.[31] Fitzgerald's neurological studies suggest that neonatal injury may result in structural and functional reorganization of the nervous system and altered adult patterns of neural connections.[32] The phenomenon of sensitization illustrates that responses are affected by previous experience, even if pain is not consciously remembered. There is now some evidence to support this view in relation to circumcision. Taddio, et al., showed that circumcision may affect pain responses some months after the event.[33]

In the United States, where routine neonatal circumcision is performed on the majority of boys, it has been shown that circumcision disrupts feeding and impairs infant-maternal attachment.[34] As a result there are difficulties in establishing breastfeeding, and, if a mother is serious about breastfeeding, she needs to be informed that circumcising her son may prevent her from doing so.

5. CIRCUMCISION MYTHS

5.1. Penile Cancer

Prevention of penile cancer is commonly claimed to be an advantage of circumcision performed in infancy. The basis of the claim is an article published in 1932 by Wolbarst.[35] Squamous cell carcinoma of the circumcised penis, however, has since been reported. When one compares the incidence of penile cancer in the United States (0–2.1 per 100,000 males) where most men are circumcised at birth, with that in Denmark (1.1 per 100,000 males), where the circumcision rate is 1.6%, the original contention that circumcision protects against cancer looks doubtful.[36] In fact, a recently published report shows that the incidence of penile cancer in Denmark has been falling in the last 50 years without any change in the circumcision rate.[37] The authors suggest that improvements in penile hygiene may be responsible for this change. It is likely that many factors other than circumcision are implicated in the genesis of penile cancer.

Since penile carcinoma is a disease of the elderly, Wolbarst was looking at the statistics for men born between 1850–1880. Penile carcinoma undoubtedly has many causes, and much has changed in the environment in the last 110–140 years. Known risk factors are smoking, number of sexual partners, poor hygiene and exposure to sexually transmitted diseases, and, particularly, human papilloma virus.

5.2. Carcinoma of the Cervix

In the past, it was claimed that circumcision protected the female partner from cervical carcinoma, and that smegma was carcinogenic. The older studies, published in the United States, on which this idea was based, were, however, flawed. Rates of cervical carcinoma, like penile carcinoma, tend to be higher in developing countries than in Western countries, and there seems little doubt that indoor plumbing — providing the means for good hygiene — is important in the prevention of both diseases. In the only study conducted where indoor plumbing was the rule rather than the exception, Kjaer, et al., investigated 645 women, 20–49 years of age from Copenhagen, with histologically confirmed cervical carcinoma or carcinoma in situ and 614 controls drawn at random from the female population of the same area.[38] To study the role of the "male factor," monogamous cases and controls, together with their husbands, were invited for further examination. In total, 41 case couples and 90 control couples were enrolled (89% and 92% of eligibles, respectively). The most significant risk determinants were a history of genital warts in the male (RR = 17.9) and the use of condoms (RR = 0.2). Circumcision status was not statistically significant. No studies have yet shown that smegma is carcinogenic. The literature shows that the best ways of avoiding cancer of the cervix and penis are to use condoms, to restrict the number of sexual partners, to practice good post-coital hygiene and to treat human papilloma virus infections in both males and females when they occur.

5.3. Urinary Tract Infections

Since 1985, a series of papers by Wiswell and his collaborators in the United States have claimed to show that circumcision protects boys against urinary tract infections.[39–44] This has become something of a cause célèbre in pediatrics in the United States. It is beyond the scope of this article to discuss in detail the methodology of these studies. It seems reasonable, however, to conclude that Wiswell's case is not proven. The published studies to date are all retrospective. No prospective, controlled study has yet been published. Even if an association is shown between the prepuce and urinary tract infections, the incidence of simple urinary tract infections is very low and the risks of circumcision would still outweigh any perceived benefit.

The other factor, never mentioned in this debate, is that circumcision does nothing for the circumcised boys, or for the girls who develop urinary tract infections. Pursuing vaccination for the various uropathogens, encouraging "rooming-in" (i.e., keeping newborn babies in the same room with their mothers), and promoting breastfeeding may end up being much more beneficial in preventing urinary tract infections than amputating normal tissue.

5.4. Sexually Transmitted Diseases

The data on the association, if any, between circumcision and sexually transmitted diseases (STD) are conflicting. Donovan, et al., studying patients attending an STD clinic in Australia, found there was no association between circumcision status and risk of infection with genital herpes simplex, genital warts, and non-gonococcal urethritis. Gonorrhea, syphilis and acute hepatitis B were too infrequent to assess.[45] In Africa, several studies have suggested that having a prepuce is a risk factor for HIV infection.[46] It would never be safe to recommend circumcision for protection against HIV, as it is no substitute for other preventive measures, such as avoidance of multiple partners, the use of condoms, and the avoidance of unprotected high-risk activities such as anal intercourse.

6. MEDICAL ETHICS

The Hippocratic oath, the foundation of medical ethics, states:

I will prescribe regimen for the good of my patient according to my judgment and my ability, and never do harm to anyone.

Circumcision of healthy children falls outside this ethical rule, since there is no proven medical benefit, and there certainly is harm.

6.1. Human Rights

It is now recognized that children have rights. Ten articles of the *United Nations Convention on the Rights of the Child* are breached by unnecessary circumcision of children.

7. PSYCHOLOGICAL CONSIDERATIONS

Wallerstein wrote in 1980:

When newborn circumcision began to be routinely practiced, the positive aspects were considered to be of such a magnitude that they completely out-weighed any possible negative aspects. To a large degree this view is still held. There has not been one article in a medical or lay journal specifically devoted to a total overview and analysis of the potentially negative psychological aspects of circumcision. The question is usually scoffed at as nonsense.[47]

The situation has unfortunately changed little in the sixteen years since those words were written. Bigelow has considered possible motives for the vogue of circumcision in the United States.[48] He suggests circumcision is one way of controlling young males. Circumcision is a form of violence acted out against a child, and this may make the individual more prone to become violent later in life, and of course to repeat this particular violent act on his sons.

Denial is a psychological defense mechanism. Bigelow, writing in the United States, suggests that our need to deny the pain and the effects and to justify the continuation of routine infant male circumcision in the United States distorts our perception of those things done to children worldwide. These rituals are not performed for the child's benefit:

they are performed to make adults feel more secure. Adults minimize and discount the pain and terror they inflict on children through circumcision when they claim that "it lasts only a little while."

Humor is a defense mechanism akin to denial, and circumcision is frequently the subject of humor, forcing the listener to block out painful associations of the practice. Bigelow goes on to consider what motivates the American circumciser: training, beliefs, and the need for power. He does not refer to financial gain, though this may also be a factor.

We also need to consider what happens to the circumciser. Physicians who perform circumcisions develop defenses that shield them from empathizing with the infant undergoing sexual mutilation. For a long time, doctors denied the neonate's capacity to feel pain. Doctors may deny that the red and bleeding glans of the newly circumcised infant penis has been harmed. They may joke about the operation. They may rationalize all the supposed benefits of circumcision in order to justify their actions. With repeated exposure to the procedure, circumcisers will no longer hear the screams of the child, and will isolate themselves from any identification with the patient. It is perhaps the effect of these defenses set up by doctors that prevents them from understanding the man who presents himself to a doctor complaining of the harmful effects of circumcision.

8. CONCLUSIONS

There are three main areas of harm resulting from circumcision of children:

- The risk of complications from the operation
- The loss of the prepuce, a specialized erogenous zone, with its unique structure and special tactile sensitivity; a reduction of total penile skin and full physiological penile skin mobility; loss of the protection for the glans and meatus; thickening and resulting desensitization of the artificially externalized surface of the glans
- The exposure of the child to pain, which is now known to have lasting harmful effects in very young children.

There are no demonstrable health benefits from circumcision, and those claimed for it do not outweigh the proven harm or risks. Both the circumcised individual and the circumciser are likely to be affected by psychological denial that prevents them from recognizing the damage caused by circumcision.

Circumcision of a healthy child does not conform to medical ethical standards. It breaches ten articles of the *United Nations Convention of the Rights of the Child.*

Since circumcision is harmful, it should not be performed on children incapable of consenting, unless there is a pressing medical necessity.

9. REFERENCES

1. Frisch M, Friis S, Kjaer SK, Melbye M. Falling incidence of penis cancer in an uncircumcised population (Denmark 1943–1990). BMJ 1995;311:1471.
2. Taylor JR, Lockwood AP, Taylor AJ. The prepuce: specialised mucosa of the penis and its loss to circumcision. Br J Urol 1996;77:291–5.
3. Money J, Davison J. Adult penile circumcision: erotosexual and cosmetic sequelae. The Journal of Sex Research 1983;19:289–92.

4. Gairdner D. The fate of the foreskin. BMJ 1949;2:1433–7.
5. Øster J. Further fate of the foreskin. Arch Dis Child 1968;43:200–3.
6. Bigelow J. The Joy of Uncircumcising! 2nd edition. Aptos: Hourglass, 1995.
7. Wright JE. The treatment of childhood phimosis with topical steroid. Aust NZ J Surg 1994;64:327–8.
8. Kikiros CS, Beasley SW, Woodward AA. The reponse of phimosis to local steroid application. Pediat Surg Int 1993;8:329–32.
9. Jorgensen ET, Svensson A. The treatment of phimosis in boys, with a potent topical steroid (clobetasol propionate 0.05%) cream. Acta Derm Venereol 1993;73:55–6.
10. Emmett AJJ. Z-plasty reconstruction for preputial stenosis - a surgical alternative to circumcision. Aust Paediatr J 1982;18:219–20.
11. Hoffman S, Metz P, Ebbehoj J. A new operation for phimosis: prepuce-saving technique with multiple Y-V-plasties. Br J Urol 1984;56:319–21.
12. Wahlin N. "Triple incision plasty." A convenient procedure for preputial relief. Scand J Urol Nephrol 1992;26:107–10.
13. de Castella H. Prepuceplasty: an alternative to circumcision. Ann R Coll Surg Engl 1994;76:257–8.
14. Cuckow PM, Rix G, Mouriquand PDE. Preputial plasty: a good alternative to circumcision. J Pediatr Surg 1994;29:561–3.
15. Fleet MS, Venyo AKG, Rangecroft L. Dorsal relieving incision for the non-retractile foreskin. J R Coll Surg Edinb 1995;40:243–5.
16. Gordon A, Collin J. Save the normal foreskin. BMJ 1993;306:1–2.
17. Ratz JL. Carbon dioxide laser treatment of balanitis xerotica obliterans. J Am Acad Dermatol 1984;10:925–8.
18. Bale PM, Lochhead A, Martin HCO, Gollow I. Balanitis xerotica obliterans in children. Pediatr Pathol 1987;7:617–27.
19. Rickwood AMK, Hemalatha V, Batcup G, Spitz L. Phimosis in boys. Br J Urol 1980;53:147–50.
20. Rickwood AMK, Walker J. Is phimosis overdiagnosed in boys and are too many circumcisions performed in consequence? Ann Roy Coll Surg Engl 1989;71:275–7.
21. Escala JM, Rickwood AM. Balanitis. Br J Urol 1989;63:196–7.
22. Herzog LW, Alvarez SR. The frequency of foreskin problems in uncircumcised children. AJDC 1986;140:254–6.
23. Williams N, Kapila L. Complications of circumcision. Br J Surg 1993;80:1231–6.
24. Gearhart JP, Rock JA. Total ablation of the penis after circumcision with electrocautery: a method of management and long-term follow-up. J Urol 1989;142:799–801.
25. Miller A. Banished Knowledge: Facing Childhood Injuries. London: Virago Press, 1991.
26. Cansever G. Psychological effects of circumcision. Br J Med Psychol 1965;38:321–31.
27. Walco GA, Cassidy RC, Schechter NL. Pain, hurt, and harm. The ethics of pain control in infants and children. N Engl J Med 1994;331:541–4.
28. Marshall RE, Stratton WC, Moore JA, Boxerman SB. Circumcision I: effects upon newborn behavior. Infant Behavior and Development 1980;3:1–14.
29. Hawdon JM. Perinatal stress. In: Aynsley-Green A, Platt MPW, Lloyd-Thomas AR (eds) Stress and pain in infancy and childhood. Bailliere's Clinical Paediatrics 1995;3(3):511–28.
30. Fitzgerald M. The postnatal development of cutaneous afferent fibre input and receptor field organisation in the rat dorsal horn. J Physiol 1985;364:1–18.
31. Anand KJS, Hickey PR. Pain and its effects in the human neonate and fetus. N Engl J Med 1987;317:1321–9.
32. Fitzgerald M, Anand KJS. Developmental neuroanatomy and neurophysiology of pain. In: Schachter NC, Berde CB, Yaster M (eds) Pain in Infants, Children and Adolescents. Baltimore: Williams and Williams, 1993:11–31.
33. Taddio A, Goldbach M, Ipp M, Stevens BB, Koren G. Effect of neonatal circumcision on pain response during vaccination in boys. Lancet 1995;345:291–2.
34. Dixon S, Snyder J, Holve R, Bromberger P. Behavioral effects of circumcision with and without anesthesia. J Dev Behav Pediatr 1984;5:246–50.
35. Wolbarst AL. Circumcision and penile cancer. Lancet 1932;1:150–3.
36. Frisch M. Personal communication.
37. Frisch M, Friis S, Kjaer SK, Melbye M. Falling incidence of penis cancer in an uncircumcised population (Denmark 1943–1990). BMJ 1995;311:1471.
38. Kjaer SK, de Villiers EM, Dahl C, Engholm G, Bock JE, Vestergaard BF, Lynge E, Jensen OM. Case-control study of risk factors for cervical neoplasia in Denmark. I: Role of the "male factor" in women with one lifetime sexual partner. Int J Cancer 1991;48:39–44.

39. Wiswell TE, Smith FR, Bass JW. Decreased incidence of urinary tract infections in circumcised male infants. Pediatrics 1985;75:901–3.

40. Wiswell TE, Roscelli JD. Corroborative evidence for the decreased incidence of urinary tract infections in circumcised male infants. Pediatrics 1986;78:96–9.

41. Wiswell TE, Enzenauer RW, Cornish JD, Hankins CT. Declining frequency of circumcision: implications for changes in the absolute incidence and male to female sex ratio of urinary tract infections in early infancy. Pediatrics 1987;79:338–42.

42. Wiswell TE, Geschke DW. Risks from circumcision during the first month of life compared with those for uncircumcised boys. Pediatrics 1989;83:1011–5.

43. Wiswell TE, Tencer HL, Welch CA, Chamberlain JL. Circumcision in children beyond the neonatal period. Pediatrics 1992;92:791–3.

44. Wiswell TE, Hachey. Urinary tract infections and the uncircumcised state: an update. Clin Pediat 1993;32:130–4.

45. Donovan B, Bassett I, Bodsworth NJ. Male circumcision and common sexually transmissable diseases in a developed nation setting. Genitourin Med 1994;70:317–20.

46. Cameron DW, Simonsen JN, D'Costa LJ, Ronald AR, Maitha GM, Gakinya MN, Cheang M, Ndinya-Achola JO, Piot P, Brunham RC, Plummer FA. Female to male transmission of human immunodeficiency virus type I: risk factors for seroconversion in men. Lancet 1989;2:403–7.

47. Wallerstein E. Circumcision: An American Health Fallacy. New York: Springer, 1980:135.

48. Bigelow J. The Joy of Uncircumcising! 2nd edition. Aptos: Hourglass 1995:89–112.

8

CIRCUMCISION: AN IATROGENIC EPIDEMIC

George C. Denniston

Doctors Opposing Circumcision (D.O.C.) was founded to provide accurate information about the consequences of circumcision and to make available the scientific facts about the uniquely specialized, uniquely sensitive erogenous tissue that circumcision destroys. In the nine months since its founding, Doctors Opposing Circumcision has grown rapidly and now has medical representatives in all fifty of the United States, and in all of the Provinces and Territories of Canada as well as Great Britain, Australia, and New Zealand — the only other countries where doctors circumcise the citizens without a religious reason. In addition, Doctors Opposing Circumcision has members in countries such as Japan, where this practice is virtually unknown.

Doctors Opposing Circumcision has a home page on the World Wide Web (http://weber.u.washington.edu/~gcd/DOC) that provides world-wide access to accurate and up-to-date scientific information about the normal human penis, the consequences of circumcision, and precisely what it is that a doctor is doing when he performs a circumcision. Doctors Opposing Circumcision is also associated with the world's first peer-reviewed virtual medical journal, *CIRCUMCISION* (http://weber.u.washington.edu/~gcd/CIRCUMCISION).

With this wide representation, Doctors Opposing Circumcision is already empowering parents in these countries to protect their children from circumcision. As more and more parents realize that doctors have organized in opposition to circumcision, they will no longer be misled into following the tragic misinformation espoused by circumcisers. Parents will then act in their son's best interest and protect him from circumcision.

1. CIRCUMCISION: AN IATROGENIC (DOCTOR-CAUSED) EPIDEMIC

Up until the Nineteenth Century, women in childbirth were at high risk of contracting and dying of puerperal fever, commonly known as *childbed fever*. A number of doctors, most notably Ignaz Philipp Semmelweis in Austria and Oliver Wendell Holmes in America, demonstrated that puerperal fever was transmitted from victim to victim by the very doctors who were supposed to be helping these women deliver their children safely.

Sexual Mutilations: A Human Tragedy, edited by Denniston and Milos
Plenum Press, New York, 1997

Despite the compelling nature of the data collected, it took many years before all doctors accepted the horrifying truth. The researchers demonstrated that the transmission of child-bed fever could easily be prevented if doctors simply rinsed their hands in a caustic solution before attending to the next woman. Once it was understood and accepted that doctors caused the fatal illness, the epidemic was eradicated.

Similarly, routine neonatal circumcision occurs in the United States at an epidemic rate. Approximately one million healthy newborns have part of their penis removed each year by doctors soon after birth. Circumcision only became a major epidemic after 1950. Approximately half of all males living in the United States have been subjected to the surgical removal of normal, healthy, sexually-sensitive penile tissue. The National Center for Health Statistics stated that, in 1994 — the latest year for which there are statistics — 62.1% of newborn infant males were circumcised nationwide for all hospitals reporting. In the Northeast, 69.6% were circumcised. In the Midwest, 80.1% were circumcised. In the South, 64.7% were circumcised, but in the western region of the United States, only 34.2% were circumcised. These statistics are the result of a randomized hospital survey and signify only the number of babies that leave the hospital circumcised. They do not include home births, birth centers, circumcisions performed in doctor's offices, or religious circumcisions. For this reason, while they may not be absolutely accurate, since they are recorded year after year at the same hospitals, they do reflect the trend in the United States.

Thousands of males, left intact at birth, including men in their eighties, have been circumcised without valid medical indications. Many children in the United States, fortunate enough to have been left intact at birth, are subjected to having their healthy foreskins amputated while they undergo other surgeries, such as tonsillectomy. The non-ritual routine circumcision of infants also occurs in Canada, Great Britain, Australia, and New Zealand, but on a considerably smaller scale.

There is no question that the circumcision epidemic is caused by doctors. Once the public recognizes that circumcision is harmful, this epidemic, too, will disappear.

Clearly, circumcision is unnecessary. This is proven by the example of the countless billions of men, who throughout history, have each led their entire life happily intact. There are billions of men living today in Europe, Asia, Africa, and the continents of North, Central, and South America who enjoy life with intact genitals and whose foreskins do not cause them to suffer from any of the complaints or diseases American circumcisionists allege will lower the quality of their life.

2. MEDICAL EXCUSES

The iatrogenic epidemic of circumcision is sustained by the invention and proliferation of alleged medical reasons. These excuses range from the prevention of masturbation, epilepsy, hysteria, alcoholism, bed-wetting, to cancer and death. In the history of medicine, there has never been so much unfounded data produced to protect a harmful medical practice. As each medical reason is scientifically disproven, new reasons for circumcision are quickly invented. The truth is that these alleged medical reasons are not valid reasons for subjecting infants to invasive penile surgery. The attempt to use science to justify the practice of circumcision is an abuse of science. There are no scientific or medical indications to validate the practice of routine circumcision. This truth was stated clearly by the American Academy of Pediatrics in 1971. Since then, a few new excuses have been invented, but even these excuses cannot justify circumcision. A doctor's license to practice medicine does not permit him or her to remove healthy organs in the name of prevention without the expressed permission of the person who is undergoing the operation.

2.1. Urinary Tract Infections (UTI)

Recently, the most commonly cited "medical reason" used to justify depriving boys of their foreskin has been the prevention of urinary tract infections. On the basis of a retrospective review of hospital charts, Wiswell, et al., claimed that 1.4% of intact sick and hospitalized infants had succumbed to urinary tract infections whereas 0.14% of circumcised infants contracted urinary tract infections.[1] Even if we grant Wiswell his figures — with which other scientists disagree — 98.4% of intact infants are not at risk for urinary tract infections. Wiswell, however, now proposes that, on the basis of this insignificant difference, the normal foreskins of 100 infants be removed on the 1.4% chance of protecting one child from an infection that is easily treated with antibiotics, and, more importantly, is often easily prevented by less invasive means.

Since Altschul's methodologically correct study of 25,000 infants did not find that intact male infants are at a statistically significant increased risk for urinary tract infection,[2] it is probable that the results of Wiswell's study of 5,261 infants reflect methodologic differences rather than anatomical realities. Altschul noted that significant differences in foreskin care may have caused the differences in results. In fact, the parents of the intact infants born in the military hospital that Wiswell studied, were incorrectly advised about the care of the intact penis. The military doctors admitted to recommending partial retraction of the immature foreskin and cleansing of the glans penis with soap. Forced retraction is a contraindicated intervention that has been demonstrated to introduce pathogenic bacteria into the urethra.[3] Washing the glans penis with soap destroys the barrier of protective microbial flora, permitting only the most virulent pathogens to survive.[4] The consequences of these actions would be an increased rate of infection.[5] If Wiswell's findings are correct, they only demonstrate that it is forced retraction and washing with soap, not normal penile anatomy, that increases the risk of urinary tract infections.

Numerous studies demonstrate that rooming-in and breastfeeding are protective against urinary tract infections.[6-7] Since these interventions have been shown to be effective, non-lethal, and non-invasive methods of preventing urinary tract infections, the principles of human rights and medical ethics require that doctors advocate breastfeeding and rooming-in rather than circumcision. The latter has not been demonstrated to be effective, and is both harmful and invasive.

Another serious flaw in Wiswell's study relates to the number of intact and circumcised boys. Wiswell's information on the circumcision status of the infants in the study was obtained from old hospital charts. A recent study by O'Brien, et al., uncovered the fact that circumcision was indicated on only 84.3% of the hospital charts of circumcised boys.[8] There is no reason to suspect that the hospital Wiswell studied had better recording methods. If 15.7% of the infants with urinary tract infection that Wiswell counted as intact were actually circumcised, it would make his data even more meaningless.

There are other serious scientific flaws in Wiswell's urinary tract infection hypothesis. It has been shown that the bag technique, the most common method of diagnosing urinary tract infection, has a 16% false-positive rate in female and intact male newborns.[9] This would substantially decrease Wiswell's proposed minor difference (1.2 percentage points). Also, studies have shown links between urethral and periurethral infections and poor perineal hygiene.[10] The medically ethical solution is to instruct mothers to clean their babies properly and to change their diapers more often. It is unethical to suggest subjecting a child to the risk and consequences of penile surgery when less invasive, less expensive, and more effective means of preventing urinary tract infections exist.

2.2. Penile Cancer

Another alleged reason for performing circumcision has been that circumcision prevents cancer of the penis. This type of cancer occurs in 1 in 100,000 men. It must be stressed that there is no scientific proof that circumcision prevents penile cancer. There is, however, compelling evidence that smoking causes penile cancer.[11] This cancer is also associated with known behavioral risk factors such as alcoholism, frequent venereal infections, poverty, and multiple sex partners.[12] It is unreasonable and unethical to suggest that the removable of normal tissue be performed on 100,000 normal male infants for the possibility of preventing one case of cancer of the adult penis. By comparison, the risk of breast cancer is now about one hundred times greater but no one suggests we remove all female breasts to prevent that formidable disease.

3. COMPLICATIONS AND CONSEQUENCES

Gairdner's classic 1949 study, published in the *British Medical Journal*, is associated with the virtual cessation of circumcision in Great Britain in the 1950s. Extrapolating figures from his data, there would be 17 infant circumcision-related deaths each year per 100,000 circumcisions.[13] This figure has a direct bearing on whether or not to advocate circumcision to prevent cancer of the penis. Even if it were scientifically shown that the presence of the foreskin, rather than risk behaviors, caused penile cancer, it is unethical to risk the death of 17 infants to possibly prevent 1 case of penile cancer in one older man.

An unknown number of circumcisions result in death in the United States each year. Although the precipitating cause is the circumcision wound, the cause of death is often reported simply as "sepsis."[14] Every neonatal death within ten days of circumcision should be suspect.

The number of infants who *almost* die from circumcision is better known. Bleeding and infection can occur any time the body's integrity is compromised. According to Dr. Julian Ansell, who favors routine circumcision, 1 in 500 circumcised boys suffers a significant complication as a result of this surgery.[15] This translates to 2,000 completely unnecessary, significant medical complications occurring each year in the United States.

Actually, the true long-term complication rate of circumcision is 100%. The artificially exposed glans penis thickens and hardens. The urinary opening usually ulcerates and contracts, becoming incapable of normal closure. The edges of the circumcision wound will adhere to the glans or form an unsightly scar on the shaft of the penis. The potential amount of tissue lost from the adult penis with infant circumcision is a greater percentage of the total genital surface area than that removed with female circumcision.

4. THE ROLE OF DOCTORS

Doctors are the agents of the epidemic of circumcision. Only a handful of doctors actually invent the "medical" myths that drive the epidemic. Many doctors, however, fail to examine these myths critically. In this way, the epidemic of circumcision spreads without check.

Doctors who circumcise justify their actions in many ways. Some doctors may be nominally opposed to circumcision but will perform the operation if the parents "insist." Many doctors claim that they can rarely dissuade parents from their decision to have their children circumcised, while others say they can almost always talk parents out of it. Doctors in hospitals frequently fail to honor parents' requests to leave the child's penis intact and circumcise the infant anyway. A doctor can make up to $1,200 an hour performing circumcisions (six circumcisions an hour at $200 each). These are some of the factors that contribute to the circumcision of little boys.

The vast majority of doctors in the United States, however, do not advocate circumcision, but the few who do have been very effective, influential and far-reaching with their misinformation. With the organization of Doctors Opposing Circumcision, this misinformation about circumcision will now be met with the facts from other members of the same profession. Already, the efforts of a small number of health professionals and other children's rights advocates have helped reduce the national rate of male infant circumcision in the United States from a high of nearly 90% in the 1970s to less than 60%. This means that tens of millions of American parents have had the courage, wisdom and information they needed to keep their baby boys intact and safe.

5. ETHICAL CONSIDERATIONS

The epidemic of circumcision continues despite ethical principles and mandates designed to prevent such abuses. In performing circumcisions, doctors violate the first tenet of medical practice — *First, Do No Harm* — and all seven Principles of the American Medical Association's *Code of Ethics*.[16]

Many doctors have actually tried to deny that circumcision is painful. Anesthesia is rarely used. Since the publication of Anand and Hickey's study on neonatal pain in the November 19, 1987, issue of the *New England Journal of Medicine*,[17] it can no longer be denied that infants feel pain. Some doctors now use local anesthesia for circumcision, but this does not mitigate the fundamental human rights violation. A medical license does not permit doctors to amputate healthy tissue, with or without anesthesia, from the body of an unconsenting person. If it is unethical and illegal to subject an animal to such pain, how can we permit this to happen to our babies?

6. HUMAN RIGHTS CONSIDERATIONS

The epidemic of circumcision is especially calamitous because circumcision represents a violation of the fundamental human rights to autonomy, security of the person, physical integrity, physical and mental health, and self-determination.

The performance of routine neonatal circumcision directly violates Article 24.3 of the United Nations Convention on the Rights of the Child, which commands that traditional practices prejudicial to the health of children be abolished. Article 5 of the European Charter for Children in Hospital states:

> Children and parents have the right to informed participation in all decisions involving their health care. Every child shall be protected from unnecessary medical treatment and investigation.[18]

To change medical practices that violate human rights, it is important to understand first that the epidemic of involuntary circumcision was instituted and is perpetuated by the medical community. Physicians created the current social demand for this surgery. Consequently, it is the duty of physicians to eradicate the practice.

7. SOLUTION TO THE PROBLEM

The solution to this tragic situation is simple. Infant and childhood circumcision must be stopped. Males should be allowed to grow up with intact genitalia. Once they have reached the age of majority, they can decide for themselves, with fully informed consent, whether they wish to have part of their penis amputated. Males should be allowed to decide for themselves whether they wish to take whatever small risk there might be — if indeed there is any — in living life with an intact penis. If we grant people the right to smoke and drink, can we ethically deny people the right to intact sexual organs?

The words of Oliver Wendell Holmes about the tragic iatrogenic epidemic of childbed fever may also apply to the equally tragic iatrogenic epidemic of circumcision:

> Whatever indulgence may be granted to those who have heretofore been the ignorant causes of so much misery, the time has come when the existence of a private pestilence in the sphere of a single physician should be looked upon, not as a misfortune, but a crime...[19]

8. REFERENCES

1. Wiswell TE, Bass JW. Decreased incidence of urinary tract infections in circumcised male infants. Pediatrics 1985;75:901–3.
2. Altschul MS. Larger numbers needed. Pediatrics 1987;80:763–4.
3. Pfaff G, Bolkenius M. Hands off the prepuce. Lancet 1984;2:874–5.
4. Birley HDL, Walker Mm, Luzzi GA, Bell R, Taylor-Robinson D, Byrne M, et al. Clinical features and management of recurrent balanitis; association with atopy and genital washing. Genitourinary Medicine 1993;69:400–3.
5. Winberg J, Bollgren I, Gothefors L, Herthelius M, Tullus K. The Prepuce: a mistake of nature? Lancet 1989;1:598–9.
6. Coppa GV, Gabrielli O, Giorgi P, Catassi C, Montanari MP, Varaldo PE, Nichols BL. Preliminary study of breastfeeding and bacterial adhesion to uroepithelial cells. Lancet 1990;335:569–71.
7. Gothefors L, Olling S, Winberg J. Breast feeding and biological properties of faecal *E. coli* strains. Acta Paediatrica Scandinavica 1975;64:807–12.
8. O'Brien TR, Calle EE, Poole WK. Incidence of circumcision in Atlanta, 1985–1986. Southern Medical Journal 1995;88:411–5.
9. Schlager TA, Hendley J, Dudley SM, Hayden GF, Lohr JA. Explanation for false-positive urine cultures obtained by bag technique. Archives of Pediatric and Adolescent Medicine 1995;149:170–3.
10. Ginsburg CM, McCracken GH. Urinary tract infections in young infants. Pediatrics 1982;69:409–12.
11. Hellberg D, Valentin J, Eklund T, Nilsson S. Penile cancer: is there an epidemiological role for smoking and sexual behaviour? British Medical Journal 1987;295:1306–8.
12. Maden C, Sherman CJ, Beckmann AM, Hislop TG, Teh, C, Ashley RH, Daling JR. History of circumcision, medical conditions, and sexual activity and risk of penile cancer. Journal of the National Cancer Institute 1993;85:19–24.
13. Gairdner D. Fate of the foreskin. British Medical Journal 1949;2:1433–7.
14. Gellis SS. Circumcision. American Journal of the Diseases of Children 1979;133:1079–80.
15. Gee WF, Ansell JS. Neonatal circumcision: a ten-year overview. Pediatrics 1976;58:824–27.
16. Denniston GC. Circumcision and the Code of Ethics. Humane Health Care International 1996;12(2):78–80.
17. Anand KJS, Hickey PR. Pain and its effects in the human neonate and fetus. New England Journal of Medicine 1987;317:1321–26.

18. Alderson P. European charter of children's rights. Bulletin of Medical Ethics. 1993;9(October):13–15.
19. Holmes OW. The contagiousness of puerperal fever. In: Medical Essays. Boston: Houghton Mifflin, 1887:169.

9

WHY DOES NEONATAL CIRCUMCISION PERSIST IN THE UNITED STATES?

Robert S. Van Howe

The United States leads the world in per capita medical spending; however, in this era of rising health-care costs and drastic budget cuts, closer scrutiny must be given to the allocation of increasingly scarce health-care dollars. Perhaps the most obvious target for scrutiny is the routine amputation of the prepuce, euphemistically known as circumcision. Shortly after World War II, the *British Medical Journal* published a landmark study by Douglas Gairdner that disproved the alleged justifications for circumcision.[1] This, coupled with the socialization of the medical system in Great Britain, resulted in a precipitous drop in the number of procedures performed. The American medical establishment has remained a fee-for-service system, despite attempts by Harry Truman to follow the British example.

In the 1960's, with the publication of Morgan's study, "The Rape of the Phallus," in the *Journal of the American Medical Association*,[2] circumcision along with tonsillectomies came under closer scrutiny in the United States. By 1971, both the American Academy of Pediatrics (AAP)[3] and the American College of Obstetrics and Gynecology[4] no longer recommended routine neonatal circumcision. Because there was no concomitant reform in reimbursement practices, these policy statements had little effect on the circumcision rates in the United States.[5] In 1989, an ad hoc Task Force Committee on Circumcision,[6] commissioned by the AAP and chaired by Edgar J. Schoen, M.D., broadened its position slightly after retrospective studies suggested an association between the foreskin and urinary tract infections.[7-10] Ironically, only after the AAP Task Force statement was issued did the rate of circumcision begin to drop more rapidly. Still, the neonatal circumcision rate in the United States remains high, ranging from 34.2% on the West Coast to 80.1% in the Midwest. The AAP and the American Academy of Family Practice are currently in the process of reconsidering their positions on circumcision. In the absence of compelling medical indications, the persistence of secular circumcision in the United States deserves examination.

Circumcision is the most commonly performed surgery in the United States. In a recent editorial in the *British Journal of Obstetrics and Gynecology*, Gonik and Barrett point

Sexual Mutilations: A Human Tragedy, edited by Denniston and Milos
Plenum Press, New York, 1997

out: "Given the uncertain nature of the scientific data and the fact that the procedure is not without pain and risk, one would anticipate fewer circumcisions."[11]

Fewer circumcisions cannot be anticipated as long as the penis and circumcision continue to be the focus of myths, misinformation, and irrationality. The following anecdote illustrates this irrational focus on the penis to the exclusion of more crucial matters. After spending hours resuscitating and assessing the extent of injuries to a boy who was born pulseless, non-breathing, with a fractured humerus and a depressed skull fracture resulting from a difficult forceps breech delivery, I visited his mother. The first question the mother asked me was, "When can he be circumcised?"

In the American medical community, the justifications for performing circumcisions are no less obtuse. An article in *Pediatric News* discussed the debate over whether obstetricians or pediatricians should be circumcising boys, and inferred that each group wished the other group would do the surgery.[12] Three responses to this article were subsequently published and are representative of the array of physician viewpoints. The first respondent said that circumcision is necessary and, in his hands, there have never been any complications.[13] The second respondent noted that, while circumcision is completely unnecessary, parents are going to find someone to perform the surgery. He claimed that, because he could do a better job than other physicians in his community, he chooses to perform it.[14] The third respondent refused to perform the surgery because he recognized it as an unethical and unjustifiable mutilation.[15]

1. RIGHTS OF CHILDREN

To understand the issue of circumcision in the United States, the position of children in our society must be examined. Remarkably, the medieval notion of women and children as chattel has persisted into the Twentieth Century. Women were not allowed to vote in the United States until after the first World War, and the fight for women's equality continues in the United States and around the world. Unfortunately, the rights of children lag further behind. Recent court cases in the United States have brought this issue to center stage. The cases of Jessica DeBoer and Baby Richard both involved babies put up for adoption at birth by their biological mother at a time of no active involvement of the biological father. After these babies had been placed in adoptive homes, the biological fathers suddenly became interested in their offspring and demanded custody. Prolonged legal battles ensued, and in both cases, the children, by then three years old and well-bonded with their adoptive families, were returned to their biological parents — whom they had never before met. In both cases, the best interests of the child were never considered, no guardian ad litem was appointed, and the rights of the biological fathers were of higher importance than the child's psychological well being.

First Lady Hillary Rodham Clinton, a long-time champion of children's rights, wrote in *Children's Rights: Contemporary Perspectives* in 1979.

> Decisions about motherhood and abortions, schooling, cosmetic surgery, treatment of venereal disease, employment, and others where the decision or lack of one will significantly affect the child's future should not be made unilaterally by parents.[16]

Because of her advocacy for children's rights, Hillary Clinton drew much criticism at the 1992 Republican National Convention from conservatives who believe parents should have absolute control over their children without government interference, and who are currently lobbying to have this become law throughout the United States.[17] Current child abuse and neglect statutes prevent the judicial system from adequately protecting children. In the United States, a small child has fewer rights than an unborn fetus and far fewer rights than animals.

2. THE PHYSICIAN'S ROLE

Although the circumcision controversy has been raging for the past thirty years in the United States, many physicians are unable to confront the issue. One factor may be the deadened emotional state that results from their medical training. With daily exposure to illness, death, and cutting of live bodies, physicians in training must create an emotional barrier between themselves and their patients in order to remain dispassionate. This deadened emotional state is especially apparent when physicians perform circumcision and openly deny that the baby is in distress. Some physicians who do acknowledge the pain and suffering caused by circumcision shift the burden of responsibility to the parents who requested the surgery.

When a patient requests elective, cosmetic surgery, the physician has the right to refuse to perform it. If a patient requests non-therapeutic, mutilative surgery, the physician has an obligation to refuse to perform it. The physician is all the more obligated to refuse third-party requests to perform a non-therapeutic, mutilative surgery on unconsenting individuals. If all physicians refused to perform routine circumcisions, the practice would cease.

3. PUBLICATION BIAS IN THE AMERICAN MEDICAL LITERATURE

The major opinion pieces advocating routine circumcision that have been published in American medical journals in the past seven years have been written by either Edgar J. Schoen,[18–22] James A. Roberts,[23–25] Thomas E. Wiswell[26–29] or Gerald N. Weiss.[30–31] The opinions of these men have been readily published in major American medical journals such as *Pediatrics*.[7,9,10,32–35] Studies by American researchers whose conclusions do not support the alleged indications for routine circumcision have traditionally been rejected for publication by American medical journals and must be published in British and foreign journals,[36–38] in minor American journals with regional circulation,[39] or "throw away" journals.[40]

Pediatrics has repeatedly published articles of dubious scientific merit, while dissenting studies and letters to the editor are refused publication. In December of 1993, *Pediatrics* published a study by Thomas E. Wiswell, M.D., on post-neonatal circumcision,[33] which I often use to demonstrate that neonatal circumcision may have more complications than later circumcision. Ironically, Wiswell, in his discussion, uses this data to support routine infant circumcision. *Pediatrics* invited Schoen to submit an editorial in the same issue[41] in which he misrepresents the conclusions of the 1989 Task Force on Circumcision. The ambiguous statements on circumcision issued by the 1989 AAP Task Force on Circumcision[6] and the misrepresentation of the findings of the Task Force frequently made by Schoen reinforce the misinformation and disinformation that has allowed circumcision to persist. This departure from scientific objectivity in the case of circumcision is uncharacteristic for *Pediatrics*, which is an otherwise highly respectable medical journal.

Physicians depend on medical journals and their own specific organizations to provide them with up to date, accurate, balanced information. By giving the pro-circumcision advocates free reign to present biased, one-sided, out-dated, inaccurate information, the editors of these journals have done a major disservice to practicing physicians and have placed them at an increased risk for litigation. Zealots of any stripe rely on proven scare tactics. One common scare tactic seen in the literature today posits that, if a child is not circumcised at birth, he is at risk for penile cancer, HIV, UTI, renal failure, brain damage, or death. Each of these risks represents extremely rare events that have never been clearly proven to be caused by the prepuce. Circumcision advocates use these scare tactics because they have the power to provoke the irrational fears of uninformed, vulnerable parents, who have insecurities about their newborns and who have a blind trust in the medical establishment. These scare tactics are likewise effective in maintaining the high circumcision rate because physicians do not have time to research the issue properly and reinforce the misinformation taught in American medical schools.

4. ANTI-SEMITISM

Because circumcision is a religious issue of primary importance in the Jewish and Islamic faiths, many physicians are unwilling to confront the mutilative aspects of circumcision for fear of offending their Jewish or Islamic colleagues or, worse yet, of being labeled an "anti-Semite." This irrational fear of encroaching upon the sensitivities of Jews has extended to the United States Department of Health & Human Services. When asked what the agency could do to limit routine non-religious neonatal circumcision, the agency replied that, "Any attempt by any public agency to discourage non-medical circumcision could be misinterpreted as an attack on those religious groups which practice it,"[42] and "it is not proper for our Government to adopt a policy that is directly or indirectly critical of a religious practice."[43]

5. ESTABLISHED PROTOCOLS

The practice of medicine is regulated by established protocols that help insure patients receive the highest standards of care. For circumcision, however, these protocols are violated. For example, professional protocols require consultation between the primary-care physician and the surgeon before any surgical interventions may take place. The pediatrician is, by definition, the primary-care physician for the newborn, yet obstetricians routinely circumcise the newborn without consulting the pediatrician.

Additionally, established protocol requires that, when tissue is removed from the body, it be sent to a laboratory for pathologic/histologic examination. If normal tissue is removed, the surgeon is required to explain why he has performed the surgery. With circumcision, this protocol is inexplicably abandoned.

The protocols for obtaining informed consent, likewise, are abandoned for circumcision. Studies investigating the type and quality of informed consent given to parents by physicians demonstrate that those physicians who did speak with the family grossly underestimated the complications of the procedure. Even when adequate informed consent is obtained, this does not lower the rate of circumcision.[44,45] Educational videotapes summarizing factors relating to neonatal circumcision have been proven to have an impact on the rate of circumcision.[46] Many now feel that video presentations of procedures should be part of the informed consent process in all elective surgical cases.

In the United States, solicitation of unnecessary or cosmetic surgery is unethical. For example, if a plastic surgeon riding in an elevator notices that a woman's nose is a little crooked, he is not allowed to offer his surgical services unless she initiates the consultation process. Physicians do, however, openly solicit circumcision. During a pregnant woman's initial visit to the obstetrician, she is usually asked if she desires circumcision for her unborn child. Likewise, when admitted to the hospital for delivery, she is routinely asked about circumcision. Asking parents to consent to an unnecessary surgery on behalf of their healthy newborn that will financially benefit both the obstetrician and the hospital is unethical.

The usual route for acceptance of a medical therapy — be it a medication or a procedure — is to test its efficacy against established therapies in treating or preventing illness. If a therapy cannot be shown to be effective, it is abandoned. This fundamental protocol has never been applied to circumcision. It should have been conclusively demonstrated that neonatal circumcision has real and significant prophylactic benefits that far outweigh the known risks before the medical establishment initiated the practice. The studies used to support circumcision and to implicate the prepuce as a cause of disease do not stand up well to scientific scrutiny. Such studies rely on weak behavior-based associations and not upon standard epidemiological methods. The surgical risks of circumcision are real, while the alleged benefits are merely speculation. It would be more logical to justify routine, prophylactic insertion of tympanotomy tubes shortly after birth. One-third of all children will have multiple bouts of otitis media with some developing hearing loss and speech delays. The savings in the cost of office visits and antibiotics would be vast. No one endorses this allegedly prophylactic surgery, however, because the idea of prophylactic surgery is unacceptable, even if one-third of all children would be benefitted.

The technique of radical circumcision as therapy for clinically-verifiable penile problems likewise deserves careful scrutiny. Topical therapies[47-52] and plastic surgical techniques[53-66] have been demonstrated to have significantly lower morbidity and better outcomes for penile problems.[59]

6. THE ROLE OF MONEY

It is not clear why third-party payers, including insurance companies and the government, continue to pay for circumcision when it has been shown repeatedly to be cost ineffective.[67-71] Insurance companies would profit by utilizing the data from current studies demonstrating that the financial advantages of stopping circumcision are dramatic.[71]

When the British National Health Service ceased payment for neonatal circumcision in 1949, the rate of neonatal circumcision dropped to less than one percent. Wiswell, a neonatalogist, has correctly pointed out that circumcision is an easy way for physicians to pad their income.[72] Currently, younger male obstetricians are more likely to perform and charge more for circumcisions than older or female obstetricians or pediatricians.[73] The charge for the procedure ranges between $50 and $350, with $115 being the average. The average reimbursement is between $93 and $98.[74] Most insurance companies hand over more cash to the circumciser than they do to the physician caring for the newborn. This willingness to pay for neonatal circumcision, but not circumcision in later life, creates an additional incentive for physicians to perform neonatal circumcision. In most states, medical assistance for poor families pays for the procedure. A busy obstetrician who pushes mothers to agree to have their boys circumcised can generate an additional $25,000 to $30,000-per-year in income. If neonatal circumcision were to cease, this loss in income would be noticed.

The Canadian experience, as documented by George Denniston, M.D., shows that, when payment stops, the procedure stops.[75] Unfortunately, some uninformed parents are willing to pay over $1,000 (Canadian) to have their sons circumcised, prompting some physicians to continue the practice.

The ripple effect of the tort system on American society should not be underestimated. Multi-million dollar lawsuit awards grab the attention of corporations, and practices subsequently change. Physicians have an obsessive fear of litigation. This fear supports the multi-billion-dollar defensive-medicine industry. Multiple tests are ordered, not because they are necessary, but for the sole purpose of having the results of those tests on the patient's medical chart to protect the physician from potential litigation. The power and prevalence of this fear should not be underestimated. This fear may have prompted the formation of the 1989 AAP Ad Hoc Task Force on Circumcision.

7. CONCLUSIONS

In her book, *Circumcision: What Every Parent Should Know*,[76] Anne Briggs tries to answer the question of why circumcision persists in the United States. She astutely notes that, while most physicians recognize that circumcision has no medical benefits, they still facilitate the parents' misperceptions about circumcision because parents understandably believe that, if circumcision had no medical benefit, physicians would refuse to perform it.

Creating barriers to the performance of the surgery will decrease its incidence. Briggs gives the example of a hospital that stopped performing inpatient circumcisions, and, although several physicians offered outpatient circumcision services, the rate dropped considerably. Ceasing the performance of inpatient circumcision gave the clear message to parents that the hospital did not explicitly or implicitly approve of circumcision.

When physicians learn there are no medical indications for prophylactic routine circumcision, and that there are no medical indications for therapeutic circumcision except in clinically verifiable cases of life-threatening disease or trauma, these unnecessary surgeries will be abandoned. The spurious argument that routine circumcision eliminates "the need to do it later" will no longer be made.

The speculations and fabrications of circumcision advocates should not be allowed to go unchallenged. The scientifically valid medical literature and the world standard of practice do not support the practice of routine circumcision. Maden's study has disproved the penile cancer myth.[77] Donovan's study has disproved the sexually transmitted disease myth.[78-79] Cuckow's study has disproved the notion of "needing it later."[59] Wright's study has disproved the phimosis myth.[47] My current research has disproved the hygiene myth (publication pending).[70] Wiswell's studies on urinary tract infection fail to demonstrate that the proven risk of circumcision is lower than the alleged risk of UTI. Finally, using the American experience as a model, the circumcised penis may be the most important vector for HIV transmission.[80]

New justifications for imposing circumcision on children will undoubtedly arise. As in the past, the new justifications for circumcisions will be to prevent those incurable diseases that make newspaper headlines. It is important that laymen and scientists insist on verifiable scientific proof for any justifications. In this way, speculation, fabrication, and bogus justifications will be eliminated. The protocols for circumcision must be the same as the protocols for any other surgery. Full information must be given, consultation must be granted prior to the procedure, full disclosure of risks and alternative treatments must be explained. Solicitation of this surgery must be prohibited. Circumcision is essentially an issue of sovereignty. As the citizens of the United States become more enlightened about individual human rights, they will demand that the American medical establishment reform itself and align itself with the universal principles of human rights and medical ethics. As a result, routine neonatal circumcision will end.

8. REFERENCES

1. Gairdner D. The fate of the foreskin: a study of circumcision. BMJ 1949;2:1433–7.
2. Morgan WKC. The rape of the phallus. JAMA 1965;193:223–4.
3. American Academy of Pediatrics, Committee on Fetus and Newborn. Standards and Recommendations for Hospital Care of Newborn Infants. 5th ed. Evanston, IL: American Academy of Pediatrics; 1971:110.
4. American College of Obstetricians and Gynecologists. Statement on Neonatal Circumcision. December 1978.
5. Patel DA, Flaherty EG, Dunn J. Factors affecting the practice of circumcision. Am J Dis Child 1982;136:634–6.
6. American Academy of Pediatrics: Report of the Task Force on Circumcision. Pediatrics. 1989;84:388–91.
7. Wiswell TE, Enzenauer RW, Holton ME, Cornish JD, Hankins CT. Declining frequency of circumcision: implications for changes in the absolute incidence and male to female sex ratio of urinary tract infections in early infancy. Pediatrics. 1987;79:338–42.
8. Wiswell TE, Miller GM, Gelston HM Jr; Jones SK, Clemmings AF. Effect of circumcision status on periurethral bacterial flora during the first year of life. J Pediatr 1988;113:442–6.
9. Wiswell TE, Roscelli JD. Corroborative evidence for the decreased incidence of urinary tract infections in circumcised male infants. Pediatrics 1986;78:96–9.
10. Wiswell TE, Smith FR, Bass JW. Decreased incidence of urinary tract infections in circumcised male infants. Pediatrics. 1985;75: 901–3.
11. Gonik B, Barrett K. The persistence of newborn circumcision: an American perspective. Br J Obstet Gynecol 1995;102:940–1.
12. Nellist CC. Is circumcision a job for ob. gyns. or pediatricians? opinions vary. Pediatric News 1994 (May):20.
13. Becker MD. Going around and around on circumcision: pediatricians talk back: Circumcision 'turf war.' Pediatric News 1994 (Aug):16.
14. Washburn ER. Going around and around on circumcision: pediatricians talk back: A job for pediatricians. Pediatric News 1994 (Aug):16.
15. Gilhooly J. Going around and around on circumcision: pediatricians talk back: Discourages 'genital mutilation.' Pediatric News 1994 (Aug):16.
16. Rodham H. Children's Rights: Contemporary Perspectives, 1979.
17. Spence A. Advocates fear parents' rights bill will trample child abuse laws. AAP News 1996 (July);12(7):1,8.
18. Schoen EJ. The status of circumcision of newborns. N Engl J Med. 1990;322:1308–12.
19. Schoen EJ. Urologists and circumcision of newborns. Urology. 1992;40:99–101.
20. Schoen EJ. The relationship between circumcision and cancer of the penis. CA Cancer J Clin. 1991;41:306–9.
21. Schoen EJ. 'Ode to the circumcised male' [letter] Am J Dis Child. 1987;141:128.
22. Schoen EJ. Is it time for Europe to reconsider newborn circumcision? letter] Acta Paediatr Scand. 1991;80:573–7.
23. Roberts JA. Is routine circumcision indicated in the newborn? An affirmative view. J Fam Pract. 1990;31:185–8.
24. Roberts JA. Does circumcision prevent urinary tract infection. J Urol. 1986;135:991–2.
25. Roberts JA. Neonatal circumcision: an end to the controversy? South Med J 1996;89:167–71.
26. Wiswell TE. Circumcision: an update. Curr Probl Pediatr. 1992;22:424–31.
27. Wiswell TE. Do you favor routine neonatal circumcision? Yes. Postgrad Med. 1988;84:98, 100, 102 passim.

28. Wiswell TE. John K. Lattimer Lecture. Prepuce presence portends prevalence of potentially perilous periurethral

    pathogens. J Urol. 1992;148:739–42.

29. Wiswell TE. Routine neonatal circumcision: a reappraisal. Am Fam Physician. 1990;41:859–63.

30. Weiss GN, Weiss EB. A perspective on controversies over neonatal circumcision. Clin Pediatr Phila. 1994;33:726–30.

31. Weiss GN. Neonatal circumcision. South Med J. 1985;78:1198–2000.

32. Wiswell TE, Geschke DW. Risks from circumcision during the first month of life compared with those for uncircumcised boys. Pediatrics. 1989;83:1011–5.

33. Wiswell TE, Tencer HL, Welch CA, Chamberlain JL. Circumcision in children beyond the neonatal period. Pediatrics. 1993;92:791–3.

34. Perlmutter DF, Lawrence JM, Krauss AN, Auld PA. Voiding after neonatal circumcision. Pediatrics. 1995;96:1111–2.

35. Blass EM, Hoffmeyer LB. Sucrose as an analgesic for newborn infants. Pediatrics. 1991;87:215–8.

36. Taddio A, Goldbach M, Ipp M, Stevens B, Koren G Effect of neonatal circumcision on pain responses during vaccination in boys. Lancet. 1995;345:291–2.

37. Cook LS. Koutsky LA. Holmes KK. Clinical presentation of genital warts among circumcised and uncircumcised heterosexual men attending an urban STD clinic. Genitourin Med 1993;69:262–4.

38. Taylor JR, Lockwood AP, Taylor AJ. The prepuce: specialized mucosa of the penis and its loss to circumcision. Br J Urol 1996;77:291–5.

39. O'Brien TR, Calle EE, Poole WK. Incidence of neonatal circumcision in Atlanta, 1985–1986. South Med J. 1995;88:411–5.

40. Mansfield CJ, Hueston WJ, Rudy M. Neonatal circumcision: associated factors and length of hospital stay. J Fam Pract. 1995;41:370–6.

41. Schoen EJ. Circumcision updated — indicated? Pediatrics 1993;92:860–1.

42. Correspondence of February 18, 1994 from Louis Emmet Mahoney, Acting Chief Medical Officer of the Public Health Service of the Department of Health and Human Services, to Frederick Hodges.

43. Correspondence of March 8, 1994 from Louis Emmet Mahoney, Medical Consultant to the Public Health Service of the Department of Health and Human Services, to Frederick Hodges.

44. Christensen Szalanski JJ, Boyce WT, Harrell H, Gardner MM. Circumcision and informed consent. Is more information always better? Med Care 1987;25:856–67.

45. Ciesielski Carlucci C, Milliken N, Cohen NH. Determinants of decision making for circumcision. Cambridge Quarterly of Healthcare Ethics 1996;5:228–36.

46. Enzenauer RW, Powell JM, Wiswell TE, Bass JW. Decreased circumcision rate with videotaped counseling. South Med J. 1986;79:717–20.

47. Wright JE. The treatment of childhood phimosis with topical steroid. Aust N Z J Surg. 1994;64:327–8.

48. Lang K. Eine konservative Therapie der Phimose. Conservative therapy of phimosis] Monatsschr Kinderheilkd. 1986;134:824–5.

49. Kikiros CS, Beasley SW, Woodward AA. The reponse of phimosis to local steroid application. Pediatr Surg Int 1993;8:329–32.

50. Jorgensen ET, Svensson A. Phimosis hos pojkar kan behandlas med steroidsalva Phimosis in boys can be treated by a steroid ointment (letter)]. Lakartidningen 1994;91:1291.

51. Jorgensen ET, Svensson A. The treatment of phimosis in boys, with a potent topical steroid (clobetasol propionate 0.05%) cream. Acta Derm Venereol 1993;73:55–6.

52. Muller I, Muller H. Eine neue konservative Therapie der Phimose. Monatsschr Kinderheilkd 1993;141:607–8.

53. Wahlin N. "Triple incision plasty." A convenient procedure for preputial relief. Scand J Urol Nephrol 1992;26:107–10.

54. Hoffman S, Metz P, Ebbehoj J. A new operation for phimosis: prepuce saving technique with multiple Y-V-plasties. Br J Urol 1984;56:319–21.

55. Leal MJ, Mendes J. A circuncisao ritual e correccao plastica da fimose. Ritual circumcision and the plastic repair of phimosis] Acta Med Port 1994;7:475–81.

56. Emmett AJ. Z plasty reconstruction for preputial stenosis a surgical alternative to circumcision. Aust Paediatr J 1982;18:219–20.

57. Emmett AJ. Four V flap repair of preputial stenosis (phimosis). Plast Reconstr Surg 1975;55:687–9.

58. de Castella H. Prepuceplasty: an alternative to circumcision. Ann R Coll Surg Engl 1994;76:257–8.

59. Cuckow PM, Rix G, Mouriquand PD. Preputial plasty: a good alternative to circumcision. J Pediatr Surg 1994;29:561–3.

60. Holmlund DE. Dorsal incision of the prepuce and skin closure with Dexon in patients with phimosis. Scand J Urol Nephrol 1973;7:97–9.

61. Diaz A, Kantor HI. Dorsal slit. A circumcision alternative. Obstet Gynecol 1971;37:619–22.

62. Ohjimi T, Ohjimi H. Special surgical techniques for relief of phimosis. J Dermatol Surg Oncol 1981;7:326–30.

63. Parkash S. Phimosis and its plastic correction. J Indian Med Assoc 1972;58:389–90.

64. Moro G, Gesmundo R, Bevilacqua A, Maiullari E, Gandini R. La circoncisione con postoplastica. Nota di tecnica operatoria. [Circumcision with preputioplasty. Note on operative technic] Minerva Chir 1988;43:893–4.

65. Gil Barbosa M, Aguilera Gonzalez C, Alipaz A, Garcia Sanchez JL. La balanolisis como sustituto de la circuncision. [Balanolysis as a substitute of circumcision] Salud Publica Mex 1976;18:893–9.

66. Ohjimi H, Ogata K, Ohjimi T. A new method for the relief of adult phimosis. J Urol 1995;153:1607–9.

67. Lawler FH, Bisonni RS, Holtgrave DR. Circumcision: a decision analysis of its medical value. Fam Med 1991;23:587–93.

68. Ganiats TG, Humphrey JB, Taras HL, Kaplan RM. Routine neonatal circumcision: a cost utility analysis. Med Dis Making 1991;11:282–93.

69. Chessare JB. Circumcision: is the risk of urinary tract infection really the pivotal issue? Clin Pediatr Phila 1992;31:100–4.

70. Cadman D, Gafni A, McNamee J. Newborn circumcision: an economic perspective. Can Med Assoc J 1984;131:1353–5.

71. Van Howe RS. Neonatal circumcision: cost utility analysis. Presented at "Strategies for Intactivists" Conference. Evanston, Illinois. April 11, 1996.

72. Lehman BA. The age old question of circumcision. Boston Globe June 22, 1987:41.

73. Garry T. Circumcision: a survey of fees and practices. OBG Management 1994 (October):34–6.

74. Medical Economics Pediatrics Edition. 1995(11);14:34.

75. Denniston GC. Circumcision in Canada: a twenty year decline. In press.

76. Briggs A. Circumcision: What Every Parent Should Know. Earlysville, Virginia: Birth & Parenting Publications, 1985.

77. Maden C, Sherman KJ, Beckmann AM, Hislop TG, Teh CZ, Ashley RL, Daling JR. History of circumcision, medical conditions, and sexual activity and risk of penile cancer. J Natl Cancer Inst. 1993;85:19–24.

78. Donovan B, Bassett I, Bodsworth NJ. Male circumcision and common sexually transmissible diseases in a developed nation setting. Genitourin Med. 1994;70:317–20.

79. Bassett I, Donovan B, Bodsworth NJ, Field PR, Ho DW, Jeansson S, Cunningham AL. Herpes simplex virus type 2 infection of heterosexual men attending a sexual health centre. Med J Aust. 1994;160:697–700.

80. Storms MR. AAFP fact sheet on neonatal circumcision: a need for updating. Am Fam Physician. 1996;54:1216–1218.

10

LEARNED HELPLESSNESS

A Concept of the Future

Michel Odent

As we approach the turn of the century, it has become increasingly common for people to review the greatest advances in science, technology, medicine and other disciplines that have occurred during the past decades. Ask anyone on the street what they believe to have been the most important advances in our understanding of health and disease and you will get a great variety of responses. My response would be that, during the Twentieth Century, the prototype of a pathogenic situation has been clearly identified. The most typical pathogenic situation is the condition of being trapped in adverse or threatening circumstances from which one can neither fight nor flee, a condition to which one can only passively submit, resulting in a deterioration of health. To be in a state of *initiative*, however, is health enhancing. The practical implications for this model are obvious, particularly in the framework of any study regarding sexual mutilation.

1. ANIMAL EXPERIMENTS

The discovery of this phenomenon began with independent scientific experiments carried out in the 1960s by Steven Maier[1] and Martin Seligman[2] in the USA, and Henri Laborit[3] in France. They found that dogs and rats became sick — for example, they suffered from stomach ulcers, weight loss, or a rise in blood pressure — after receiving a series of electric shocks. It was not the electric shocks in themselves that made the animals ill, but the submissive state the animals were in at the time they received the shocks. Their health, however, was not endangered if they had the opportunity to fight with another animal in the cage or if they had a means of escape, even though all the groups studied received the same number of electric shocks.

There is an altered hormonal balance during "uncontrollable adverse events." "Learned helplessness," as defined by Maier and Seligman, or "inhibition of action," as

Sexual Mutilations: A Human Tragedy, edited by Denniston and Milos
Plenum Press, New York, 1997

defined by Laborit, describe situations associated with low levels of adrenalin — the hormone which triggers sudden bursts of energy that enable one to fight or flee. Typically, in this situation, high levels of hormones like cortisol are produced which tend to depress basic adaptive systems. When we have lost all hope and have given up, a self-destructive process starts.

2. EXPLORING THE MEDICAL LITERATURE

In the framework of a study of specifically human issues, the first question is: Can the results of such experiments with rats and dogs be transposed to humans? For obvious reasons, similar experiments (ethically debatable even with animals) are not feasible with humans, but it is possible to find studies in the medical literature evaluating the health effects of situations of initiative versus situations of "inhibition of action" among humans.

Significant findings have been made in the field of occupational medicine. An important example is offered recently by a large Swedish study. During a 14-year period,[4] 12,517 men were followed. They were assigned scores according to their occupational histories and the degree of control they had in their work place. Then they were divided into four categories according to the scores. At the end of the 14 years, 521 deaths from cardiovascular diseases were identified. In the final multivariable analysis, after adjustment for age, smoking, exercise, education, social class, nationality and physical job demands, it appeared that workers with low work control had a risk of dying from cardiovascular disease multiplied by a factor of 1.83. In general, the results of these studies confirm that the boss who takes the initiative is in a healthier situation than his subordinates who have no control.

Another example of "learned helplessness" is the situation of being repeatedly bullied at school. In Newham, East London, 2,962 primary school children (mean age 8) were interviewed during the academic year 1992–93.[5] Of these, 22% reported that they had been bullied. Symptoms of altered health — for example, disturbed sleep, headaches, tummy aches, and sadness — were significantly more frequent among bullied children. The risk of health problems correlated with the frequency of bullying.

Tortured prisoners are in a typical situation of "inhibition of action." Legal and moral arguments against torture have been heard for centuries. Cicero, Seneca, and St. Augustine pointed out the moral perversity of torture, but, until recently, the lasting effects on health have neither been recognized nor studied in depth. Today, there exist centers that specialize in the health consequences of torture, such as the Treatment and Rehabilitation Unit for Survivors of Torture and Trauma in Queensland, Australia.

The life-long diseases of those who were tortured as prisoners are not the direct consequence of their injuries, but rather the consequence of their state of submission when they were tortured. High blood pressure, increased risk of cancer, increased vulnerability to infectious agents, emotional disturbances, sleeping problems, gastric ulcers, headaches, and other signs of depression are among the most common sequelae of torture.

In daily life, those situations of "inhibition of action" in which humans find themselves are usually more subtle, such as being dominated by an authoritarian spouse or the death of a loved one. Whenever there is the feeling of being trapped by circumstances, health is endangered.

3. MISSING THE LINKS

A careful review of the medical literature suggests that there are definite links between topics that may appear to be unrelated according to current classifications. These links are usually ignored because the concepts of "helplessness" or "inhibition of action" have not attracted the attention of either the health profession or the general public. The works of Maier, Seligman and Laborit have been overlooked because these authors have correctly avoided the vague, overused, and misleading word "stress." Stress is a generalized state that can be considered almost synonymous with life events. The terms "learned helplessness" or "inhibition of action" accurately describe the situation of submission to uncontrollable events, as opposed to situations of initiative. Both conditions may be stressful, but only submission is pathogenic.

The concepts of "helplessness" or "inhibition of action" may have also been ignored because health professionals are highly specialized. Doctors specializing in occupational medicine would not be expected to read medical articles about bullied children, tortured prisoners, or sexual mutilation.

4. THE CASE OF NEONATAL CIRCUMCISION

The life-long health consequences of sexual mutilations, such as neonatal circumcision, must be examined in this framework. From the child's perspective, sexual mutilation necessarily represents a situation of "inhibition of action" during the "primal period." This early phase of life is not accessible to what is commonly called conscious memory. Other recent advances in the field of epidemiology do confirm the existence of life-long health consequences resulting from early events. The earlier an event occurs, the more profound and long-lasting its consequences. There exist a tremendous number of studies now that establish significant correlations between the beginning of life — and, in particular, events in the perinatal period — and health later on in life. Jacobson,[6] for example, established a link between the use of certain drugs (opiates in particular) by a woman in labor and the risk for her child to become drug addicted twenty years later. Another Swedish study found a link between adverse events in the perinatal period (infectious disease such as measles or birth complications) and the risk of developing Crohn's disease later on in life.[7]

In 1986, in the book *Primal Health*,[8] I proposed a new vocabulary to facilitate the exploration of the long-term consequences of early events. "Early events" occur during the "primal period," which encompasses fetal life, the perinatal period, and early infancy. The "primal period" is the time when our basic adaptive systems — those involved in what we commonly call health — reach maturity. These basic adaptive systems are interconnected and should be perceived as one all-important network. This network (which was traditionally separated into the nervous system, the endocrine system and the immune system) is called the "primal adaptive system." Health is the quality of the workings of the "primal adaptive system." Any event happening during the "primal period," the stage of formation of the basic adaptive systems, will have long-term consequences. Theoretically, long-term health consequences of neonatal circumcision are plausible. Until now, the only systematic study demonstrating a "middle term" effect of neonatal circumcision focused on the pain response during vaccination in boys.[9] A Canadian team noticed that boys had higher pain scores than girls when they were vaccinated with diphtheria-pertussis-tetanus

(DPT) around the age of five months. After systematic studies, it appeared that only circumcised boys had higher pain scores.

5. CONCLUSIONS

The concepts of "inhibition of action" and "learned helplessness" offer an opportunity to include neonatal circumcision in a larger framework of cross-cultural beliefs, rituals, and practices that challenge the maternal protective instinct during the short "sensitive period" following birth. Such practices include denying the newborn colostrum, early baptism in cold water, tight swaddling, foot binding, "smoking" the newborn baby, or piercing the ears of baby girls.

It is incumbent upon researchers to explore the possible long-term health consequences of sexual mutilations inflicted upon infants and children at different ages. The most logical way to evaluate the long-term health consequences of any procedure is the "prospective randomized controlled study." In the case of sexual mutilation, there are obvious ethical obstacles to such an approach. Epidemiologists, however, have many tools designed to respect ethical barriers while still producing scientifically valid research. They are never in a state of inhibition of action.

6. REFERENCES

1. Maier SF, Seligman MEP. Learned helplessness: theory and evidence. J Exp Psychol General 1976;105:3–46.
2. Seligman MEP, Beagley C. Learned helplessness in the rat. J Comp Physio Psychol 1975;88:534–41.
3. Laborit H. L'inhibition de l'action. Paris: Masson, 1980.
4. Johnson JV, Steward W, Hall EM, et al. Long-term psychological work environment and cardiovascular mortality among Swedish men. Am J Public Health 1996;86:324–31.
5. Williams K, Chambers M, Logan S, Robinson D. Association of common health symptoms with bullying in primary school children. BMJ 1996;313:17–9.
6. Jacobson B. Opiate addiction in adult offspring through possible imprinting after obstetric treatment. BMJ 1990;301:1067–70.
7. Ekbom A, Adami HO, Helmick CG, et al. Perinatal risk factors for inflammatory bowel disease: a case-control study. Am J Epidemiol 1990;6:1111–9.
8. Odent M. Primal Health. London: Century Hutchinson, 1986.
9. Taddio A, Goldback M, Ipp M, et al. Effect of neonatal circumcision on pain responses during vaccination in boys. Lancet 1995; 345:291–92.

11

LONG-TERM CONSEQUENCES OF NEONATAL CIRCUMCISION

A Preliminary Poll of Circumcised Males

Tim Hammond

Male foreskin amputation, euphemistically termed "circumcision," has persisted in various cultures with the unsubstantiated belief that it is a trivial or benign practice. This has been due in large part to the silence of the victims. Indeed, when male genital mutilation occurs at puberty, a male's silence during the cutting is a measure of his manhood. Today, men's silence about these mutilations is being broken and they are demanding to be heard.

Since altering form inevitably alters function, circumcision, at any age, carries distinct physical, sexual and psychological consequences. The earlier the age at which the mutilation occurs, the more profound the physical and psychological damage. The earlier the age at which the mutilation occurs, however, the less likely victims are able to recognize the damage later. Furthermore, the pain inflicted by the surgery is so great that the conscious mind suppresses memories of the event.

Although estimates of the immediate complication rates of neonatal circumcision have been suggested in the medical literature, the American medical profession has not yet established an accurate and consistent method of recording these complications. The purpose of this study was to inquire into the nature and existence of *long-term* consequences of neonatal circumcision.

1. METHODS

In 1993, the National Organization to Halt the Abuse and Routine Mutilation of Males (NOHARMM) sent a questionnaire to circumcised males who had contacted either the national office of NOHARMM in San Francisco, California, or various foreskin restoration support services that work closely with NOHARMM. The survey was directed at this particular group of non-intact (circumcised) men because they may be the most aware

Sexual Mutilations: A Human Tragedy, edited by Denniston and Milos
Plenum Press, New York, 1997

of the long-term consequences of neonatal circumcision. Three-hundred-thirteen (313) circumcised males participated in the survey.

2. RESULTS

2.1. Demographic Data

Of the 313 circumcised men participating in the study, 1% were under 19 years of
age, 13.1% were between the ages of 20 and 29 years, 26.8% were between the ages of 30
and 39 years, 33.9% were between the ages of 40 and 49 years, 16% were between the
ages of 50 and 59 years, and 9.3% were over 60 years of age. The average age of respondents was 42 years.

Of the men participating in the study, 89.1% were circumcised in infancy, 6.1%
were circumcised between the ages of 1 and 12 years, 1.0% were circumcised between the
ages of 13 and 17 years, and 3.8% were circumcised after 18 years of age.

The ethnic and religious backgrounds of respondents were disproportionate to the
percentages of those backgrounds found in the United States. Of the respondents, 96.8%
identified themselves as "White," 0.3% were African-American, 1.3% were Hispanic,
0.3% were of unspecified Asian origin, 0.3% were Native Americans, 4.2% were Jews,
and 1.0% "other." The religious identification of respondents was similarly disproportionate: 77.3% identified themselves as Christian, 4.2% identified themselves as Jews (which
is greater than the overall percentage of Jewish males in the United States), 18.5% identified themselves as Atheist or Buddhist.

2.2. Reported Circumcision-Caused Harm

Of the 313 circumcised men participating in the study, 96.2% suspected or were
confident that circumcision had resulted in a reduction of the normal male capacity for
sexual response and pleasure. The percentage breakdown of categories of circumcision-
caused harm are as follows:

Sexual Harm: 84%
Emotional Harm: 83.1%
Physical Harm: 81.5%
Psychological Harm: 75.1%
Low Self-Esteem: 74.4%
Problems with Intimate Relationships: 44.7%
Problems with Addictions/Dependencies: 25.6%

A remaining 13.1% of respondents variously attributed their non-intact state to their
problems with masculine identity, self-confidence, and fear of doctors.

Of the 313 circumcised men participating in the study, 55.3% attributed the following physical problems to their circumcision:

Insensitivity of the glans penis: 55.3%
Excess stimulation required to reach orgasm: 38.0%
Prominent scarring: 29.1%
Insufficient residual shaft skin to cover the erect penis: 26.8%

Specific psychological consequences of circumcision were recorded by respondents in the unstructured essay statement requested by surveyors. A statistically significant number of identical responses were recorded. Of the 313 respondents, 69.0% felt general dissatisfaction with their condition, 62.0% felt mutilated, 60.7% felt they were unwhole, 60.4% felt resentment over what had been done to them, 60.1% felt abnormal and unnatural, 60.1% felt that their human rights had been violated, 54.3% felt anger about circumcision, 53.0% felt frustration over their non-intact condition, 49.5% felt violated or raped, 47.3% felt inferior to genitally intact males, 42.5% felt that their circumcised penis was an impediment to sexual relations, and 33.9% felt that they had been betrayed by their parents for allowing them to be circumcised.

Despite the severity of the psychological and physical harm attributed by respondents to their circumcision, 61.1% had not sought treatment at the time of the survey. Of the respondents who had not sought treatment, 39.3% believed that there was no recourse available, 19.8% were too embarrassed, 15.7% feared ridicule, 12.5% cited mistrust of doctors, and 3.5% felt that it was not important enough.

3. DISCUSSION

The disproportionate participation of men between the ages of 30 and 49 may be due in large part to two important factors. First, this is the time of life when men, in general, begin to reassess their lives and to question past experiences and assumptions. Second, this is also the time when non-intact men begin to become more aware of progressive sensitivity loss of the glans.

The results of this survey document that circumcision can adversely impact the overall psychological well-being of non-intact males. This survey demonstrates that neonatal circumcision can have negative consequences on the future sexual well-being of non-intact males. More than 60% of respondents who had gained knowledge about the functions of intact male genitalia recognized that circumcision had harmed them. Circumcised males reported that they had to resort to prolonged periods of intense and excessive thrusting to stimulate the residual nerve endings in the penis to trigger orgasm. These men reported that the unnatural dryness of their circumcised penis often made coitus painful for them and their partners.

Most circumcised men in the United States have not discussed or reported the inevitable damage inherently caused by this amputative genital surgery. Their silence may be due to the widespread societal ignorance of natural male genital anatomy and normal male genital functions. This ignorance is undoubtedly a result of the massive circumcision campaigns of the past. The results of this survey suggest that, before the damage of genital alteration can be recognized as such, the natural genital anatomy and function must be understood. The physical defects and sexual dysfunctions of which many non-intact males may be aware are often misperceived as a "birth defect" or part of the aging process, rather than as a direct consequence of their circumcision. Since many circumcised men in the United States have never seen a naturally intact human penis, they may wrongly perceive the dark, circumferential circumcision scar on the remnant of their penis to be a feature of "normal" anatomy.

While the overall complication rate here for neonatal circumcision is unknown, the estimated rates of 0.02% to 1.07% alleged by some authors[1] stands in sharp contrast to the long-term psychological and physical complication rate of 92.7% reported by respondents. The medical profession has not addressed this issue.

Most non-intact males, erroneously believing circumcision is a universal practice, may not feel that circumcision has left them with a diminished penis because they have no means by which to compare their experience. Among respondents, however, the heightened awareness of the adverse consequences of neonatal circumcision led to a firm conviction that the practice was a violation of the human rights to physical integrity, and self-determination, i.e., body ownership. Nearly half (49.5%) of respondents indicated feelings of violation. Over 60% of respondents felt that their human rights had been violated by neonatal circumcision. Such feelings increased with the age of the respondent.

Despite their strong feelings and intense focus on circumcision as a central issue in their lives, most respondents felt pressured to remain silent. In the United States, males are not encouraged to verbalize their feelings, in general, but, additionally, there is a very strong taboo against verbalizing feelings about the penis. This can arouse suspicion in other males that the person discussing his penis may be homosexual. The powerful taboos against homosexuality present in many cultures, including the United States, silences most men. They fear that violation of the taboo will lead to social ostracism, imprisonment, or violence. In some cultures, it may lead to government-authorized torture or death.

Despite these pressures, many circumcised men are breaking these taboos and are finding the courage to begin verbalizing their feelings and seeking ways to heal psychological damage caused by circumcision. To address the feelings of body dysmorphia caused by the recognition that the penis has been damaged, a growing number of non-intact men are engaging in the process of foreskin restoration. Those who feel that circumcision represents a violation of individual sovereignty find therapeutic benefit in working for social change. A significant minority seek justice through litigation. The psychological healing, social activism and foreskin restoration now being undertaken in the United States by men are documented in the award-winning film, *Whose Body, Whose Rights?*[2]

4. CONCLUSION

The results of this survey demonstrate that neonatal circumcision has profound psychological and sexual consequences for a significant number of men. The types of physical harm caused by neonatal circumcision remain largely unrecognized by the general population of non-intact males due to society-wide ignorance of the normal anatomy and functions of the intact human penis. Becoming aware of normal human male genital anatomy and function was the most important factor in recognizing the types of physical harm caused by neonatal circumcision. From this survey, it appears that subsequent to this recognition it is common for circumcised men to acknowledge that family members and respected people in the community, for example, doctors or religious leaders, are responsible for permitting this harm to occur. Many circumcised men fail to seek professional assistance because of their well-founded mistrust of the medical profession, or because they are unaware of the existence of the many peer resources now available. Others are reluctant to verbalize their feelings for fear of ridicule. Some non-intact men who have sought psychological counselling have been subjected to ridicule or misunderstanding from mental health workers. Until recently, men who understood that they had been psychologically and sexually damaged by circumcision suffered in silence. Those who have verbalized their dissatisfaction with circumcision have risked violating cultural taboos about discussing the penis or questioning their society's traditional practices. The psychological impact of recognizing one's harm, as well as the potential social disapproval from disclosing one's feelings, can be managed successfully through personal foreskin restoration, peer support groups, and altruistic activism to end the practice of neonatal circumcision and spare future generations of males from experiencing the same types of harm.

REFERENCES

1. Gee WF, Ansell JS. Neonatal circumcision: a ten-year overview: with comparison of the Gomco clamp and the Plastibell device. Pediatrics 1976;58:824–7.
2. Whose Body, Whose Rights? Produced by Tim Hammond and directed by Lawrence Dillon. 56 min. Dillonwood Productions, 1995. Videocassette. [Institutional distribution: University of California Extension Center for Media and Independent Learning, 2000 Center Street, Fourth Floor, Berkeley, CA 94704 USA. Catalog #38342.]

12

SIMILARITIES IN ATTITUDES AND MISCONCEPTIONS ABOUT MALE AND FEMALE SEXUAL MUTILATIONS

Hanny Lightfoot-Klein

Enlightened Westerners, existing in a world far removed geographically and psychologically from the strange and disturbing practices of sexual mutilation in Africa, may be tempted to disregard them as something that does not concern the West. The practice of female circumcision, which many Westerners regard as barbaric and irrational, however, has had its parallels throughout history in secular male circumcision, as practiced in the United States. The reasons given for female circumcision in Africa and for routine male circumcision in the United States are essentially the same. Politically, the underlying similarity between male and female sexual mutilations is that both are perpetrated by force on the generally unanesthetized, helpless bodies of unconsenting infants and children.

1. METHODS

Interviews with people who unquestioningly accept sexual mutilation were conducted from 1979 to 1984 in the Sudan and from 1984 to 1995 in various parts of the United States and Europe. Subjects were engaged in casual, non-confrontational conversation.

2. RESULTS

The responses that were elicited transcend cultural barriers and fall into several well-defined categories. The words of the people interviewed are directly transcribed here without emendation.

Sexual Mutilations: A Human Tragedy, edited by Denniston and Milos
Plenum Press, New York, 1997

2.1. Minimization of Damage and Pain

Africa: "She loses only a little piece of the clitoris, just the part that protrudes. The girl does not miss it. She can still feel, after all. There is hardly any pain. Women's pain thresholds are so much higher than men's."

United States: "It's only a little piece of skin. The baby does not feel any pain because his nervous system is not developed yet."

2.2. Beautification

Africa: "The parts that are cut away are disgusting and hideous to look at. It is done for the beauty of the suture."

United States: "An uncircumcised penis is a real turn-off. It's disgusting! It looks like the penis of an animal. It generates smegma and smegma stinks."

2.3. Medical Indications

Africa: "Female circumcision protects the health of a woman. Infibulation prevents the uterus from falling out. It keeps her smelling sweet so that her husband will be pleased. If is not done, she will stink and get worms in her vagina."

United States: "An uncircumcised penis causes urinary infections and penile cancer.

2.4. Maintaining Hygiene

Africa: "An uncircumcised vulva is unclean and only the lowest prostitute would leave her daughter uncircumcised. No man would dream of marrying an unclean woman. He would be laughed at by everyone."

United States: "An uncircumcised penis is dirty and only the lowest class of people with no concept of hygiene leave their boys uncircumcised. A circumcised penis is more hygienic and oral sex with an uncircumcised penis is disgusting to women."

2.5. Preventing Future Problems

Africa: "Leaving a girl uncircumcised endangers both her husband and her baby. If the baby's head touches the uncut clitoris during birth, the baby will be born hydrocephalic. The milk of the mother will become poisonous. If a man's penis touches a woman's clitoris, he will become impotent."

United States: "Men have an obligation to their wives to give up their foreskin. An uncircumcised penis will cause cervical cancer in women. It also spreads disease."

2.6. Improving Sex

Africa: "A circumcised woman is sexually more pleasing to her husband. The tighter she is sewn, the more pleasure he has."

United States: "Circumcised men make better lovers because they have more staying power than uncircumcised men."

2.7. Universality

Africa: "All the women in the world are circumcised. It is something that must be done. If there is pain, then that is part of a woman's lot in life."

United States: "Men in all of the civilized world are circumcised."

2.8. Medicalization

Africa: "Doctors do it, so it must be a good thing."

United States: "Doctors do it, so it must be a good thing."

2.9. Denial of Long-Term Harm

Africa: "Yes, I have suffered from chronic pelvic infections and terrible pain for years now. You say that all of this is the result of my circumcision? But I was circumcised over 30 years ago! How can something that was done to me when I was four-years-old have anything to do with my health now?"

United States: "I have lost nearly all interest in sex. You might say that I'm becoming impotent. I don't seem to have much sensation in my penis anymore, and it is becoming more and more difficult for me to reach orgasm. You say that this is the result of my

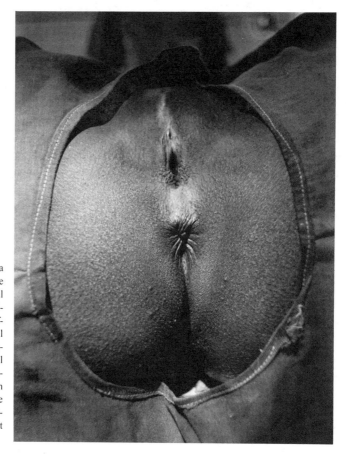

Figure 1. Genital-rectal area of a 25-year-old married Sudanese woman, showing introitus, urethral opening, and pharaonic circumcision scar. This photo was taken after she had received general anesthesia in preparation for an exploratory operation. Her vaginal opening was too narrow and inelastic to permit the introduction of instruments needed to examine her internally. Many women infibulated like this are unaware that anything is wrong with them.

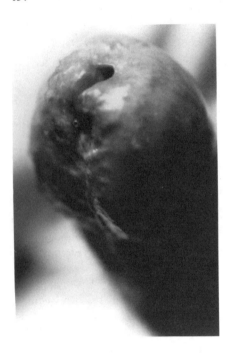

Figure 2. Ventral view of a surgically externalized glans penis of a 28-year-old American male circumcised at birth. Frenulum has been excised. The glans is deeply pitted and scarred as a result of tearing the adherent, immature neonatal foreskin from the glans. The man was unaware that anything was wrong with him. No American physician had ever indicated to this man that anything was wrong. (Photograph courtesy of John A. Erickson)

circumcision? That doesn't make any sense. I was circumcised 35 years ago, when I was a little baby. How can that affect me in any way now?"

3. DISCUSSION

The similarities revealed through these interviews confirm the theory that male circumcision in the United States and female genital mutilation in Africa occur for the same reasons. The fact that greater amounts of erogenous tissue are removed in female genital mutilation is irrelevant. It is highly unlikely that one would find many volunteers among those who shrug off the removal of the male foreskin as being insignificant, were they asked to prove their point by allowing a comparable amount of skin to be removed — even with anesthesia — from their own genitals. Regardless of the amount of tissue actually removed, the essential similarity lies in the fact that the African and American supporters of female and male sexual mutilation, respectively, minimize and trivialize the amount of tissue removed.

Perhaps the most disturbing similarity is the apparent casualness with which the decisions on what constitutes an acceptable degree of mutilation are often made. One is left with the impression that what is being talked about is an insensate piece of fabric rather than a live human being capable of feeling pain.

In the United States, no differences in attitude were noted from region to region, in different age groups, or in males or females. The wide distribution of routine circumcision and the proliferation and standardization of supporting myths through the popular press and medical establishment may account for this lack of diversity of opinion among the supporters of male circumcision. Similarly, in the Sudan, no differences of opinion were noted among the supporters of female circumcision that could be attributed to age, geographical location, or gender.

The sole distinction in attitudes toward sexual mutilation was found along class lines in both countries. These distinctions were observed in the Sudan and the United States among parents of high social class, high levels of education, comfortable standard of living, usually living in urban centers, removed from the extended family, and with a high level of equality in the rights, education, and social freedom of females within the household. People who fall into this class are more likely to reject the myths of their lower-class compatriots and decide not to subject their children to circumcision.

Both Sudanese and Americans falsely allege that there are positive health benefits from female and male circumcision, respectively. Both groups promise that sexual surgery results in cleanliness and absence of genital odors, as well as greater sexual attractiveness and social acceptability. The affected individuals in both cultures have come to view these surgeries as something that was done *for* them, and not something that was done *to* them. While the African rationalizes that women's pain threshold is far higher than that of men, Americans also rationalize that a newborn infant does not feel the pain of unanesthetized surgery.

The economic element of both practices, in Africa and the United States, cannot be ignored. In each case, it is a matter of those who profit from these surgeries by "selling" them to the gullible, conformist, easily-cowed consumer in cultures that are hostile to sexuality.

4. CONCLUSION

Interviews with people in both Africa and the United States who unquestioningly accept sexual mutilations have provided revealing sociological data to corroborate the theory that the reasons given for female circumcision in Africa and for routine male circumcision in the United States are essentially the same. Both groups claim that their respective sexual mutilation practices are minimal, painless, beautifying, medically indicated, hygienic, prophylactic, sexually improving, universal, medicalized, and harmless.

Both excised African women and excised American men are reluctant to believe that they have lost anything. In their denial, they convince themselves of the illusion of their intactness by allowing, openly or tacitly, their own daughters and sons, respectively, to undergo the same procedure. They justify their attitudes through the belief that these surgeries are a matter of tradition and/or scientific or medical necessity. In light of these attitudes, any statement that sexual mutilation is harmful is resisted by excised women and men in an attempt to assure themselves of their normality, and to alleviate the guilt they would have for having condoned the circumcision of their own children.

The thrust of any program concerned with the abolition of these practices should therefore include accurate information on such topics as genital anatomy, hygiene, and sex education in order to change attitudes and dispel misconceptions that lead people to accept sexual mutilation without question.

13

FEMALE GENITAL MUTILATION

Berhane Ras-Work

Female genital mutilation is a cultural practice without religious foundation or justification despite the misconception and misinterpretation to the contrary on the part of the
victims and perpetrators.

The ignorance of many women about religious teachings and interpretations has led
them to believe that their status is unequal to that of men and that their subordination is a
dictate of God. This belief is so deeply rooted, especially among traditional societies, that
women accept cruel and degrading treatment as part of their obligation.

Human societies that are strongly marked by a patriarchal system are also characterized by various forms of violence against women to control their sexuality and fertility.
Female genital mutilation is an extreme form of violence, injurious to millions of women
and girl children. According to the estimate of the World Health Organization, over 100
million women are affected by this practice.

1. WHAT IS FEMALE GENITAL MUTILATION?

Female genital mutilation, commonly known as female circumcision, is a practice
which involves the cutting away of part or the whole of the external female genital organs.

1.1. Who Performs the Mutilation and How Is It Performed?

The practice is usually performed, under very unhygienic conditions, by an un-
trained elderly woman — *Ouddo* in Somalia, *Daya* in Egypt, *Khafedha* in Sudan — using
razor blades, pieces of glass, or knives. These same women, in most countries, are traditional birth attendants and traditional healers. In Mali, Nigeria and Sierra Leone, practitioners perform female genital mutilation as an income-generating activity. In the Sudan,
Somalia, Djibouti and Nigeria, some mothers are known to take their daughters to clinics
to make sure that the operation is performed under medical supervision. In remote no-

Sexual Mutilations: A Human Tragedy, edited by Denniston and Milos
Plenum Press, New York, 1997 137

madic areas where a professional circumciser is not available, old grandmothers or aunts operate on the girls. In some communities, a barber is called upon to do the operation.

At the time of the operation, the girl is held by at least three persons, usually close relatives; one woman holds the trunk and hands of the girl, while the other women firmly hold her legs apart. The buttocks of the girl are usually supported by a piece of wood and the circumciser sits or squats between the legs of the girl. If the circumciser is a professional traditional woman, she comes with her special knife, otherwise a razor blade is used for the purpose. She begins the operation by excising the whole clitoris, the labia minora one at a time, and the internal faces of the labia majora one at a time. After that, she inserts about four pre-selected thorns through the remains of the labia majora. Then she winds a narrow string made of horse's hair or the bark of a tree around the thorns to make them hold tightly. Finally, she puts the resin of a plant known as *Malmal* on the wound so that the thorns, the skin of the girl, and the resin stick together. To complete the procedure, the legs of the girl are both extended and tied together from the hips down to the ankles. Then she is taken to her hut to lie down on a mat.[1]

1.2. Types of Female Genital Mutilation

To date, the types of identified and documented genital mutilation are: *sunnah*, clitoridectomy, excision, infibulation, defibulation, re-infibulation, the Gishiri cut, and Angurya cut.

1.2.1. Sunnah. Although *sunnah* means purification according to the Islamic religion, in this context it implies the removal of the prepuce of the clitoris. In some countries like Indonesia and Malaysia, small incisions are made in the prepuce of the clitoris without totally removing it.

1.2.2. Clitoridectomy. Clitoridectomy is the total removal of the clitoris. The midwife punctures the clitoris to expose it to the maximum. Then the clitoris is rubbed until it stands erect, after which it is pulled and chopped off with a blade or a knife.[2]

1.2.3. Excision. Excision involves removing the clitoris and the labia minora, and then rubbing the wound with local herbs for healing.

1.2.4. Infibulation (Pharaonic Circumcision). The word "infibulation" is derived from the Latin word *fibula*, meaning a clasp. Infibulation at present means the cutting off of the whole of the clitoris, the whole of the labia minora, and the adjacent parts of the labia majora, and stitching the two sides of the vulva, leaving a small opening for urination and menstruation.

1.2.5. Defibulation. Defibulation is performed on a bride to allow intercourse, or on a young mother at delivery.

1.2.6. Refibulation. Refibulation is performed on women who have lost their infibulation, on young mothers after delivery, or on wives during a long absence of their husbands.

1.2.7. Gishiri Cut. This operation is performed by a traditional birth attendant on women with prolonged labor. The traditional birth attendant uses a knife to cut through the soft tissues for the purpose of enlarging the passage. Cases of infection, vesico-vaginal and recto-vaginal fistulas are reported as a result of such a cut.

1.2.8. Angurya Cut. This traditional surgery is performed on female infants to remove the hymen loop. It is believed that, if the hymen is not removed, it will continue to grow and seal the vaginal orifice. Under normal circumstances, however, the loop disappears within a few weeks after the birth of the baby. So far, only Nigeria has reported the existence of the Gishiri and the Angurya cut in some communities.[3]

2. WHAT ARE THE CONSEQUENCES OF FEMALE GENITAL MUTILATION?

2.1. Short-Term

2.1.1. Hemorrhage. Hemorrhage occurs when the clitoris is completely removed and the blood vessels of the clitoris (the vein and also the deep dorsal artery of the clitoris) rupture. The hemorrhage may lead to serious collapse or death.

2.1.2. Acute Infections. Infections are related to the operating equipment used. The equipment may be such items as knives, razor blades, or straw. The two most serious and common infections are tetanus and general septicemia, and, at present, the risk of HIV/AIDS is also prevalent.

2.1.3. Bleeding of Adjacent Organs. Sexual mutilations are often performed without anesthesia, consequently, the young girl suffers much pain and agitation. This may lead to clumsy operations, which sometimes cause bleeding of the urethral meatus.

2.1.4. Violent Pain. The lack of anesthesia during sexual mutilation always causes excruciating pain. This may result in very serious shock, especially since the young girl is in a state of anguish.

2.2. Long Term

2.2.1. Chronic Complications. Chronic complications are the most frequent and spectacular, resulting from extensive scars in the clitoral zone after excision. These scars open up during childbirth and cause the anterior perineum to tear, leading to hemorrhage, which is often difficult to stop.

2.2.2. Hematic Complications. This condition, which refers to the inability of menstrual blood to exit because of the complete coalescence of the labia, is a serious complication of genital mutilation.

2.2.3. Fistula Cases. One of the most serious consequences of female genital mutilation is vesico-vaginal and recto-vaginal fistulas, leading to incontinence, due to obstructed labor resulting from circumcision scars. The woman suffering from fistulas is usually ostracized and shamed by society. Repair of fistulas is delicate and costly.

2.2.4. Functional Manifestations. Obviously, the mere notion of surgical interference in highly sensitive genital organs constitutes a serious threat to the child, and the painful operation is a source of major physical as well as psychiatric disturbances, depending largely upon the child's inner defenses and the prevailing psychological environment. The functional psychiatric manifestations may take various clinical forms and cause behavioral reactions. The extent of psychological damage needs to be studied.

2.2.5. HIV/AIDS. Considering the unhygienic conditions under which female genital mutilation is performed, the practice presents a risk to the spread of HIV/AIDS. A group of researchers in Ethiopia studied the possible link of genital mutilation and HIV/AIDS and, from the information gathered, it is evident that there is a definite risk, especially in cases where female genital mutilation is performed as an initiation rite and the same unwashed, unsterilized knife is used to operate on many girls.

3. AGE

The age at which a girl undergoes genital mutilation varies from region to region, and, within the same country, from community to community. For example, in Ethiopia, among the highland population, a baby girl is circumcised when she is seven days old. Among the lowlanders near the Somali border, girls are infibulated at the age of six or seven years. In West African countries, where female genital mutilation is performed as an initiation rite, the age range varies from thirteen up to marriage. Among the Ibos of Nigeria, excision is done just before marriage. The Abohs in Mid-Western Nigeria excise a woman just before her first child is born.

4. THE REASONS ADVANCED FOR THE PERSISTENCE OF FEMALE GENITAL MUTILATION

The reasons for the continuation of female genital mutilation vary according to the socio-cultural context where it exists. The major justifications are:

- Moral or religious
- Virginity: bride price or family honor
- Anatomic/aesthetic
- Need for social integration
- Prevent child mortality
- Hygiene

4.1. Religious

The most frequent reason advanced for the practice of female genital mutilation is religion. Those who practice female genital mutilation usually believe that Islam makes the practice obligatory. Christianity is also cited as a justification. Most women in the countries where the practice exists believe that, as good Moslems or Christians, they need to go through the ritual of female genital mutilation. A group of women from Guinea-Bissau expressed this belief, saying:

As good Moslems we must be circumcised. That way we will be ensured to have a proper Moslem burial ceremony. As wives we need to be cleaned by the circumcision ritual in order to be able to prepare food for our husbands.[4]

Very high religious leaders, however, have stated that neither the Koran nor the Bible oblige women to undergo the operation. A very high Islamic scholar from Alhazar University says:

It is reported that the Prophet Mohammed upon seeing a woman circumcising a girl said: 'Circumcise, but do not go deep, this is more illuminating to the face and more enjoyable to the husband.'[5]

It is believed that the origin of the practice predated Islam, and it reached the countries where it exists before the spread of this religion.

4.2. Virginity

Virginity is a strong reason cited by mothers and grandmothers for preserving the practice of female genital mutilation. Professor Corréa of Senegal elaborates on this point as follows:

The resplitting of the clitoris by eliminating the sexual sensitiveness of the young girl protects her from sexual instability and excesses, if not debauchery, and makes it possible for her to conserve her virginity until marriage. Infibulation, which is in fact a complementary variant of excision, was formerly practiced almost worldwide and is still today in some countries — Sudan, Somalia, Djibouti — to provide an additional security for the young girl and to make her remain sexually intact until the evening of her marriage. Young girls thus protected are reputed to have very high moral values an added advantage on which parents can capitalize by demanding a substantial dowry.[6]

4.3. Aesthetic Reasons and Social Integration

Among some communities, it is believed that the clitoris of a young uncircumcised girl gives her the semblance of a man. At birth, every individual is supposed to be endowed with a male and female soul, which affects the organs of procreation. The female soul of a man is located in the foreskin, while the male soul of a woman is located in the clitoris. To be integrated into the society, the man should lose his foreskin through circumcision and the woman should lose her clitoris through excision.

The young uncircumcised girl is still considered today as a second-class citizen, impure, a *bilekoro*, according to a typical expression in Mali. Such a young girl can neither marry nor even be allowed to prepare the family meal until she agrees to be circumcised.

The practice is inculcated in the minds of girls by family members and peer groups throughout their socializing process. In Sierra Leone, female genital mutilation forms a part of the initiation ceremony of womanhood. After the physical operation, the girls undergo training on how to be good wives, mothers, and members of their society.

Dr. Olayinka Koso-Thomas, in her book, *The Circumcision of Women*, describes the ceremony of graduation:

At the end of their training, dressed in their best clothes and finest jewelry, the new initiates parade the streets of the town or village. There is dancing, singing, heavy drinking and merriment, with relatives, fiancees and friends joining in the celebration.

After the parade, the initiates return to the bush and are sworn to secrecy concerning the activities of the society. Their heads, which were plastered with a mud "Devil's cap" are washed; the girls have now attained womanly status. They can either go home to their parents or to their husband's home, where more singing, dancing and heavy drinking continues till the early hours of the next day. The initiates receive gifts from relatives or fiancees.[7]

The initiation that takes place in the Sande bush is kept as a binding secret among the initiates who form a secret society. An uninitiated girl is neither considered eligible for marriage nor is she accepted by her community. She becomes an outcast and is not allowed to engage in any kind of business.

The reasons commonly advanced for maintaining female genital mutilation do not have religious or scientific backing. Female genital mutilation does not guarantee virginity or reduce promiscuity. It does not ensure fertility. In fact, it can cause sterility due to the resulting infections. Ignorance is a major factor for the persistence of the practice. Parents subject their children to female genital mutilation with the best of intentions, not knowing a better alternative to marriage and the security it provides. Additional factors which perpetuate female genital mutilation are:

- Benefit and status of circumcisers
- Lack of strong government policy and actions to eradicate the custom
- Low economic and educational status of women

4.4. Benefit to Circumcisers

Circumcisers are respected among their societies as skilled traditional surgeons and herbalists. In many countries, they are the traditional birth attendants who render services to mothers during child delivery. They are paid in cash and kind, such as chicken, eggs, rice, and money. They enjoy high social status.

The eradication of female genital mutilation entails the deprivation of these practitioners from their income and status. In order to effectively campaign against these practices, alternative sources of income have to be secured for this group.

5. HISTORY OF FEMALE GENITAL MUTILATION

Several speculative theories have been advanced for the origin of female genital mutilation. Shandal, in his 1963 study, *Circumcision and Infibulation of Females*, states: "A large number of circumcised females were found among the mummies of ancient Egyptians, but a few infibulations were encountered." It is also believed that female genital mutilation was performed on Egyptian women to mark a class distinction.

Dr. A. H. Taba, in his paper on female circumcision, states: "In the Fifth Century B.C., female circumcision was practiced by the Phoenicians, Hittites, and Ethiopians, as well as by the Egyptians. This practice was transported from Egypt to the Sudan, the Horn of Africa and moved along the Sahel belt with the migration of the population."[8] The origin and history of female genital mutilation is eclipsed by the passage of time, and more extensive anthropological research is necessary to identify and define its source.

6. GEOGRAPHICAL DISTRIBUTION OF FEMALE GENITAL MUTILATION

Female genital mutilation is said to have been practiced worldwide at one time in history for various reasons, all related to women's sexuality. At present, its prevalence is largely observed in Africa. According to reports presented in different seminars, the practice exists in the following countries.

6.1. Excision (Clitoridectomy)

Benin, Burkina Faso, Cameroon, Central African Republic, Chad, Côte D'Ivoire, Djibouti, Egypt, Ethiopia, Gambia, Ghana, Guinea, Guinea-Bissau, Kenya, Liberia, Mali, Mauritania, Niger (small part of the country), Nigeria, Senegal, Sierra Leone, Sudan, Tanzania, Togo, Uganda, and Yemen.

6.2. Circumcision (*Sunnah*)

The above-mentioned countries plus Australia, Bahrain, parts of India, Indonesia, Malaysia, the United Arab Emirates, and Yemen.

6.3. Infibulation

Djibouti, Egypt (Nubians), Ethiopia, Mali (among a few ethnic groups), Somalia and Sudan.

6.4. Gishiri and Angurya Cuts

These are practiced only in Nigeria. Female genital mutilation is also reported to exist in Europe among the immigrant populations in England, Finland, France, Italy, Netherlands, Sweden, and the United States. The type of operation existing in these countries depends on the origin and cultural background of each immigrant family. It could vary from circumcision to infibulation (among Somalis, Sudanese, and Ethiopians). It was reported that some doctors in England (Harley Street) practice female genital mutilation under medical conditions.

In a few countries in Africa, all three forms of genital mutilation are practiced. Ethiopia is one such country. The extent of the mutilations practiced depend on the geographical location of the communities and of the degree of awareness among the population. In Djibouti, Somalia, and Sudan, a few of the educated families either excise or circumcise while the majority are infibulated.

7. PROGRESSIVE EFFORTS MADE TO ERADICATE FEMALE GENITAL MUTILATION

7.1. International and Regional Levels

7.1.1. World Health Organization (WHO). The first major step taken to deal with female genital mutilation was the 1979 Khartoum Seminar on Traditional Practices, organized by the World Health Organization Regional Office for the Eastern Mediterranean (EMRO). Representatives from ten countries — Burkina Faso, Djibouti, Egypt, Ethiopia, Kenya, Nigeria, Oman, Somalia, Sudan, South Yemen — attended the meeting.

One of the subjects discussed as a harmful traditional practice was female genital mutilation. The complications caused by female genital mutilation were noted, and recommendations were made for its progressive eradication. In general, the seminar proposed the establishment of a national commission to coordinate activities including legislation, intensification of general education, and sensitization of midwives and traditional birth attendants. The adoption of a clear-cut policy was also recommended.

In 1982, the World Health Organization issued a statement on its position regarding female genital mutilation (female circumcision). In this statement, female circumcision was recognized as having serious health consequences. The recommendations made at the Khartoum meeting were re-emphasized, and the World Health Organization expressed its readiness to support national efforts aimed at eradicating the practice. Strong advice was expressed to health workers not to perform female genital mutilation under any circumstances.

WHO/EMRO adopted a resolution at its 35th session, stating that women's health must be safeguarded by ensuring the elimination of harmful traditional practices. In September 1989, the World Health Organization Regional Committee for Africa (AFRO) adopted unanimously a resolution recommending that concerned members adopt appropriate policies and strategies to eliminate female circumcision. The Director was asked to provide support and to report at the 40th session on the progress of work in this area.

In May 1992, at the World Health Organization Technical Discussion on Women, Health, and Development, the issue of female genital mutilation and other traditional practices was raised, and a proposal was made stating that more courageous steps must be taken by the national and international communities to eliminate mutilating practices.

At the Safe Motherhood Conference in Niamey, February 1989, organized by the World Bank, United Nations Fund of Population Activities, World Health Organization, and the United Nations Children's Fund (UNICEF), a call for the eradication of harmful traditional practices was included in the final declaration.

The World Health Organization initiated and funded a research study on the influence of female genital mutilation on the choice of contraceptive methods, which was undertaken by the Inter-African Committee in Djibouti and Sierra Leone.

7.1.2. United Nations Children's Fund (UNICEF). UNICEF co-sponsored a Regional Seminar on Traditional Practices, held in Dakar in 1984. It provided financial, moral, and technical assistance to the Inter-African Committee and its national affiliates. It gave financial support for research on traditional practices undertaken in Burkina Faso, Chad, Ethiopia, Niger, and Sudan. It also financed activities, such as seminars and workshops in countries such as Benin, Ethiopia, Sierra Leone, and Uganda. The UNICEF Executive Board paper E/ICEF/1992/L.5 confirms the UNICEF policy regarding the genital mutilation of girl children.

7.1.3. United Nations (UN) and Non-Governmental Organization (NGO) Forum. The Copenhagen Conference on Women's Decade, held in 1980, brought the subject of female circumcision to international attention. At the Non-Governmental Organization Forum, held parallel to the Conference, concerned Western women discussed and condemned the practice of female genital mutilation as a barbaric custom. Africans regarded this interference as Western cultural imperialism and reacted to it negatively.

The actual Conference document on the revision and evaluation of progress achieved, document A/CONF.94/9, refers to the subject of female genital mutilation in the sub-heading, "Cultural practices affecting women's health."

The Second United Nations/Economic Commission for Africa (UN/ECA) Regional Conference on the Integration of Women, held at Lusaka (Zambia), 3–7 December 1979, condemned sexual mutilation, but called for a cautious approach to the international campaign. It called upon Africans to find suitable solutions to the problem.

7.1.4. United Nations, Human Rights, Other Conventions, and Legislation. Human rights are based upon the principles of equality and non-discrimination. These rights are articulated in several conventions such as the *United Nations Charter,* the *Universal Declaration of Human Rights*, the *International Covenant on Civil and Political Rights,* the *Convention on the Elimination of All Forms of Discrimination Against Women*, and the *Convention on the Rights of the Child.* Female genital mutilation violates basic human rights principles to health, life, freedom from cruel and/or degrading treatment, freedom from slavery and servile status, and freedom from discrimination.

The *Convention on the Rights of the Child*, Article 24.3, states: "The States Parties of the present convention shall seek to take all effective and appropriate measures with a view to abolishing traditional practices prejudicial to the health of children."

7.1.5. Female Genital Mutilation at the United Nations/Human Rights Center. The subject of female genital mutilation was introduced by non-governmental organizations to the Working Group on Slavery and Slavery-Like Practices in 1981. On 13 March 1984, the Commission on Human Rights, by its resolution 1984/48, recommended the setting up of a special Work Group of experts on traditional practices, and the Economic and Social Council (ECOSOC) endorsed the recommendation by its resolution 1984/34, May 24, 1984. The members of the Working Group assigned as experts were Mrs. Halima Embarek Warzazi of Morocco and Mrs. Murlidhara Bandari of India. Mrs. Wassila Tamzali of the United Nations Educational, Scientific, and Cultural Organization (UNESCO), Mrs. Marjorie Newman-Black of UNICEF, and Mr. Robert Cook of the World Health Organization were invited to join the Group and provide their expertise.

The Non-Governmental Organization Working Group held its first session 18–25 March 1985, in the presence of several non-government organizations, to study the practice of female genital mutilation, the preference of the male child, and traditional birthing practices. Female genital mutilation was considered a priority, and it was dealt with from socio-cultural, medical, and human rights aspects.

The conclusion reached was that female genital mutilation is a complex problem that has an evolutionary aspect. The Group called on governments to adopt policies and legislative measures for its eradication. It also recommended educational measures to be undertaken and requested governments to support local efforts being made by individuals and organizations. It recommended the organization of international, regional, and national meetings for the exchange of information. The report of the Working Group, document E/CN.4/1986/42, was presented to the United Nations Commission on Human Rights at its 42nd session.

The Commission, by its resolution E/CN.4/1986, requested the relevant specialized agencies of the United Nations system and interested non-governmental organizations to provide assistance to the governments in their efforts to fight harmful traditional practices.

For the purpose of a follow-up, Mrs. Halima Warzazi of Morocco was appointed as a rapporteur to study the situation of traditional practices and report back to the Sub-Commission at its 43rd session in August 1991.

A Regional Seminar on Traditional Practices was organized by the United Nations Human Rights Center in Ouagadougou (Burkina Faso), 29 April to 3 May 1991. Another Regional Seminar was organized for Asia, from 4 to 8 July 1994, in Sri Lanka. The recommendations made at these two seminars formed the basis for a plan of action drawn by the Special Rapporteur to be adopted by the Sub-Commission on Prevention of Discrimination and Protection of Minorities.

7.2. National and Regional Instruments

7.2.1. Sudan. In 1946, the British government, then in power in the Sudan, legislated against infibulation. Since this action was considered as another colonial imposition, the practice went underground and continued to be performed, thus creating a worse situation. Complications such as infections and hemorrhage resulting from the infibulation could not be reported for fear of legal repercussions.

7.2.2. Egypt. In 1959, an order by the Ministry of Health was issued prohibiting female circumcision in government hospitals and health centers. In spite of this order, the practice continued both in and outside health centers.

7.2.3. Europe. France, Great Britain and Sweden have laws prohibiting female genital mutilation. The British and Swedish legislation regarding female genital mutilation are clear about the prohibitions of the practice. The French Penal Code, Article 312, stipulates that a person who has committed an act of violence involving mutilation or resulting in death — even without the intention of doing so — is still liable to criminal proceedings. As a result of this law, African mothers have been prosecuted for having circumcised their daughters.

Article 18.3 of the African Charter on Human and People's Rights reads:

- The State shall ensure the elimination of every discrimination against women and also ensure the protection of the rights of the woman and the child as stipulated in international declarations and conventions.

7.2.4. The African Charter on the Rights and Welfare of the Child. This document protects children from harmful traditional practices.

7.2.5. The Abuja Declaration. The United Nations Economic Commission for Africa organized a conference in Abuja (Nigeria) in November 1989 to review the "Role of Women in Africa in the 1990s." Among other issues, traditional practices such as early marriage and pregnancy, female circumcision, and nutritional taboos were discussed and proposals for action were made. The proposal calls for research, training, dissemination of information, and legislation to eradicate harmful traditional practices. The setting up of regional and sub-regional structures was also recommended for the follow-up.

7.3. Statements of Leaders and Policy Makers. President Jomo Kenyatta of Kenya supported the preservation of culture as a defense for one's identity against colonial aggression. In his book, *Facing Mount Kenya,* he supports the initiation ritual of circumcision. In 1990, his successor, President Arap Moi, issued a ban on the practice, stating that such customs do not belong to modern times.

President Thomas Sankara of Burkina Faso also denounced the practice of female genital mutilation on 20 December 1983, stating:

> It also shows an attempt to confer an inferior status on women by branding them with this mark which diminishes them and is a constant reminder to them that they are only women, inferior to men, that they do not even have any rights over their own bodies or to fulfillment, either bodily or personal.[9]

President Abou Diouf of Senegal stated:

> These practices, however, raise a problem today because our societies are in a process of major transformation and are coming up against new socio-cultural dynamic forces in which such practices have no place or appear to be relics of the past: What is therefore needed are measures to quicken their demise.[10]

At the United Nations Seminar in 1991, the First Lady of Burkina Faso, Madame Chantal Compaoré, said:

> We in Africa still have some backward and unacceptable customs and traditions. One of the objectives of the August Revolution in Burkina Faso was to combat all the social and cultural impediments which are holding the country back. The practice of female circumcision is the most pernicious impediment to the psychological and physical flowering of women and children.[11]

The International Conference on Assistance to African Children, held in November 1992 in Dakar (Senegal), treated the issue of female genital mutilation as a threat to African children. The final document, adopted as the "Consensus of Dakar," Paragraph 28, reads:

> Furthermore, we commit ourselves to ensure the protection of the female child from all forms of harmful traditional practices and in particular to the elimination of such practices as female genital mutilation, and early and forced marriages.

Recently, female genital mutilation has gained prominence in various international conferences. The World Conference on Human Rights, held in June 1993 in Vienna, condemned gender-based violence and accepted the principle that women's rights are human rights and, as such, should be respected fully, regardless of cultural diversity or economic disparity. The indivisibility and non-selectivity of the principles of human rights prohibits the violation of human rights on the basis of culture or religion.

The International Conference on Population and Development, and its program of action, condemns the practices of female genital mutilation and early marriage, along with other harmful traditional practices, and several measures are proposed to governments and non-governmental organizations to work toward their elimination.

The World Summit for Social Development, held in Copenhagen in 1995, reaffirmed the call for the elimination of violence against women, including female genital mutilation.

The Fourth World Conference on Women, held in Beijing in September 1995, witnessed the international awareness about violence against women, in general, and female genital mutilation, in particular. Several statements by high-level officials, including the

Secretary-General of the United Nations and delegates, called for the elimination of female genital mutilation as a gender-based violence.

8. CONCRETE ACTIONS TO STOP THE PRACTICE

The campaign against female genital mutilation was initiated by committed and convinced individuals who considered the practice of female genital mutilation to be a health hazard and a violation of the human rights of women.

Gradually, as more and more public awareness developed, organizations were formed with the aim of eradicating female genital mutilation. In 1977, the Non-Governmental Organization Working Group on Traditional Practices was set up in Geneva with a membership of international organizations enjoying consultative status with the United Nations Economic and Social Council. The Coordinator of the Group and a representative were assigned to undertake missions to several African countries to study the extent of the problem and to begin dialogues with nationals on the best approach to adopt in handling the problem. The various visits and meetings resulted in building collaborative efforts. The Working Group initiated educational activities in Burkina Faso, Egypt, Kenya, Mali, and Sudan, and raised funds for such local initiatives.

A vital role of the Group has been lobbying at the various relevant meetings, such as the World Health Assembly, the UNICEF Board meetings, the sessions of the Commission on Human Rights, and the Commission on the Status of Women. Members of the Group made statements, submitted communiqués and appealed to governments to take action. Briefing sessions with African delegates were held during the World Health Organization Assembly in 1983 and 1984 at the request of members of the Working Group. Members of the Group took an active part during the two sessions of the United Nations Working Group on Traditional Practices held in 1986. They advocated the appointment of a Special Rapporteur on traditional practices, and, at present, they work closely with this Special Rapporteur, Mrs. Halima Embarek Warzazi.

During the drafting of the *Convention on the Rights of the Child*, it was the non-governmental organizations that lobbied for the inclusion of Article 24.3, calling upon the States Parties to protect children from practices prejudicial to their health.

In 1984, the Working Group, in collaboration with the Government of Senegal, the World Health Organization, United Nations Fund for Population Activities, and UNICEF, organized a Regional Seminar in Dakar, to which twenty African countries sent representatives to examine the issues of female genital mutilation, early marriage, nutritional taboos, and practices related to childbirth. A unanimous agreement was reached to eradicate harmful traditional practices and to follow this decision by establishing the Inter-African Committee on Traditional Practices Affecting the Health of Women and Children.

The Working Group continues its campaign against female genital mutilation through advocacy and fundraising. The World Health Organization and UNICEF participate in its activities with an observer status.

9. INTER-AFRICAN COMMITTEE (IAC)

The Inter-African Committee is a regional body set up in 1984 with the following mandate:

- To reduce the morbidity and mortality rates of women and children through the eradication of harmful traditional practices. To promote traditional practices which are beneficial to the health of women and children.
- To play an advocacy role, by raising the importance of taking action against harmful traditional practices at international, regional and national levels.
- To raise funds and support local activities of national committees and other partners.

Since its creation, the Inter-African Committee has set up national committees in the following 26 countries: Benin, Burkina Faso, Cameroon, Chad, Congo, Côte D'Ivoire, Djibouti, Egypt, Ethiopia, Gambia, Ghana, Guinea, Guinea-Bissau, Kenya, Liberia, Mali, Mauritania, Niger, Nigeria, Senegal, Sierra Leone, Somalia, Sudan, Tanzania, Togo, and Uganda.

The main focus of its activities are:

9.1. Training and Information Campaign (TIC)

Training and Information Campaign workshops are aimed at providing intensive and meaningful health education with the help of visual aids. The subjects discussed are related to female genital mutilation, early childhood marriage, human reproduction, pregnancy, childbirth, breastfeeding, and hygiene, as well as to nutritional taboos.

The program consists of four sets of training workshops, to be conducted consecutively in five months. After each Training and Information Campaign program, 28 persons will have been trained to be able to conduct sensitization programs on the harmful effects of female genital mutilation and other traditional practices, and an additional 136 persons will have attended workshops to spread information regarding the issues.

9.2. Training of Traditional Birth Attendants

As traditional birth attendants can play an important role in the campaign against harmful traditional practices, it is necessary to provide them with an effective training program and to encourage them to campaign for the abolition of female genital mutilation and other such practices.

For the Inter-African Committee, the aim of the traditional birth attendants training is, first to train head trainers for a short period, and to ensure that the required information pertaining to the practice is transmitted to other traditional birth attendants working in rural areas and mothers in the communities. A head trainer gives a one-day training for future trainers. Each will, in turn, train fifty traditional birth attendants in rural areas, thus creating a multiplying effect. When each traditional birth attendant program is completed, fifty traditional birth attendants will have been trained to play a key role in rural areas in the campaign against female genital mutilation and other harmful traditional practices.

9.3. Alternative Employment Opportunities

Practitioners or circumcisers are highly respected individuals whose skills are indispensable to the community. Their service is paid for in cash or in kind and they enjoy special social status in the community. The campaign against female genital mutilation has to include changing the attitudes of practitioners and finding them alternative sources of income for their livelihood.

The Inter-African Committee runs two Alternative Employment Opportunities projects for circumcisers, one in Ethiopia and another in Sierra Leone. In both projects, a selected number of women have identified income-generating activities such as baking (Ethiopia) and dyeing (Sierra Leone), and are working in groups to run their projects. Members of these groups have abandoned the practice of female genital mutilation and other harmful traditional practices. They are used as agents of change within the communities.

Such projects have to be designed and implemented in order to convince practitioners to give up some of their old habits and practices, and to provide beneficial services.

9.4. Research

The Inter-African Committee conducts research in the area of traditional practices, particularly female genital mutilation. Several research papers are produced showing the extent of the problem. These documents are valuable, particularly for designing strategies for intervention.

9.5. Production of Education Materials

The Inter-African Committee produces and distributes a number of educational materials to be used in the different programs of education and information.

9.5.1. Anatomical Model. An anatomical model of the lower part of the female body with seven removable parts showing (a) the normal state of the female genital organs, (b) the result of *sunnah*, (c) the result of excision, (d) the result of infibulation, (e) keloid formation, (f) normal delivery, and (g) delivery of an infibulated or severely excised woman.

9.5.2. Flannelgraphs. A set of five folders contain schematic designs to be stuck on a piece of flannel for group teaching based on a small diagram contained in each folder. The series is comprised of (a) the female genital organs, (b) fertilization, (c) pregnancy, (d) birth, (e) complications during childbirth, and (f) a consideration of female genital mutilation.

9.5.3. Simple Viewer with a Set of Slides. The slides are shown in connection with the flannelgraphs, and are made from realistic designs that demonstrate (a) infibulation, (b) keloid formation, (c) incision at delivery, (d) delivery by pulling out the child, and (e) a child injured at birth.

9.5.4. Multi-Media Training Modules and Materials. The training modules and materials are targeted to reach four major groups: (a) women in influential positions and those participating in activities of women's organizations, (b) secondary school students and youth groups, both male and female, (c) teachers, religious and community leaders, and (d) paramedical staff. The modules include transparencies, slides, cassettes and stories with pictures.

9.5.5. The Inter-African Committee Video (Beliefs and Misbeliefs). Beliefs and Misbeliefs, a 43-minute video, which explains the dangers of female genital mutilation, and shows the activities of the Inter-African Committee in Africa. The film is available in English and French.

9.5.6. The Inter-African Committee Newsletter. The newsletter of the Inter-African Committee is published twice a year in English and French and is widely distributed.

9.5.7. The Inter-African Committee Information Leaflet. The *Inter-African Committee Information Leaflet* of the Inter-African Committee is available in English and French.

The Inter-African Committee organizes international and regional conferences to examine the problem, to determine new strategies, and to formulate activity plans. Such a conference was held from April 11–15, 1994, for the purpose of evaluating a decade of Inter-African Committee activities. Representatives of 24 countries participated and the First Ladies of Burkina Faso, Ghana and Guinea graced the conference with their presence. The full report of this conference is available from the Inter-African Committee.

9.6. Inter-African Committee /United Nations High Commissioner for Refugees Joint Project

A joint project between the Inter-African Committee National Committee in Ethiopia (NCTPE) and the United Nations High Commissioner for Refugees (UNHCR) among refugees and indigenous Somali displaced persons in the Jijiga refugee camp has been in progress since 1993.

The Somalis are known for practicing the worst form of female genital mutilation — infibulation — and the purpose of this project should be seen in the light of one more effort to minimize and ultimately eradicate this harmful traditional practice. In addition, the project promotes beneficial traditional practices such as breastfeeding and improved child care.

The strategy used is to sensitize the socially-influential target groups by means of short-term training and seminars. The beneficiaries of the project are traditional birth attendants and opinion leaders, in addition to the refugee/returnee communities in the different camps within the Jijiga area. An estimated two hundred opinion leaders in nine of the camps could be reached in this process. In addition, an estimated fourteen participants benefited from a seminar on the hazards of female genital mutilation that was held for non-government organization representatives.

9.7. Advocacy

The advocacy of the Inter-African Committee, in cooperation with other non-government organizations, is showing gradual progress.

At the United Nations level, the appointment of a special rapporteur on traditional practices is an outcome of this lobbying. The fact that the Inter-African Committee has an official relationship with the United Nations, Organization of African Unity, and the World Health Organization allows its voice to be heard on behalf of African women and children who are the victims of prejudicial treatment.

At the national level, the national committees in Djibouti, Ethiopia, Ghana and Nigeria have succeeded in impacting policy changes by including articles that prohibit harmful traditional practices. This is a welcome sign.

The Inter-African Committee and its national committees are making efforts to free women and children from socially-sanctioned violence, such as female genital mutilation. These efforts alone could not have produced results if it were not for the collaboration of other organizations and concerned individuals.

10. PROPOSALS

Despite the widespread violence against women, particularly in relation to culture and misinterpretations of religion, women themselves have to be empowered through information and education to protect their human rights. In this domain, the following proposals are made:

- Educate women through various means to value themselves and to develop self-esteem.
- Explain and clarify misconceptions about religion.
- Disseminate information about the functions of the female body and project positive images about the reproductive role of women.
- Educate the community about the contribution of women towards the development of the community and the nation.
- Give value to the image of the girl child through education, including religious teachings.
- Adopt legislation which will allow women to inherit property, including land, in order to allow them to be economically self-sufficient.
- Adopt measures to abolish practices such as female genital mutilation.
- Conduct research to collect gender-desegregated data.
- Coordinate efforts with concerned organizations, international, national, and government institutions to integrate activities related to abolishing violence against women in their plans and programs of work.

11. REFERENCES

1. Dr. Mahdi Alie Dirie. Female Circumcision in Somalia: Medical and Social Implications, 1986:21–22.
2. Dr. M. Karim, Egypt. Circumcisions and Mutilations: Male and Female. 1992.
3. Inter-African Committee. Report on Regional Conference, Addis Ababa. 1990:59–60.
4. Inter-African Committee. Report on mission to Guinea-Bissau. September 1988.
5. Dr. Mahdi Ali Dirie. Female Circumcision in Somalia: Medical and Social Implications. 1986.87.
6. Inter-African Committee. Report on Seminar on Traditional Practices, Dakar, Senegal. 1984:5658.
7. Dr. Olayinka Koso-Thomas. The Circumcision of Women: A Strategy for Eradication. 1987:23.
8. EMRO Technical Publication No. 2 on Traditional Practices Affecting the Health of Women and Children: p. 43.
9. UN Document E/CN.4/1986/42.
10. UN Document E/CN.4/1986/42.
11. UN Document E/CN.4/Sub.2/1991/48.

14

EPIDEMIOLOGICAL SURVEYS ON FEMALE GENITAL MUTILATION IN ITALY

Pia Grassivaro Gallo, Franco Viviani, M. Livio, R. Corsaro, F. De Cordova, G. Fortunato, S. Beccacini, and Sirad Salad Hassan

A work group was set up at the Department of General Psychology at the University of Padua, coordinated by Professor Pia Grassivaro Gallo, which brought together several Italian scholars interested in studying female genital mutilation practices in Italy.

The group has been working since 1988 in response to the impact of immigration from areas where female genital mutilation is practiced, and, in particular, in response to a press campaign stimulated by statements attributed to the Ministry of Health that indicated that female sexual mutilation was being practiced in Italian public health units. At present, the work group has conducted several extensive investigations into the problem of female sexual mutilation in immigrant communities in Italy, the results of which are described below.

1. FEMALE SEXUAL MUTILATION IN ITALY

In 1988, the work group investigated the position of the Italian government regarding female genital mutilation. The resulting studies, *Italy faces problem of female genital mutilation by African immigrants,*[1] *Les mutilations genitales feminines des Africains en Italie,*[2] published in 1991 and 1992, respectively, were conducted to investigate the suspicion that female genital mutilation was taking place in Italian health units. This suspicion was first raised by the press and denied by the government during the winter of 1988. The government stated: "... there are no ethnic groups in Italy who would ask for such operations."

A study of the presence of African migrants in Italy at the time, and interviews with Italian and African health professionals at reception and support centers and with families and young people coming from countries with a tradition of excision and infibulation confirmed the hypothesis of the existence of "risk factors" for female sexual mutilation.

We have not found objective proof of female sexual mutilation being performed in Italian hospitals, but the staff interviewed admitted that they were accustomed to dealing with the post-operative consequences of female genital mutilation and that the number of mutilated women in the obstetric wards of Italian hospitals was steadily growing.

Qualitatively significant aspects of the African presence in Italy (interethnic solidarity, reuniting relatives) suggested the possibility of a covert practice of female sexual mutilation. According to health-care professionals in touch with African immigrant communities, the mutilations were already likely to be performed in Italy. Some members of the African communities themselves admitted to the practice of sending little girls home to be excised or infibulated. This practice seemed to be common among Egyptians and Somali immigrants.

2. ITALIAN MEDICAL PERSPECTIVES

In 1995, the work group published a study, *An epidemiological survey of obstetricians and gynecologists who encounter the problem of excision in African immigrants in Italy,*[3] based on interviews with 318 Italian obstetricians and gynecologists who, attending two national congresses and who were actively working in the health departments of various Italian regions, permitted us to create a map of female sexual mutilation in Italy. Female sexual mutilation was found to be present throughout Italy. It was found to a lesser degree in the northern border regions, in some central areas (Basilicata and Molise), and in the main islands.

Forty-six percent of the health-care professionals interviewed had experience with mutilated females. The problem appears to be more serious in Italy than in any other European countries studied. The problem of female sexual mutilation has intensified since 1990. It was also difficult to estimate the number of mutilated women living in Italy at the time. Some of the physicians had examined hundreds of women, most of whom came from the Horn of Africa. An estimate of the number of excised African women living in Italy suggests that there are at least 27,000 mutilated women living in Italy (data from the Ministry of Interior, January 1, 1994).

In general, patients required health care as a result of the consequences of the operation they had undergone; very few of the women requested circumcision in its various forms (defibulation, refibulation, excision, etc.) From this, it can be inferred that a substantial underground market exists in order to meet the demand for these surgeries.

The worrying presence of small girls, even two-year-old babies, suffering from the immediate consequences of mutilation, indicating that female sexual mutilation is carried out in Italy and with sometimes "perfect" surgical techniques, leads us to ask whether female sexual mutilation is being carried out in public health units.

In contrast to other European countries, Italy is unique for the type of health-care professional that mutilated women seek out when in trouble. Generally, they choose public health units (such as in Rome or Milan) known to specialize in the care of non-Europeans or who have on their staff physicians who have experience in developing nations or physicians of bi-racial, Italian/African background, familiar with female sexual mutilation.

A synthesis of these results was presented at the International Symposium on Female Genital Mutilation, held in Padua in 1994. Its aim was to discuss female sexual mutilation occurring in Europe in order to formulate a common policy regarding this problem.

The work group feels that the problem of female sexual mutilation should first of all be understood and scientifically examined. This cognitive approach is the most productive one at present. A hostile attitude would certainly not be constructive.

In the course of deeper investigations, we looked into the condition of the mutilated African women living in Italy. Some psychology students at Padua University who were writing their graduation thesis on developing nations helped to carry out these field surveys.

3. CULTURAL PARADOXES

In 1994 and 1995, the following two surveys were conducted. First, we reexamined the data of the first study on the experience of Italian obstetricians and gynecologists. Second, we completed the African perspective with interviews with Somali immigrant women and created a bibliography of the different areas where female sexual mutilation is performed.

Our study, *Female Genital Mutilation: An Analysis of the Cultural Paradox,*[4] conducted in 1994 and 1995, examined the possibility of identifying interethnic ethics to help understand and solve the differences between Western and African cultures.

We compared the opinions about female sexual mutilation described according to Somali, Sudanese, and Senegalese cultures with the opinions of Italian obstetricians. The data was collected from questionnaires and interviews conducted at national Italian congresses in 1993. The results of this study show that two different points of view about the tradition of female sexual mutilation appear to coexist.

The different approaches to the subject that can be adopted, according to the Western or the African perspective, represent a cultural paradox. The paradox comprises seven areas of difference: operation; sanitary aspect; pedagogical role of the doctor; linguistic connotation about the practice; mutilated patient's body perception; legal regulation; and social aspect and cultural connotation of female sexual mutilation.

4. CONFLICTS BETWEEN AFRICAN WOMEN AND ITALIAN DOCTORS

Our study, *The Therapeutic Relation Between the Italian Gynecologist and the Excised Patient,*[5] represents an in-depth analysis of excised women according to a point of view that favors the Italian health-care professional. For the latter, female sexual mutilation is a preoccupying phenomenon in terms of social implications, technical difficulties, lack of understanding of the cultural aspects, and absence of specific legislation.

The Italian obstetrician and the excised woman focus on the negative aspect of the therapeutical relationship and on the general lack of appropriate professional training. Both expressed the desire that this problem be solved. Only the doctor was responsible for the resulting relationship with the excised woman. The cultural mediator or the relatives of the woman do not completely accomplish the objective.

Disagreement between the obstetrician and the mutilated patient occurs over the preference for the gender of the health-care professional. While the African patient, for cultural and traditional reasons, seems to prefer a female doctor, Italian female doctors feel more uncomfortable than their male colleagues. They may be more emotionally involved when confronted with this uniquely female problem.

5. DEFIBULATION

In *Defibulation: a biological test useful to evaluate the integration of sexually mutilated women in Western countries,*[6] we attempted to determine when and why African women come to choose to be defibulated. Preliminary results were obtained from interviews with 43 Somali women; these demonstrate that immigrants rarely practice defibulation without a medical motivation. Defibulation may be performed:

- For health related problems; this is the most common reason.
- Between the wedding and its consummation: this is done to avoid the instrumental opening of the scar, an event that terrorizes both the woman and her partner.
- During delivery: In Italy, the mutilated woman usually remains open.

Other than these cases, defibulation is rare. We have known only five young women who became well-known in their communities for having undergone defibulation. Three live in immigrant communities in Padua, Brescia, and Florence, and the other two live in America and in Switzerland. These appear to be "outsiders," who are not in conformity with the average Somali woman. Their degree of literacy is very high; they are very independent; they usually work for a living in the foreign country; they have peculiar families that often accept their choice; they do not care about the negative social consequences of their decision since they will carefully select their future husband. Even after years, they are glad to have chosen to be defibulated. Apparently they are not banished from the Somali community in Italy. It is not known whether these "open" women will be accepted in Somalia.

6. RISK FACTORS FOR EXCISION

Our 1996 study, *Female Genital Mutilation in Evolutive Age in Italy (Preliminary Report),*[7] documented the presence of young immigrant girls in Italy whose cultural background placed them at risk for excision. As in our 1993 study, 46% of Italian obstetricians interviewed had treated sexually mutilated African patients. Eighteen of the 157 health-care professionals had cared for 271 mutilated women. Of these, 42 patients were young girls (2 to 16 years of age). These young patients were originally from East Africa, and now residing in different Italian regions, including Sicily. A single case of female genital mutilation was found in a young Italian girl from La Spezia (Liguria).

Additional information on the impact of the practice of female sexual mutilation in Italy was gathered from two patients treated for the immediate consequences of infibulation at two hospitals (Padua and Milan). Both girls had been operated on in Italy by competent personnel using surgical techniques that could only be found in a professional health care setting.

Other cases in Florence were referred to health units for the treatment of minor complications; another girl was treated in Rome for psychological trauma and advanced state of agitation.

From the above cases, the following determinations can be made:

- At least two African girls have been mutilated in medical settings in Italy;
- Some girls are operated on at home (in Florence and Trieste) and also on the Somali Refugee Transit Camps in Aprilia-Roma, by traditional birth attendants;
- Six girls belonging to two Somali families living in Florence were sent to Djibouti and Kenya, respectively, to be infibulated.

7. REFERENCES

1. Grassivaro Gallo P, Livio M. Italy faces problem of excision by African immigrants. Win News 1991;17:37.
2. Grassivaro Gallo P, Livio M. Les mutilations feminines des Africans en Italie. Rivista di Antropologia, 1992;70:175–83.
3. Grassivaro Gallo P, Livio M, Viviani, F. Survey on Italian obstetricians and gynaecologists: FGM in African immigrants, in: FGM: a Public Health Issue Also in Italy. Padova: Unipress, 1995:11–12.
4. Grassivaro Gallo P, De Cordova F. Analisi di un paradosso culturale: le MGF. Tesi di Laurea in Psicologia, AA. 1994/95, Universite di Padova.
5. Grassivaro Gallo P, Fortunato G. L'ostetrico italiano e la paziente escissa. Tesi di Laurea in Psicologia, AA. 1994/95, Universite di Padova.
6. Grassivaro Gallo P, Beccacini S. La defibulazione: un test biologico per valutare l'integrazione della immigrata infibulata. Tesi di laurea in Psicologia, Universite di Padova, (in press).
7. Grassivaro Gallo P. Sirad Salad Hassan. FGM in ete evolutiva presenti in Italia. 1er. Congres Europeen de Psychopatologie de l'Enfant et de l'Adolescent . Venise, Octobre, 1996.

15

FEMALE GENITAL MUTILATION IN GERMANY

An Update from (I)NTACT

Christa Müller

Before 1995, the subject of female genital mutilation was largely unknown in Germany. Other than a few articles in women's magazines, the German press did not report on this subject. There are several reasons for this silence. Female genital mutilation concerns women and, as such, is of minor importance to German society as a whole. Female genital mutilation is also primarily an African problem, and Africa is quite distant from Germany. Female genital mutilation is a subject that necessarily relates to sexuality, and the social taboos about such issues remain quite strong, even in Germany. Finally, journal editors have repeatedly justified their refusal to report on female genital mutilation because the subject is not topical, as it has been practiced for thousands of years.

Similarly, the scientific and academic communities, including ethnologists, have paid little attention to the subject of female genital mutilation. As recently as the early 1990s, many female students had to battle with their professors if they wanted to write a seminar paper or Masters thesis on female genital mutilation or a related topic. They did not always succeed. Consequently, there is very little German literature dealing directly with female genital mutilation.

The ignorance of female genital mutilation as a human rights issue may stem from the fact that the various human rights and major aid organizations in Germany had long excluded the issue of female genital mutilation from their work because they did not wish to interfere with the culture, religions and traditions of other nations. This view has now changed, or is currently changing. Whether at UNICEF, Terre des Femmes, or Amnesty International, female genital mutilation is becoming an increasingly important issue. The human rights violation of female genital mutilation became known to a large part of the German population for the first time in 1995 as a result of media reports from the World Conference on Women in Beijing.

Sexual Mutilations: A Human Tragedy, edited by Denniston and Milos
Plenum Press, New York, 1997

1. THE FOUNDING OF (I)NTACT

While on a state visit to Benin in western Africa in early 1995, the wife of the then president, Mrs. Vieyra-Soglo, requested that I meet her. As the president of a leading women's organization in Benin, she informed me about the spread of female genital mutilation in the northern part of her country. She requested financial and organizational support for an education and information campaign her organization was conducting.

In the first few months of my involvement, I attempted to tell as many people as possible about female genital mutilation and to collect donations to support the women in Benin. In only a few months, 80,000 German Marks were raised, and this sum will be supplemented with public funds.

Recognizing that female genital mutilation is also practiced in other countries, and that the women there need assistance as well, the organization, Internationale Aktion Gegen die Beschneidung von Mädchen und Frauen (International Action Against the Circumcision of Girls and Women), otherwise known as (I)NTACT, was founded in January 1996. (I)NTACT is an association whose purpose is to fight against forced female genital mutilation. (I)NTACT's activities focus primarily on raising money in Germany, which is then made available to African organizations for their work in the fight against female genital mutilation. Donations totalling more than 100,000 German Marks have been collected to date, and some of this money has already been sent to Africa. The campaign for donations will be stepped up over the next few months. (I)NTACT will not itself implement any campaigns or measures in African countries. The association will, however, respond to queries and offer self-help support, and is open for inquiries from African organizations in need of support.

2. POLITICAL ACTION

(I)NTACT's involvement is chiefly directed towards African countries; however, simply providing financial support for African organizations is not sufficient to fight the tradition effectively. Action is needed at the political level as well.

In its dealings with the African countries concerned, the German Federal Government has so far refrained from taking a specific stand on female genital mutilation but instead has spoken out generally against human rights violations and violence towards women. To date, there has been no government financing of education projects to combat female genital mutilation. In response to a query, however, the Federal Ministry for Economic Cooperation has declared its willingness to support such projects by non-governmental organizations in the future.

Together with members of parliament, (I)NTACT is attempting to move the Federal Government to take a clear position towards African nations, condemning female genital mutilation as a human rights violation, and to make financial aid for development increasingly contingent on improvements in the circumstances of women, and specifically on fighting female genital mutilation.

3. FEMALE GENITAL MUTILATION IN GERMANY

(I)NTACT has come to an agreement with Terre des Femmes — an organization concerned with female genital mutilation in Germany — to concentrate its activities in Africa; however, now that (I)NTACT is confronted with daily queries from Germany, we are under increasing pressure to address the situation in Germany as well.

There are no reliable figures for the number of women living in Germany who are affected by female genital mutilation. Projections (based on the number of female immigrants from each country and the percentage of women affected by female genital mutilation in that country) suggest that approximately 20,000 immigrant women who have been genitally mutilated live in Germany.

Although there are reports that the genital mutilation of girls does take place in Germany, no case has yet been proved. It is known, however, that daughters of African immigrants are taken to their home countries during the summer vacation and return circumcised.

As the German legal system has not been confronted with any cases of female genital mutilation in practice to date, there is not yet a specific law prohibiting female genital mutilation. It is, however, prohibited under the existing legislation on bodily harm and child abuse. It is a criminal offence both for anyone to perform such an operation and for parents to allow or cause it to be performed.

(I)NTACT expects that proven cases of female genital mutilation in Germany will become public in the next few months. (I)NTACT will do all it can to ensure that such cases come to light. A separate law banning female genital mutilation is needed for such cases, primarily, because the legislative process would sensitize doctors and judges — who have barely touched upon the issue in the past — to respond appropriately in practice.

Doctors are becoming aware of the severity of the surgery and refraining from performing it on ethical and medical grounds. Judges are also imposing severe penalties on those who perform the surgery. They are no longer maintaining that the law should not interfere with harmful cultural or religious practices.

There should also be a law which provides that girls under eighteen years of age living in Germany may not be taken to their home countries to be circumcised. Experience in other countries has shown that it is the long-term psychological consequences that are particularly severe for the girls and women concerned. Living in a Western culture, they will at some time realize that they have irretrievably lost something possessed by women in their adopted culture. Likewise, in the event of marriage or sexual relations with men of Western cultures, there may be added difficulties in the partnership due to sexual incompatibility caused by mutilated or missing sexual organs.

(I)NTACT will work at various levels to have the German Federal Parliament pass a law that prevents or, as the case may be, penalizes genital mutilation in Germany or in any other country of girls under eighteen who live in Germany (18 being the age of majority).

4. RIGHT OF ASYLUM

It is necessary to rethink the German legislation on asylum so that greater consideration is given to humanitarian questions in the asylum-granting process, especially in regard to the right of asylum or residence for women or their daughters who are at risk of mutilation on returning to their home countries. As female genital mutilation was relatively unknown until recently in Germany, the risk of mutilation was not seen as a reason not to send women or children back to their home countries. In one case, this went so far that lawyers and judges initially declared a German woman to be hysterical because she wished to refuse her Sudanese husband the right of access to her child for fear that the girl would be abducted and smuggled to the Sudan and subjected to genital mutilation.

We are currently dealing with the following case: In 1991, a young Sudanese woman gave birth to a daughter whose Sudanese father does not acknowledge paternity. A residence permit was granted to the mother and child until September 1996. This young woman's return to Sudan with an illegitimate child would mean social isolation and doubtless severe hardship as well, and her child would certainly be at risk of sexual mutilation. A petition is currently before the Rhineland-Pfalz State Parliament to obtain a right of residence for the Sudanese woman and her daughter. The fact that the young woman supports herself and her child by working may help towards the success of the petition.

Special medical care is needed for female immigrants who are sexually mutilated and live permanently in Germany. This care must take into account the physical and psychological consequences of their circumcision. In contrast to other western European countries where genitally mutilated women can go to special clinics for childbirth, health care for these women is deficient in Germany and urgently requires remedy.

5. CONCLUSIONS

The issue of female genital mutilation will gain importance in Germany over the next few years. The organization (I)NTACT is a very new movement that is only at the very beginning of its work. At the same time, the organization can already point to some successes. These lie only partly in attracting donations. It has been more important to inform large parts of the German population about this violation of human rights and to generate awareness. Only through education, in western cultures and in Africa, can the fight against female genital mutilation succeed.

16

REDEFINING THE SACRED

Miriam Pollack

Gathered here at the end of the Twentieth Century, we peer into the dawning of the coming millennium, fearful and hopeful of what the human journey will be. Pondering the same questions, Elie Weisel, holocaust survivor and internationally renowned writer, recently concluded a speech in San Francisco with a story about a man who had gotten lost deep in a forest.[1] Finally, another man appeared who was also lost and asked, "How do I find my way out of here?" The first man answered, "I don't know, just not the way you came in." Certainly, the Twentieth Century is not something we want to repeat. The question remains, "How do we get out of here?" In order to understand and commit ourselves to a new direction, we also need to have some notion of how we got lost. What needs to change if we are to not only survive together on this planet, but, indeed to flourish? The patterns of violence towards each other and towards this earth are too familiar: pollution, starvation, crime, and wars. We could enumerate these forces which threaten our biological and social survival for hours and argue for days which have greater priority.

In our Western habit of thought, we assume the necessity of hierarchical thinking. We tend to rank and prioritize everything, spending much energy in the process. An alternative approach is to focus on the whole rather than the parts, to ask what do all of these crises have in common. What is the connection between pollution and, say, circumcision? Do we have to choose which violence is greater, or can we understand that the question crying out from all of these crises is the same? The question is where is our reverence for life? Where is our reverence for life when we poison the very earth, water and air that sustains us, and where is our reverence for life when we welcome our beautiful babies into this world with a knife to their genital organs or visit this surprise upon them as older children?

An estimated 100 million women and girls have been genitally mutilated in Africa.[2] The number of boys and men who have experienced forced foreskin amputation is approximately 500 million.[3] In the United States today, the only country in the world where male circumcision is practiced by the medical establishment for non-religious or tribal reasons, 62.1% of all newborn males are circumcised.[4]

Female genital mutilation and male foreskin mutilation are quite different in scope and in consequence. Can we really speak about them in the same breath? Female genital mutilation destroys the clitoral hood; additionally, it usually includes the excision of the clitoris, often the external labia, and sometimes the inner labia as well. The remaining opening is stitched closed, leaving minimal room for the passage of menstrual blood. Before a woman's first sexual experience, she must be cut open by her husband and he is thus assured of her sexual "purity." This violent assault on the most tender parts of a girl's body inevitably produces long-lasting profound psychological scars and increases her risks for severe disease, infection and serious childbirth complications which put her life and her babies' lives in jeopardy. How can we compare such violence to male circumcision?

There are many of us who come from male circumcising traditions who are horrified by female genital circumcision and see no connection whatsoever to male circumcision. I understand this. I used to feel this way. As a Jew, I felt what **we** did was not damaging. It was *kosher*, ordained by G-d, by an ancient tradition, justified by thousands of generations of Jews persecuted for our identity, and what **they** did was primitive, barbaric, horrifying. For a long time, I felt oh-so-superior, but that very comfortable distance has eroded, however, as I have attempted to untangle the ancient skeins of thread which encase the sacrosanct ritual of *brit milah* in Judaism.

You might be wondering what a Jewish woman is doing speaking at a symposium on circumcision. There are Jews who will say and have said, "She couldn't be very connected to her Jewishness. She's just one more example of a sick, self-hating Jew." Non-Jews may ask, "If she's really Jewish, can she be serious about challenging male circumcision?" I am Jewish. I am not religiously observant in the orthodox sense of the word, but most of what has formed my values, my spiritual understanding and receptivity, such that it is, my sense of history, to say nothing of my sense of humor and predilection for certain foods is Jewish. I speak Hebrew with some fluency, feel very connected to Israel and have put much energy into creating a Jewish home for my children. I also spent over twenty years as a professional Jewish educator. Judaism is not peripheral to my life. It is and has always been central to my consciousness.

The focus of this presentation will be male circumcision. I will not be dwelling on female circumcision only because I cannot presume to speak about it from the authority of experience. That does not mean that I consider it less important or less worthy of our most urgent attention and support. If hierarchy of suffering were the primary organizing criterion of this conference, certainly female genital mutilation would have to come first. We are not, however, gathered here to engage in competitive suffering. Rather, we are here to be a witness to each others' pain, to hear each others' stories, to inform our hearts, above all. If we can do this together, we will begin the great task, which I believe is a sacred task, the task of cultural transformation. Spontaneously, this energy will flow out of Lausanne, gathering momentum and no one will be able to stop it, as long as we can keep listening to each other telling our own stories. I offer you mine.

When my boys were born, 18 and 14 years ago, I very carefully prepared for nonviolent home births. As it turned out, both of them were born by unnecessary Caesarean sections. Despite my weakened and traumatized state, I know that, had anyone entered my hospital room, announced that they had come to cut either of my babies anywhere on their bodies, I would have fought them with all the strength in my possession. I would have killed rather than let my babies be hurt, and, yet, less than two weeks after they were born, like a good Jewish woman, I was on the phone arranging for their ritual circumcisions, a celebration. The *brit milah* was the only way I knew for these boys to be welcomed and bonded to the people and faith that has carried and inspired me all of my life. What was the big deal? The foreskin was inconsequential and the babies' cries, they assured me, were insignificant.

But it was a big deal. I was utterly unprepared for the shrieks and cries of my babies. My second son cried as if he were being slaughtered. This continued for twenty minutes, a time beyond any notion of eternity. My heart froze. My milk stopped. All of my mother-knowing instincts cried out in grief, but it was too late. Something terribly wrong had happened to my babies, something I had implemented with the best of intentions and the worst kind of ignorance. Silently, I stewed about this for thirteen years. Silently, I listened to their screams, which have been permanently embedded in my bones, and, silently, I began asking why we Jews are encouraged to question, to question everything, even G-d, but are implicitly forbidden to question circumcision.

I began to question and I began to learn about the true function of the foreskin. At birth the foreskin is attached with *living* tissue to the glans, not scar tissue, as I had been led to understand. Why else would the glans of a newly circumcised infant look like raw meat? This delicate, highly sensitive organ must be cut, ripped and scraped from the head of the penis in order for it to be removed. For the many people who witness the shrieks, flailing head, and convulsed limbs of an infant being circumcised and, still, are incapable of understanding that this little being is in excruciating pain, it may be illuminating to know that medical research on infant circumcision by Anand and Hickey of Harvard Medical School and Children's Hospital has established that, not only is this child in pain, but that "hormonal, metabolic, and cardio-respiratory changes (are) similar to but greater than those observed in adult subjects." Furthermore, these researchers went on to observe that:

> Other responses in newborn infants are suggestive of integrated emotional and behavioral responses to pain and are retained in memory long enough to modify subsequent behavior patterns.[5]

Circumcision is a trauma of enormous magnitude for the infant. The implications for his emotional and personality development, his ability to trust, his ease with intimacy and sexuality later in life are quite serious, even if they cannot be quantified and centrifuged through scientific methodology. Certainly, this understanding alone should give us pause before we consent to a knife being taken to our children's genitals. But there is more.

The foreskin is not inconsequential. There are at least five very important functions which the foreskins serves. First, it shields the infant glans from contamination of urine and feces, and, throughout life, it maintains the glans as the internal organ it was intended to be. Secondly, without the foreskin, the sensitive mucous membrane of the glans becomes dried up and is keratinized, a process of unnatural thickening occurs, inevitably reducing sensitivity.[6] Thirdly, the foreskin stretches to cover the penis which increases by 50% in diameter and length upon erection.[7] Without this reserve of skin, the circumcised penis is pulled taut when erect, and sometimes is bowed, causing discomfort during erection or intercourse.[8] Fourthly, because the foreskin represents one-third or more of the most erogenous tissue of the penis, having a greater concentration of fully-developed, complex nerve endings than the glans, the pleasurable function of this delicate tissue is subtracted from this male's sexual experience.[9] Finally, the presence of the foreskin facilitates pleasurable intercourse by reducing friction between partners and enhancing the pleasure dynamic of the couple.[10] As in all other aspects of biology, altering form inevitably alters function.

The Hebrew people did not invent circumcision. It was a pre-Judaic rite existing at least as early as 3000 B.C. The ritual of male circumcision entered Judaism in ancient times and has remained a central element in Jewish faith and identity. For religious Jews, the command given in Genesis 17:9–14 is a sufficient expression of the will of G-d and the mandate to perpetuate it in this form is beyond question. In this section of the Torah, G-d gives to Abraham the injunction that circumcision shall be a sign of the covenant throughout all the generations of males, even the slaves of the household, for Abraham is about to father a new nation. Traditionally, circumcision is what connects the Jewish males to their contemporary community of Jewish men, as well as to their ancient lineage of Jewish forefathers and to the Jewish G-d whose voice is represented in the masculine gender.

The circumcision we practice today, however, is, in fact, quite different from the circumcision practiced by our Biblical ancestors. Prior to the time of Hellenic and later Roman influence, Jewish circumcision consisted of cutting off that part of the foreskin which extended beyond the glans leaving much of the foreskin intact. When some Jewish men desired to compete Greek style, nude, in the athletic competitions, they were roundly ridiculed for their mutilated penises. To the Greeks, exposing the glans was a sign of vulgarity, and cutting the body in order to please G-d was unthinkable. Emperor Hadrian outlawed circumcision as well as castration. Circumcision became a signal for persecution. Many Jews tried to hide their circumcision in order to assimilate into Greek culture or, later, to elude persecution by the Romans.

In order to prevent Jews from hiding their circumcision by various methods of stretching and tying their remaining foreskins, in about 140 C.E., the rabbis demanded that, in order for a circumcision to meet the standard of Jewish law, radical circumcision, or *periah* must be performed. *Periah* consists of the complete stripping and shearing of the foreskin.[11]

As the foreskin amputation became more radical, so too the function of circumcision within the Jewish community became radicalized. Circumcision was no longer simply, or, perhaps, not so simply, a religious rite, it became a tribal act of defiance to what was to become a millennia-long confrontation with oppressors and anti-Semites who attacked Jews, spiritually and physically, for no other crime than the crime of being Jewish. If the world defines being Jewish as criminal, or deviant, capitalist in the East or communist in the West, whatever the epithet, the Jewish response from Hellenic times to the present has been tenacious: to uphold Jewish identity at all costs. Thus, circumcision has become a *sine qua non* of Jewish spiritual survival. Whether we are religious or non-religious Jews, it is laminated to our psyches by generations upon generations of trauma. At this point, challenging circumcision is experienced as a frontal attack on Jewish survival.

Much as I admire the courage it took to defy the Jew-haters throughout the centuries, I question some of the reactive dynamics inherent in this response. While being under siege is hardly a time to reconfigure the foundational structures of one's identity, from the vantage point of a less threatened existence, we Jews may question whether it was more important to irreversibly mark and mutilate our Jewish sons, making them easy targets for oppressors, rather than risk their survival, perhaps at the price of assimilation, with an intact body. How many thousands of Jewish boys and how many thousands of Jewish men have been lost throughout the ages because they were unable to "pass" when their lives depended on it? Was this the sacred intention of the covenant?

Furthermore, if circumcision is equated with Jewish identity, we must wonder at all the circumcised Jewish males who are walking around with no particular connection to their Jewishness and we also must ask about the multitudes of Jewish women who have survived and kept their identities intact for millennia without any need of altering their bodies. Clearly, circumcision is serving functions far more subtle and more powerful than simply the physical and spiritual survival and identity of the people of Israel.

To an even more profound degree, circumcision is about gender and power.[12] The Biblical injunction to circumcise speaks to a man about men. But circumcision is also a woman's issue, for on a subtle but very potent level, circumcision is about the primary disempowerment of the mother. At no other time is a woman so in touch with her most elemental and powerful mammalian instincts as after a birth. If a woman's culture tells her that, in order for her new male baby to be a man, to be part of the masculine community and bond with the male G-d, the men must cut her male baby on his most sensitive male organ, this mother is inevitably in conflict with her entire life-giving feminine biology. When a woman is made to distrust her most elemental instinct to protect her newborn child, what feelings can she ever trust? If her primal need to defend her new baby at any cost is ridiculed or trivialized, how easy will it be for her to ever find her authentic feminine voice?

The ancient knife of circumcision is poised at the male organ of our male babies, but it is just as surely aimed with equal precision at the heart and soul of the mothers. Mother wounding and subordination is an inevitable, although rarely acknowledged, consequence of circumcision. From this vantage point, the message embedded in the ritual of circumcision becomes very clear: woman, you have very limited power over this male child; he belongs to the men.

The violent disruption of the maternal infant bond is not an accidental consequence of this ancient male bonding rite. It fits the pattern of a multitude of rituals that are prevalent cross-culturally in patriarchal societies which serve to disrupt the very delicate early hours and days of maternal infant bonding: tight restrictive swaddling, foot binding, early baptism in cold water, smoking of the newborn and mother, ear piercing within the first hour of birth, and more. Circumcision is one of the most violent of these rituals.[13]

When the mother is disempowered at the birth of her son, the relationship between husband and wife is artificially distorted, and that child's manhood is also transformed. Is it any wonder that, 18 years later, the mother is often forced to relinquish him again? She has been signaled from birth by the circle of men with the knife: "Woman, you cannot protect this male child." This drama is repeated by military conscription, the combative and violent initiation into manhood. Once again, the mother must suppress her natural protest as her male child is ushered by the men into a large circle of men, not with knives, but with weapons of immense destruction. In this sense, circumcision foreshadows conscription.

The subordination of the mother and the mother's deepest maternal instincts to protect her newborn are intrinsic elements of any circumcision tradition. In Judaism, however, the primacy of the mother is also a highly viable force. The survival of the matrilineal tradition and its ongoing power in the lives of our people is apparent when we look at *halachah*, Jewish law. According to Orthodox Jewish law the answer to the question of Jewish identity is quite basic: if one is born of a Jewish mother, one is a Jew. Circumcision, according to Savina Teubal in her book, *Sarah, the Priestess: The First Matriarch of Genesis*, arose to compete with matrilineal culture.[14] It permitted the transfer of inheritance through patrilineal descent, bonding the male child to the men of his community throughout time and space and to the male G-d.

A tragic contemporary story dramatically illustrates this tension. In the July 11, 1996, issue of the *Jerusalem Report*, journalist Ze'ev Chafets, in his article, "'I Did the Family a Favor,'" tells of the story of two-and-half-year old Dor Bohadanah.[15] Dor, his mother and brother were walking along a sidewalk in Sderot, Israel, when a car and truck collided, landing on the sidewalk. Dor's mother and brother were injured and little Dor was crushed to death in his stroller. In the midst of the funeral, as Dor's body was about to be lowered into his awaiting grave, Rabbi Bar Hen, a government official appeared. Blocking their way, he informed the grieving family and friends that, indeed Dor could not be buried in a Jewish cemetery because his mother, who came to Israel as a young girl from Romania, is not a Jew according to *halacha*, Jewish law. Dor had been born in Israel of Jewishly-identified parents, and ritually circumcised, but, because his mother was not a *halachically* kosher Jew, little Dor had to be buried *hoots la-gader*, outside the fence, alone in a place apart from his people. In Israel, civil matters regarding birth, death, and marriage are under the aegis of the Ministry of Religion, so there was no recourse for this decision. Circumcision was not sufficient to secure the identity and final resting place for this little Jew. Religious and tribal identity arguments are not sufficient to explain the function of circumcision in Judaism.

While I was still feeling secure in my cultural superiority vis-à-vis the female circumcising communities, I attended the Second International Symposium on Circumcision held in San Francisco in 1991. A video presentation of female circumcision was shown with full close-up color views and complete audio reproduction. It was easily one of the most viscerally wrenching experiences I have ever had. The entire audience of conference attendees sobbed and shook as we witnessed the shrieking, terrorized young girls having their clitorises cut off and often their labia incised and removed, and always in the presence of their mothers. With enormous indignation, I wanted to scream, "Where is your love for your daughter? Where is your primal need to protect your beloved child?" Suddenly, I understood: these mothers love their daughters just as we love our sons, and they, like we, are convinced that what is being done to their children is for their own good. The elemental instincts of protection of children pale before the greater forces of tribal belonging, connection to one's family, community and ancestors, their naming of holiness and the consensus of what makes one lovable. Physically, psychologically and sexually, female circumcision is far more devastating than male circumcision, and yet the socially, culturally, and religiously motivated forces which demand that a knife be ritually incised into a child's genitals are not so different.

We use the word "circumcision," but this is a euphemism. What we are really talking about for females as well as males is culturally and religiously sanctioned sexual mutilation and child abuse. I do not believe any parent consciously inflicts this trauma on her or his child. Our capacity to deny and rationalize, however, is limitless and, perhaps, psychically necessary, lest we open ourselves to the immense grief that inevitably follows the awakening to the profound injury we have caused to our most beloved treasures: our beautiful, perfect babies.

This treatment of the newborn is not consistent with traditional Jewish values. Judaism places infinite value on life, particularly human life. The principal of *pikuah nefesh* is fundamental to Judaism, that is, for the sake of saving a life, even the Sabbath may be desecrated. *Sh'mirat ha-guf*, the protection of one's body, is a high Biblical priority. Tattooing, cutting the flesh, and amputation are all forbidden. Consciousness of animal suffering permeates both Biblical and Talmudic thought as expressed by the concept *tsa-ar ba-alei hayim*, or compassion, for living things. In the Fourth Commandment, animals as well as humans are commanded to rest on the Sabbath and, according to the Talmud, Sabbath observance may be broken to ease the suffering of an animal. The laws of *kashrut* are specific and elaborate pertaining to permissible animal slaughter with the intention of reducing and regulating animal pain if we are to be a meat-eating people. The precept of *ba-a tashhit* also informs Biblical and Rabbinical thought. We are not to destroy the fruit trees, even during a war. The notions of *shmitah* and *yovel*, the Sabbatical and Jubilee years, require that every seventh year, and again in the fiftieth year, the earth be allowed to rest from deliberate economic use. The message seems to be clear: we are stewards of this earth and it is our task to protect it and, more than that, *l'havdeel bain kodesh v'chol*, to make distinctions between the holy and the profane, so that we may consciously and continuously sanctify life.

Circumcision is antithetical to this very powerful life-affirming tradition. Its true intention was not unknown to the rabbis and is best revealed in the words of Rambam, the acronym for Rabbi Moses Ben Maimonides, the great Twelfth Century Jewish philosopher, physician and Judaic scholar, so revered in Jewish tradition that it is said, "From Moses to Moses there was no one like Moses." Here is what Rambam wrote in his well-known and widely influential work, *The Guide of the Perplexed*.

> Similarly with regard to circumcision, one of the reasons for it is, in my opinion, the wish to bring about a decrease in sexual intercourse and a weakening of the organ in question, so that this activity be diminished and the organ be in as quiet a state as possible. It has been thought that circumcision perfects what is defective congenitally. This gave the possibility to everyone to raise an objection and to say: How can natural things be defective so that they need to be perfected from outside, all the more because we know how useful the foreskin is for that member? In fact this commandment has not been prescribed with a view to perfecting what is defective congenitally, but to perfecting morally. The bodily pain caused to that member is the real purpose of circumcision. None of the activities necessary for the preservation of the individual is harmed thereby, nor is procreation rendered impossible, but violent concupiscence and lust that goes beyond what is needed are diminished. The fact that circumcision weakens the faculty of sexual excitement and sometimes perhaps diminishes the pleasure is indubitable. For if at birth this member has been made to bleed and has had its covering taken away from it, it must indubitably be weakened. The Sages, may their memory be blessed, have explicitly stated: It is hard for a woman with whom an uncircumcised man has had sexual intercourse to separate from him (Genesis Rabbah LXXX). In my opinion this is the strongest of reasons for circumcision.[16]

There they are, the twin fears: the fear of woman and the fear of pleasure. Circumcision is the antidote that both assuages and perpetuates these ancient terrors. This is the achievement and true purpose of circumcision. It achieves this by violently breaching the maternal–infant bond shortly after birth, by mutilating and marking the baby's sexual organ, by disempowering the mother at the height of her instinctual need to protect her infant, by bonding the baby to the men and the male G-d, and by psychosexually wounding the manhood still asleep in the unsuspecting baby boy. Circumcision is fundamental to patriarchy, but it is not holy. Neither is it consistent with the ancient life-affirming values which Judaism embodies.

Our traditions and tribes are living entities. They transmit meaning and beauty to our lives. Simultaneously, they also perpetuate patterns that are destructive and violent, patterns that are minimally dealt with because they are normative to the culture. This is true of genital mutilation. It is also true of anti-Semitism. If we are to engage in a thorough critique of circumcision, it would be a grave omission to not address the issue of anti-Semitism, for male circumcision is very much at the nexus of the trauma of Christian-Jewish relations.

Overt anti-Semitism may seem like an isolated, abhorrent chapter of past history and not something that is part of our mandate to discuss in this discourse over ending sexual mutilation. The sad reality, however, is that the virus of anti-Semitism is quite alive, having gone through numerous mutations in the past two thousand years, and needs to be understood if Jews and non-Jews are to engage in any meaningful dialogue with the Jewish community, even indirectly.

While the roots of Western anti-Semitism can be found in Greco-Roman history, modern Western anti-Semitism is primarily rooted in the New Testament. The Christian assertion that Jews killed Jesus has long been disproven by scholars. It is not controversial in academic circles to assert that, indeed, it was the Romans who killed Jesus. A lie repeated for millennia, however, is not easily untold. Furthermore, the Jewish rejection of Jesus as the messiah has been highly problematic for Christianity and has given rise to a theological rage and condemnation with very direct historical consequences. Jews are depicted in the New Testament, particularly in the gospel of John and the writings of Timothy as a corrupt, primitive people. "Reputedly, Jesus himself tells 'the Jews' that they are not children of God but are, by deliberate choice, children of the devil."[17]

From such sentiments, it was not a great leap for the Church to articulate a policy of supersessionism toward Judaism. The Church saw itself as the "New Israel," replacing and superseding the Jewish people in relationship to God. The Christian sacred texts were named the New Testament, the Hebrew scriptures, the Old Testament. Christianity was the new force of love and light, a theological progression from what the Church portrayed as the Old Testament's obsession with "law" and "vengefulness." The continued independent vitality of both the Jewish people and Jewish spirituality deeply threatened the Church's theological investment in supersessionism and has had disastrous consequences for both communities. For Christians, it meant the severance of Jesus from his Jewish historical roots with a concomitant distortion of personhood. For Jews, this hostility towards Judaism has created millennia of survival trauma which, in its most overt forms, has been physical annihilation and/or spiritual annihilation through aggressive proselytism to Jews. In its more covert forms, it is a very subtle message of invalidation, so subtle that many Jews feel the necessity of invisibility in order to gain acceptance in the broader community, even though they may be unaware of the negative messages they continuously receive.

Very early in the Church's history, this antipathy towards Judaism was transformed from the theological to the political realm through the instrument of legislation. In the year 315, the very first law passed under Christian influence in the Roman Empire condemning to the flames Jews who attempted to prevent other Jews from converting to Christianity or enticed Christians to convert to Judaism. During the Middle Ages, the Jew became the epitome of unbelief and was widely equated with the devil. Jews were accused of using Christian blood to prepare *matzah*, practicing sorcery, poisoning Christians, desecrating the host and ritual murder. "The most vivid impression to be gained from a reading of medieval allusions to the Jew is of a hatred so vast and abysmal, so intense, that it leaves one gasping for comprehension."[18] Martin Luther seemed to be an exception to this vicious propaganda, speaking positively of Jews and seeking their approval, until it became clear to him that the Jews still were not interested in conversion, whereupon he turned upon them with the most vitriolic speeches, which the Nazis, 400 years later, implemented quite literally.[19]

Raul Hilberg, one of the foremost documentarianists of the Holocaust, writes the following in this epic work, *The Destruction of European Jews*:

> The missionaries of Christianity had said in effect: You have no right to live among us as Jews. The secular rulers who followed had complained: You have no right to live among us. The German Nazis at last decreed: You have no right to live....The process began with the attempt to drive the Jews into Christianity. The development was continued in order to force the victims into exile. It was finished when the Jews were driven to their deaths. The German Nazis, then, did not discard the past; they built upon it. They did not begin a development; they completed it.[20]

It is significant that Hitler was never excommunicated by the Catholic Church, and Hermann Goering died as an Evangelical.[21] In 1965, at the historic Vatican Council II, the Jews were officially pardoned for the crime they never committed, namely deicide. Today, fifty years after the defeat of Nazism, the Holocaust is still considered, basically, a "Jewish issue," anti-Semitism is on the rise, and covert messages to Jews to keep their Judaism more or less "in the closet" abound.

It is against this background that Jews are hearing our critique of circumcision. Is it any surprise, then, that the anti-circumcision movement is so often met with a charge of anti-Semitism? It is precisely because of this historical background of oppression that some Jews may cling to circumcision. It is essential that activists in the movement against circumcision become educated about the historical relationship of Christians and Jews, sensitized to anti-Semitism, and outspoken in our condemnation of this violence in all of its subtle and more aggressive forms.

Misperceptions that Jews are responsible for the high circumcision rate among non-Jews in the United States, or that Jews advocate routine circumcision of non-Jews to acquire covertly Christian converts may not be intended to be malicious, but neither are they simply erroneous. They echo, with all the dangers of the old canards of exaggerated Jewish power, Jewish conspiracy theories, and are not so very far removed from that lingering image of the Jew as the embodiment of evil. Jews, unlike Christians, do not actively seek converts and once a non-Jew has decided he or she wants to become Jewish, the process is long and arduous. The proliferation of such misperceptions inevitably contribute to the creation of a hostile atmosphere towards the Jewish community, rightfully causing Jews, even secular Jews, to close ranks against such positions. Such misperceptions will not serve the movement to end circumcision.

What would Christianity look like without anti-Semitism? What would Judaism be without circumcision? How would the African and Asian cultures function without female or male genital mutilation? These are daring visions which go to the heart of our identities and challenge all of us to rethink our notions of the sacred, both sacred text and sacred ritual. Who names what is sacred? Can it be altered, transformed, redefined and still carry the transcendent, bonding power and beauty of our traditions?

Male and female circumcision within Jewish, Moslem and African communities are issues that need to be confronted primarily by members of those groups. As a white Jewish female, I could not presume to tell African women how to oppose genital mutilation. I can, however, tell them that I would stand by them, offer support, which is for them to define, and honor their need to stay connected to their heritage, while at the same time battling desperately against it.

My arena is Judaism and the Jewish community. I would encourage Jews to ask more questions about this "sacred" ritual. To those Jews who say that ending circumcision would be ending Judaism, I would point out that Judaism is an evolving vital organism which has survived 4,000 very harsh years precisely because of its ability to change. Animal sacrifice was an integral part of worship during the Biblical period. Few today would countenance such acts as connected with sacred worship. The biggest shift of all came when, not only was the Temple destroyed, but our homeland was devastated and we were driven out. For 2,000 years, Jews maintained their identity without land. Jewish civilization was put in a suitcase: culture, languages, literature, music, and religion became portable because they were held in people's heads and hearts, not in the Jewish penis.

Recently, a well-known rabbi spoke about his need to remind converts that they are entering into a religion that is not perfect, but is perfectible. Even though this comment was not made in the context of circumcision, I feel it is eminently applicable to Jewish women in the process of reweaving the fabric of Jewish tradition. Specifically, we need ceremonies to hearken to the voice of Sarah so that we may not only honor and celebrate the traditional moments of children's separation from mothers, such as weaning and *bar mitzvah*, but also we need to create ceremonies which will support and celebrate a woman's transformation into motherhood: ceremonies that will validate and affirm her natural and elemental life-giving and life-protecting instincts as the essence of holiness, deserving of community support and blessing. We must envision a Judaism that can welcome all of our children, non-violently, into the *brit b'lee milah*, a covenant without circumcision, a covenant that will bless, celebrate and protect the sacredness of this child's sexuality. We need to support and affirm men's struggle to revise the old notion of masculinity, which is rooted in fear of women. We invite men to explore ways to ritualize and celebrate masculinity and the critical passages of male bonding in ways that are life affirming, non-violent, and protective of the sacred wholeness of men. Only in these ways will we begin the restoration of the holy and establish *tikkun*, healing, between the sexes.

Ultimately, we all must know that it is not possible to violate or suppress the sexuality of one gender without doing harm to the other. Certainly, there are very important differences which need to be acknowledged between male and female circumcision, but fundamentally we know this: raising a knife to the genitals of a child is not holy. It is not sacred. Just as the angel intervened to stop Abraham from slaughtering Isaac according to his understanding of G-d's command to sacrifice his beloved son, so too it is time for us to intervene and oppose the knife aimed at our babies' tender and innocent genitalia. To do so is to affirm that which is holy and life-affirming within our tradition. To do so is to reclaim the power of naming the sacred. To do so is to bless and protect our children's sexuality. To do so is to sanctify life. *L'hayyim*!

REFERENCES

1. Weisel E. Presentation. Temple Emanuel, San Francisco, California, May 9, 1996.
2. Toubia N. Female circumcision as a public health issue. New England Journal of Medicine 1994;331:712–6.
3. Wallerstein E. Circumcision: The Uniquely American Medical Enigma. Symposium on Advances in Pediatric Urology, Urologic Clinics of North America 1985;12,1:123–32.
4. National Center for Health Statistics, Department of Health and Human Services. 1994.
5. Anand KJS and Hickey PR. Pain and its Effects in the Human Neonate and Fetus. New England Journal of Medicine 1987;317(21):1326–9.
6. Ritter T. Say No To Circumcision. Aptos, CA: Hourglass, 1992:11–1,2.
7. Masters W and Johnson VE. Human Sexual Response. Boston: Little, Brown, 1966:192.
8. Ritter T. Say No To Circumcision. Aptos, CA: Hourglass, 1992:5–2.
9. Ritter T. Say No To Circumcision. Aptos, CA: Hourglass, 1992:18–1.
10. Bigelow J. The Joy of Uncircumcising. Aptos, CA: Hourglass, 1992:16–17.
11. Kohler K. Circumcision. The Jewish Encyclopedia. New York: KTAV, 1964:93.
12. Pollack M. A Jewish Feminist Perspective. In: Weiner K, Moon A, eds. Jewish Women Speak Out: Expanding the Boundaries of Psychology. Seattle, WA: Canopy Press, 1995:181.
13. Odent M. Colostrum, Prepuce and Civilization. Paper presented at the Second International Symposium on Circumcision, San Francisco, CA, 1991.
14. Teubal S. Sarah, The Priestess: The First Matriarch of Genesis. Athens, OH: Swallow Press, 1984:66.
15. Chafets Z. Out of Order: "I Did the Family a Favor." Jerusalem Report July 11, 1996:20.
16. Maimonides M. The Guide of the Perplexed. S. Pines, Trans. Chicago & London: University of Chicago Press, 1963:609.
17. Eckardt R. Your People, My People: The Meeting of Jews and Christians. New York: Quadrangle/New York Times Book Co., 1974:10.

18. Trachtenberg J. The Devil and the Jews: The Medieval Conception of the Jew and its Relation to Modern Anti-Semitism. Cleveland and New York: World Publishing Company (Meridian Books), 1943; Philadelphia: Jewish Publication Society of America, 1961:12.

19. Trachtenbert J. The Devil and the Jews: The Medieval Conception of the Jew and its Relation to Modern Anti-Semitism. Cleveland and New York: World Publishing Company (Meridian Books), 1943; Philadelphia: Jewish Publication Society of America, 1961:12.

20. Hilberg R. The Destruction of European Jews. Chicago: Quadrangle Books, 1961:3–4.

21. Eckardt R. Your People, My People: The Meeting of Jews and Christians. New York: Quadrangle/New York Times Book Co., 1974:25.

17

CHALLENGING CIRCUMCISION

A Jewish Perspective

Jenny Goodman

It is now June 1996, and I am joyfully expecting my first baby at the end of this month. I do not know the sex of the baby, and I believe I may be one of the first Jewish women of my generation who does not need to whisper the silent prayer, "Please God, let it be a girl." I am calm and comfortable in the knowledge that no one will ever take a knife to this baby's flesh in the name of religion, and that my child will be every bit as Jewish as I am, or as Jewish as he or she chooses to be, with no mutilating mark upon the body. I am confident that my people have such an abundance of life-enhancing and mind-opening traditions, that our identity and sense of cultural self-hood will happily survive our outgrowing of circumcision, a relic which has always felt to me like an aberration at the heart of an otherwise life-affirming religion.

I have attended brit milah ceremonies many times. Unlike most women, I did not turn away; I watched. Even where I saw the adults celebrating and honoring the ancient covenant, I saw the baby, unaware of all such concepts, in terrible pain. I saw a helpless infant held down and screaming while a highly sensitive part of his body was suddenly and needlessly cut away. For the baby there could be no meaning, no warning and no comfort, only trauma and terror.

I started speaking to people in my community about my concerns. Most of the people I speak to take circumcision for granted; they believe it is healthy, harmless, hygienic, and/or divinely commanded. They believe it is a "little snip" that does not hurt, leaves no trace in the memory, and causes no scars in the soul of mother or child. They believe that their cultural identity and sense of belonging will crumble if they stop cutting pieces off their babies' bodies. Each ethnic group sees circumcision as a unique cultural marker, despite the fact it is practiced by Jews, Muslims, Africans and Australian Aborigines alike, and is therefore unique to none of them. In all groups, challenging the practice evokes great fear. It is the fear of being different; not like Dad, not like their peers. Ironically, in the Jewish world, circumcision is held up as an essential way of keeping males within the fold, even while young men are actually leaving the faith in

Sexual Mutilations: A Human Tragedy, edited by Denniston and Milos
Plenum Press, New York, 1997

droves. If circumcision is the key to Jewish identity, where does that leave the 52% of Jews who are female?

In debates about circumcision, I talk about the facts: the intense pain, and the risks of haemorrhage, infection, and mutilation which inevitably accompany any surgery, even in the best hands. I talk about the physiological evidence for severe pain and trauma during circumcision: the rise in the baby's heart rate, breathing rate, blood pressure, adrenalin level and steroid hormone level. I explain that, contrary to popular opinion, there are no medical benefits, but that there are considerable complications, and that the best form of hygiene is simply to wash. I present the ethical arguments against injuring a defenseless person. I talk about the disempowerment of mothers and the damaging of the mother-infant bond: mothers feel they have to violate all their maternal instincts which urge them to cherish and protect the child; if they do not do so they will be cast out of their tribe, spiritual exiles. They feel torn apart by this dilemma. I also name the effects on sexual experience described by men circumcised in adulthood. Finally, I describe the alternative, gentle, celebratory ways we could welcome newborn babies into our culture and our world.

The response to all these points, from Jewish and Muslim people, is remarkably consistent. It consists of no logical argument at all, and very little actual response to what I have said. It consists, in a word, of fear. Religious fundamentalists say, "We are commanded by God, we have to do it, and that's the end of the story." They feel profoundly threatened. Secular and liberal people among these ethnic communities feel equally terrified, but cannot fall back on literal interpretation of biblical commandments. They say such things as, "But we've always done it, we've been doing it for thousands of years. You can't ask us to just stop now, it's an integral part of our identity."

I reply by emphasizing that all spiritual traditions evolve and change — indeed, they only survive by changing. I emphasize that a thousand years does not justify hurting a child. At this point, people very often say to me: "You're right, I can't argue with you. What you say is unanswerable, but I know I'd still have my son circumcised — I just couldn't not. It's not a rational thing. I just feel I must."

This is culturally conditioned terror, a form of admittedly compulsive behavior on the part of people who at some level do want to stop. The fact is, however, that the change is already happening: some Jewish people have chosen a new, non-violent path; a small but growing number have faced the apparent conflict between loyalty to tribe and loyalty to child, and have decided to leave their children whole and uninjured. Most importantly, these people are still part of their respective communities.

Does circumcision cause lasting psychological trauma? Personally, I believe that unconscious scars must remain in the adult man; this can neither be proved nor disproved, although I have spoken to several men who have experienced a painful reliving of their circumcision during psychotherapy. Even without this, however, the ethical argument is strong enough to stand alone. The infliction of pain and damage on a helpless child is absolutely wrong even if there were no memory, no residue, no consequences. To people who tell me that "the pain is momentary, it's over in a flash," I say, "I disagree with you, but even if you were right, is it acceptable to hurt your fellow human beings, even for a second, on the basis that they'll probably forget about it?"

Circumcision is perpetuated down the generations by denial, repression, numbness, and compulsive repetition. In other words, "It did me no harm, it'll do him no harm." It is a special man who has the courage to acknowledge his own loss, to say, in the face of tribal history, universal peer pressure and his parents, "Yes, I have been damaged. I won't pass this damage on down the line. The wounding stops with me." It is unnecessary to require that everyone have such courage. It is enough that we encourage each other to stop, on the basis that times have changed, that we now have new information about babies' sensitivity and experience that we did not have a generation ago (except silently in every mother's heart, of course). Most of all, we need to reassure people that their child will not be alone, will not be the only one, will not be exiled. We are really dealing with the parents' own fear of differentness, expressed as a fear for their child.

When I began speaking out publicly on this issue, I was afraid I would be attacked, and called a traitor to my people. This has certainly happened, but I have also had an amazing amount of support, sometimes from unexpected quarters. Many Jewish grandmothers, in their seventies and older, have told me: "You know, I always thought it was a dreadful thing to do, but I never said a word, because I thought I was the only one. I thought it was my problem that it worried me. In my day," they continue, "we didn't question circumcision, we didn't question anything, but if you young people want to challenge it — well, go ahead and good luck to you!" Since Victor Schonfeld's film, *It's A Boy!*, was shown on television in September 1995, some of these older Jewish women have taken the pressure off their adult sons and daughters; they are no longer insisting on circumcised grandchildren.

A few weeks after the film was broadcast, a woman sat in my living room and sobbed. She recalled how her son had nearly bled to death after his ritual circumcision at eight days. She was so traumatized that she never had a second child: she could not face the dilemma, should she have a boy again, of whether to repeat the deed or not. Despite the fact that her son had almost died, circumcision remained a dilemma for her. She could neither circumcise another son nor face having an uncircumcised son. Consequently, she had no more children. She was very sad. Such is the power of the tribe.

This mother is Jewish, but I have met Muslim mothers and non-Muslim African mothers who have equally harrowing stories. This is an issue that unites women across all ethnic divides. All of us are injured when we allow a man to take a knife to our child, to claim him as one of the men. We betray ourselves and our babies.

In the Jewish world, certain emotionally powerful "arguments" are brought up again and again in response to my challenging of circumcision. Even in the cattle cars on the way to Auschwitz, it is said, we circumcised our sons, with whatever implements were available. Even in the face of death we honored this commandment. And you, you would have us stop now? The implication is that I am dishonoring the memory of the millions who died. It is intended to silence me, by eclipsing my concern by comparison with such huge collective horror. My response is that our tremendous historical suffering does not cancel out the continuing pain of our baby boys. Those who died in the camps were doing what they thought best, circumcising their sons even in the depths of hell. This does not prevent us from taking what we now know to be the most ethical course of action; leaving our little ones intact and touching them henceforth only with gentleness.

The other powerful historical "argument" is that persecutors of the Jews, from the Romans onwards, have tried to outlaw circumcision as part of general anti-Semitic oppression. Challenging circumcision, even when the challenger is Jewish, is therefore perceived as anti-Semitic. Furthermore, retaining circumcision in the face of great oppression has become a symbol of our defiant survival against all the odds. That is why people react so vehemently when circumcision is questioned; they feel on some level that their very survival is being imperilled. The significance of circumcision in the collective Jewish psyche is undeniable; unfortunately, however, what is merely symbolic for educated adults is horribly real and immediate for the baby being circumcised.

A long time ago, we are told, Abraham heard the voice of God, commanding him to circumcise his sons. Whatever voice he may have heard was true and profound for him, and he was conscience-bound to follow it. I, on the other hand, hear a different voice, and I too am conscience-bound to follow it. Whether it be the voice of the Goddess, of Nature, of humanity, of the innocent child; whatever voice it is, it rises from the womb and from the heart, and it speaks words very similar to those God commanded Abraham as Abraham was about to sacrifice Isaac: "Lay not thy hand upon the boy, neither do anything to him."

The prophet of Isaiah commands: "Circumcise the foreskin of your heart." This is the only kind of circumcision that makes sense to me today — to melt the shell of insensitivity around our hearts, so that we open our ears to our children's screaming, and do not hurt them anymore.

People are only able to circumcise little children because ultimately, at some hidden level, they still do not see them as fully human. They permit themselves to do to an infant what they would not dream of doing to another adult — the forcible restraint, the exercise of sheer physical power to cause an injury. In law, they would be guilty of assault if they did this to an unconsenting grown-up person.

In our legal and ethical systems, in our hearts, we — globally — still do not recognize the full humanity of the human baby. I am happy to say this situation is beginning to change. Thanks largely to the pioneering work of Michel Odent, obstetrics — that great bastion of the patriarchy — is slowly acknowledging that the newborn baby is at least as aware, as alive, as exquisitely sensitive as you and I. In other words, is a fully human being. This change in obstetrics has, of course, not gone nearly far enough, although I believe it has gone further in Britain than in the United States, and is helping to change adults' perceptions and treatment of babies in the culture at large.

The struggle around childbirth is intimately linked with the struggle to end circumcision. A young Jewish mother recently told me that if she had had a hospital birth with high-tech invasion and interference, she might well have consented to circumcision as just another medical violation in a seemingly inevitable chain of such violations. Feeling strong and clear and empowered after a gentle, natural birth, underwater and in the sanctity of her own home, she felt, however, fully able to refuse any potential attack upon herself, upon her baby, or upon the bond between them.

The fight against circumcision is not a "single issue" cause. It is about awakening the adult world to see even the tiniest baby as a full person, deserving of all human rights, respect, and dignity. It is about challenging all of us to keep lowering the age threshold at which we recognize full humanness, a shift that is part of historical progress towards a truly civilized society. This battle is part of a larger battle to humanize and rehumanize the world.

18

THE WOUND REVEALS THE CURE

A Utah Model for Ending the Cycle of Sexual Mutilation

Jeannine Parvati Baker

Dominator societies inflict the greatest wounds on children during the perinatal and pubescent periods. Experiences at this age are deeply imprinted. Whether they are intact or mutilated, all members of a dominator society are affected by its cycle of war on infants and children. The sequelae of sexual abuse of males and females, whether by genital mutilation or otherwise, leaves distinct psychological wounds. There are, however, ways to heal those wounds in order to end the cycle of mutilation.

The ancient adage, "The wound reveals the cure," which is often associated with the Greek Goddess of health, Hygieia, summarizes the primary approach I use in protecting infants and children from genital harm. Unless we determine the primal motivations of those who would perpetrate sexual mutilation, merely staying the hand of the circumciser will not guarantee the child a safe environment in which to grow. Healing the trauma buried in parents who would subject their children to sexual mutilation has been the most effective strategy for safeguarding the integrity of the child and the family.

1. REVEALING THE WOUND

The core values of any culture are imprinted through rite-of-passage ceremonies. The members of dominator societies are bound to the sado-masochistic tendencies of the group by rites that inflict pain to what should be the most pleasurable, sensitive tissue of the body. They show the symptoms of traumatic childhood rites in their war-like behavior and, most especially, in the reenactment and perpetration of sadistic initiation rituals on infants and children. These groups do not value the physical integrity of the baby as it comes into the world, rather, they feel obliged to alter or "fix" the body of the newborn to make it conform to an artificial and unattainable ideal.

Cultural patterns of violence are inherited through the ways we are treated by those entrusted to protect us. Those who have had technocratic perinatal flesh-wounding rituals

Sexual Mutilations: A Human Tragedy, edited by Denniston and Milos
Plenum Press, New York, 1997

imprinted on them in hospital neonatal wards, often become compelled to reenact these rituals on their own children.

1.1. Judging the Baby

Many obstetric and pediatric rituals likewise perpetrate the original wounds. There are many erroneously lauded medical procedures that deceive members of dominator societies into hurting their children, "for their own good." Aggressive Western medicine is analogous to tribal markings and scarifications found in pre-industrialized, non-Western societies.

An example of this tendency is found in the modern American hospital practice of grading each baby on a scale of one to ten, according to a standard created by Virginia Apgar, to assess health in the immediate post-partum period. This symptom of the dominator society is characteristic of groups that believe that even babies are in need of judging and correction. Each baby is laid upon a Procrustean bed of the mythical and unattainable norm and "fixed" to make it fit. Each of us has been imprinted with a score of nine or less, for there is rarely a baby who receives a perfect score of ten at birth.

One of the most disturbing modern examples of the symptomatic tendency to regard babies as inherently imperfect, is the sexual mutilation of boys, euphemistically called "circumcision," that regularly occurs in the United States. Infant boys who are delivered into familial or obstetrical situations where such tendencies exist are subjected to having their penis graded, judged, and surgically "fixed" to make it conform to the image of the artificial, surgically-created adult circumcised penis.

The medical profession in the United States gives validation to this process, not only by actively judging and "fixing" the child, but by upholding and perpetuating the myth that the circumcised penis, rather than the intact natural penis, is the standard against which all penises should be judged. Pictorial and descriptive representations of the penis in American medical literature almost always depict the penis as being circumcised. The reduced anatomy and truncated functions of the circumcised penis are held up as the ideal, while the balance of the complete anatomy and functions of the natural penis are ignored, denied, or dismissed as redundant.

Circumcised fathers validate this process by judging their newborn son's penis against their own penis and, in obedience to the demands of the dominator society, by uttering the deceptively simple command imprinted on them by their own wounding and cultural conditioning, "I want my baby to be fixed to look like me."

2. SEXUAL WOUNDING IN MORMON SOCIETY

Mormonism was founded in the 1830s by Joseph Smith. His followers moved westward from New England, eventually arriving in the Utah Territory. In 1848, they founded Salt Lake City, making it the headquarters for the Mormon church and the capital of the state of Utah. Mormonism is one of the few religions whose scriptures directly forbid circumcision.

2.1. Circumcision in Mormon Scripture

The Book of Mormon, first published in 1830, is considered by Mormons to be the direct word of God. It contains the essence of the Mormon position on circumcision. In

the "Book of Moroni," God delivers directly to Mormon, the father of Moroni, the following words:

1. Listen to the words of Christ, your Redeemer, your Lord and your God. Behold,
   I came into the world not to call the righteous but sinners to repentance; the
   whole need no physician, but they that are sick; wherefore, little children are
   whole, for they are not capable of committing sin; wherefore the curse of Adam
   is taken from them in me, that it hath no power over them; and the law of circumcision is done away in me.[1]

The companion volume to the *Book of Mormon* is the *Doctrine and Covenants*,
which Mormons believe to be the direct revelation of God to Joseph Smith. The covenants
and commandments contained in this book are as binding to Mormons as those in the
Book of Mormon. Section 74 of the *Doctrine and Covenants* comprises an explanation of
the Apostle Paul's first Epistle to the Corinthians (7.14) and is believed to have been
given to Joseph Smith by direct revelation from God on January 1832.

2. Now in the days of the apostles the law of circumcision was had among all the
   Jews who believed not the gospel of Jesus Christ.
3. And it came to pass that there arose a great contention among the people concerning the law of circumcision, for the unbelieving husband was desirous that
   his children should be circumcised and become subject to the law of Moses,
   which law was fulfilled.
4. And it came to pass that the children, being brought up in subjection to the law
   of Moses, gave heed to the traditions of their fathers, and believed not the gospel of Christ, wherein they became unholy;
5. Wherefore, for this cause the apostle wrote unto the church, giving unto them a
   commandment, not of the Lord, but of himself, that a believer should not be
   united to an unbeliever, except the law of Moses should be done away among
   them,
6. That their children might remain without circumcision; and that the tradition
   might be done away, which saith that little children are unholy; for it was had
   among the Jews,
7. But little children are holy, being sanctified through the atonement of Jesus
   Christ; and this is what the scriptures mean.[2]

2.2. Contradictions in Doctrine and Practice

Despite this doctrinal interdiction against circumcision, Utah, with its large Mormon
population, has the second highest circumcision rate in the United States.[3] Faith in these
scriptures was evidently insufficient to halt the spread of the obstetrical practice of routine
circumcision of newborn boys in Utah hospitals in the 1950s and 1960s. The practice has
remained in force to the present day.

3. A MODEL FOR CHANGE

The majority of the population of Utah lives in the major urban centers of Salt Lake
City and Ogden, but a sizable minority continues to thrive in vast rural sections of the
state. Since 1982, I have been serving the central part of the state of Utah as midwife and

birth instructor. Upon my arrival, I found that the circumcision rate among Mormon families in this rural area was no less than in the populous urban areas. As an advocate for safe birth, family unity, and child safety, it was necessary for me to develop strategies to meet these goals in this specific cultural milieu.

3.1. Interview Process

Interviewing prospective clients enables me to determine the extent to which the natural maternal and paternal instincts to nurture and protect the child has been compromised by the influence of the dominator society. Although modern Americans are generally deficient in knowledge about birth and have been conditioned to turn to the perceived experts for help and delivery (in every sense of the word), I cultivate an approach that affirms and stimulates the parents' naturally-active role in birth.

I explain to the mother that I will neither cut her flesh nor the flesh of her baby. Through a series of gentle questions, the parents' commitment to breastfeeding and protecting their baby from genital cutting can be ascertained. By encouraging the parents to answer openly and to tell me about their lives, I can determine where defenses have been erected that may lead to non-nurturing behaviors. I find it instructive to listen to the language used by the mother and to check if she has any flesh wounds characteristic of dominator societies, such as surgical scars or deliberate piercings. The more she uses victimizing and sabotaging language and the more flesh wounds, the more likely she is to allow her child to be circumcised. As a tool for greater insight, I question the mothers about menstruation: do they look forward to menstruation, or do they dread it. I find that these questions and observations are excellent methods for finding the primal causes of the sexual mutilation of infants.

When asked, "What about circumcision?," a typical young Mormon mother will generally reply that, if the child is a boy, she will want him circumcised. I find that further questioning will often reveal that it is the father who, in fact, wants the baby circumcised, simply because he was circumcised in infancy. I then bring the relevant passages from *The Book of Mormon* and *Doctrine and Covenants* to the parents' attention. Invariably, Mormons are surprised to learn that circumcision is not a religious requirement, since they, apparently, have never read these passages. Many Mormon parents are relieved by the information and feel validated. They often respond with the affirmation that Joseph Smith was indeed a true prophet. Obedience is an exalted principle in Mormon society, and Mormon clients want to feel obedient. I reveal to them that, by protecting their baby from circumcision, they have the personal pleasure of feeling obedient to a higher principle.

This same technique is used by activists to eradicate female sexual mutilation in Muslim and Christian societies in Africa. At-risk women are shown that neither the Koran nor the Bible requires female genital cutting. This gives them the strength to protect their daughters from cutting rituals.

If this revelation is not enough to revive the protective and nurturing instinct, I ask them, "How does it serve you to circumcise your baby?" This question generally brings deep-seated, powerful cultural imprinting to the surface. Generally, the mother or father answering the question will take on a different persona and will speak with a voice and manner unlike their own. After they have spoken, I will ask "Who in you is now speaking?" The most frequently encountered reply is that the client's mother or father is speaking. I further encourage the client to continue speaking, and to convince me of their need to circumcise their child.

It is important, at this point, to work with the circumcised father. After listening to the father's justifications for wanting to have his baby circumcised, I will ask him a leading question, such as, "When have you felt like this before, that you wanted to hurt a baby?" While the answers to this question vary tremendously, it serves to stimulate the father to examine his motivations. If he repeats that he wants the baby to look like him, I employ humor and ask him, "If you had a long nose, would you want the baby to have rhinoplasty so that he looked like you?" Alternatively, I ask the father if *he* would be willing to have plastic surgery to make his nose match the baby's nose. Such questions allow the father to see that he has no vested interest in circumcising the baby, and that such an action would not serve him. These questions also allow him to discover his own protective and nurturing instincts.

3.2. Effecting the Cure

The most effective response to whatever emerges from the interview process is support and care. It is counterproductive to argue with the justifications that emerge for circumcision in the interview process. The underlying feature of every justification that emerges for circumcision is fear. Fear is the tool used by the dominator society to mold the behavior of its members. The supportive interview process outlined above can be used to transform the parents' fear into power and excitement about the life-affirming and life-enhancing process of birth.

Once the mother has transcended her fears, she is prepared to have an ecstatic birth. In my experience, women who have an ecstatic birth will not want to hurt their baby. The more positive the birth experience is for the mother, the stronger her natural nurturing, protective instincts will emerge. I listen to peoples' stories and allow them to trust me. I remind the parents that they are whole and lead them to extend wholeness to their family.

4. CONCLUSIONS

The effectiveness of this method is reflected in the 0% circumcision rate among my clients in central Utah. While the Mormon experience is unique, the methods used here to eradicate the cycle of genital cutting may have cross-cultural applications. A healing model of building trust, listening, and transforming fear into power can resurrect the natural instinct in humans to protect, respect, and nurture their children.

5. REFERENCES

1. Moroni 8.8. The Book of Mormon. trans. Joseph Smith. first published 1830. Salt Lake City: The Church of Jesus Christ of Latter-Day Saints, 1921:516.
2. Section 74.2–7. Doctrine and Covenants. Salt Lake City: Deseret News Company, 1880:260–1.
3. National Center for Health Statistics. Department of Health and Human Services Washington DC. 1993.

19

NURSES FOR THE RIGHTS OF THE CHILD

An Update

Mary Conant and Betty Katz Sperlich

In the fall of 1993, after a long internal struggle with our consciences, we decided that we could no longer assist with infant circumcision. In October of that year, we wrote a letter to the staff and administration at St. Vincent Hospital, Santa Fe, New Mexico where we work, stating that we would no longer participate in infant circumcision: "Ethically, we find ourselves unable to assist with the procedure." Twenty-two other nurses at the hospital joined us in signing the letter and in refusing to take part in infant circumcision. Our actions resulted in media attention, including a documentary by Barry Ellsworth, *The Nurses of St. Vincent: Saying No to Circumcision.*

By the summer of 1994, the atmosphere at our work place had profoundly deteriorated due to tensions surrounding circumcision. Instead of ignoring the situation, the hospital administration agreed to our request to resolve the conflict with the assistance of a professional mediator. The group that met for mediation consisted of conscientious objector nurses (nurses who do not assist with circumcision), "consenting nurses" (nurses who participated with circumcisions), hospital administrators, physicians, and union representatives. The resulting legal document, called a "Memorandum of Understanding for Circumcision Procedure" (MOU), officially recognizes our status as conscientious objectors to infant circumcision. The MOU excuses all St. Vincent Hospital nurses who declare themselves conscientious objectors to circumcision from all duties related to circumcision, including obtaining informed consent, preparing the instruments, taking the baby from his mother, strapping the baby down to the circumcision board, assisting with the mutilation itself, assisting with the immediate post-operative care, and disposing of the amputated sexual parts.

In accordance with our ethical position to respect the genital integrity of infants of both sexes, the MOU is not gender specific. The MOU supports our position that the child's right to the body he or she was born with is absolute. Other nurses throughout the country can use the MOU as a model for obtaining official recognition as conscientious objectors to circumcision in their own hospitals.

Sexual Mutilations: A Human Tragedy, edited by Denniston and Milos
Plenum Press, New York, 1997

Achieving the MOU was a difficult struggle. Ironically, one of the ground rules of the mediation process was that the ethics of circumcision could not be discussed. We also faced insult and ridicule from some members of the negotiating team. Nevertheless, the MOU was achieved. The fact that the MOU exists is a credit to the skills of Ann Lown, our spokesperson.

Immediately after the MOU was signed, Carole Ann Alley, one of the R.N. Conscientious Objector nurses on the MOU mediation team, resigned from St. Vincent Hospital. She is the only nurse we know who has resigned from a hospital for ethical reasons specific to circumcision, stating that she "could no longer accept blood money." Carol Ann Alley's letter of resignation, dated January 31, reads in full:

> With the approval and signing of the Memorandum of Understanding, this letter can now be written. I would like first and foremost to congratulate all involved parties for your courage, stamina, and hard work to reach a common ground. Since mediation began last summer, the best in all of us was required for this agreement to become a reality. Perhaps now a civilized and professional relationship can be a part of the daily work day at St. Vincent's Hospital.
>
> On a more personal note, my role at St. Vincent's has come to a close. Working, and striving to meet halfway is not acceptable when the violation of human rights continues. Ultimately, this trespass has made it impossible for me to continue being a nurse at your hospital.
>
> In an even larger picture, we as a nation persist in disregarding the basic human rights of our newborns. Unlike other species, our infants are born intimately dependent on us for their survival and well-being. To make a decision, without the infant's consent, on the surgical removal of a portion of his sexual organ, is violence. Who do we think we are?
>
> Mediation, and the signing of the MOU is one more step in consciousness raising. Perhaps now, as time, awareness, and education continue, we may one day be able to say that our children share and hold the same basic rights that we do.

By the summer of 1995, it became clear to us that we needed an identity apart from St. Vincent Hospital. In June 1995, Mary Conant, Mary-Rose Booker, and Betty Katz Sperlich founded Nurses for the Rights of the Child (NRC), a non-profit organization dedicated to protecting children's right to bodily integrity. After founding this organization, we no longer felt constrained in speaking out against the sexual mutilation of children.

For example, after we held our press conference in June 1995 to announce the founding of Nurses for the Rights of the Child, one of the circumcisers at our hospital became very angry and said that a donation of several thousand dollars for remodeling the hospital's labor and delivery area — including a new circumcision room — had been rescinded because of us. Apparently, the donation was *not* rescinded because the hospital continued to perform circumcisions, rather, it was rescinded because we had broken a taboo against publicly discussing circumcision.

In Spring 1996, we shamed circumcisers at St. Vincent Hospital into using local anesthetic. We accomplished this by confronting circumcisers who were circumcising infants without providing anesthesia. In one instance, after listening to the screams of a baby being circumcised, we approached the baby's pediatrician and informed her that her patient had just been subjected to unanesthetized surgery, and that this constituted torture. We also sent hospital officials and section chiefs copies of the 1987 study by Anand and Hickey, "Pain and its Effects in the Human Neonate and Fetus,"[1] as well as the position statement of the American Academy of Pediatrics Committee on Fetus and Newborn,

"Neonatal Anesthesia."[2] We realize that anesthesia is not the central issue: anesthesia masks the pain, not the mutilation. We could not ethically allow unanesthetized surgery to continue. The eradication of circumcision is a gradual process. Some circumcisers must first recognize that unanesthetized circumcision is torture before they can recognize that circumcision is a human rights violation.

In recent years, the number of circumcisers at the hospital has dropped from about twenty circumcisers to six. We see this as a step in the process of delegitimizing circumcision. Some of the circumcisers stopped performing the procedure altogether, while others retired or moved away. Several circumcisers moved the surgery to their offices, which opens the surgery to more public scrutiny. Office circumcision decreases the number of circumcisions because parents sometimes cancel post-natal circumcision appointments once they have an opportunity to bond with the baby and do not want him to be hurt. Often they accept his intact genitalia, or they simply find it inconvenient to take the baby to the office.

1. BREAKING THE CYCLE OF VIOLENCE: ACCOMPLICES AND WITNESSES SPEAK OUT

In the United States, infant male circumcision is a brutal custom that is passed on from one generation to the next. Nurses for the Rights of the Child is dedicated to breaking this cycle of violence. The eminent Swiss psychologist Dr. Alice Miller, discusses the cycle of violence in her book, *Banished Knowledge*:

> What eventually happens to the person who was mutilated as a child? When a small child is tortured by ignorant adults, won't he have to take his revenge later in life? He is bound to avenge himself unless his subsequent life allows the old wounds to heal in love, which is seldom the case. As a rule, children who were once injured will later injure their own children, maintaining that their behavior does no harm because their own loving parents did the same.[3]

We have observed that a primary reason parents give for having their newborn son circumcised is that the father himself is circumcised. Frequently, a father will say, "Well, I'm circumcised and I'm fine, so I guess we'll have him done."

According to Dr. Miller, an enlightened witness can break the cycle of violence:

> It depends on whether an informed witness can help the victim to become aware of the cruelty experienced, that is, to feel and see the cruelty inflicted on him.[4]

1.1. Nurses for the Rights of the Child

Nurses for the Rights of the Child is dedicated to awakening the public to the brutalities of circumcision. We were accomplices in the circumcision room. Consequently, we are in a unique position to give testimony. Our work includes educating and informing the public that the surgical alteration of the genitals of an unconsenting infant or child, whether in the name of medicine, religion, or social custom, is a human rights violation. We empower, support and advise other nurses to stop the socially sanctioned genital mutilation of minors. We promote the human rights principles of the United Nations Convention on the Rights of the Child. We also cooperate with others who are working in this country and abroad to promote the rights of children to bodily integrity.

1.2. Saying No to Circumcision

When they come now
in dreams
those round and fleshy wondrous
baby boys
we meet eagerly and with affection
new spirit and earth guide,
a trusting miracle of welcome
I am no longer handmaiden
of amputations, mutilations
too gross and grievous to be rational.
The nightmare agony of mute witness
has shifted —
now when the flayed, the mangled, the dismembered appear
my voice cries out the wounding,
mine are the hands of healing.

Patricia Worth, conscientious objector nurse, St. Vincent Hospital, Santa Fe, New Mexico. August 1, 1996.

2. REFERENCES

1. Anand KJS, Hickey PR. Pain and its effects in the human neonate and fetus. NEJM 1987;317:1321–9.
2. Committee on Fetus and Newborn, Committee on Drugs, Section on Anesthesiology, Section on Surgery. Neonatal anesthesia. Pediatrics 1987;80:446.
3. Miller A. Banished Knowledge: Facing Childhood Injuries. New York: Doubleday. 1990:139.
4. Miller A. Banished Knowledge: Facing Childhood Injuries. New York: Doubleday. 1990:140.

20

NOCIRC OF AUSTRALIA

George Williams

1. NOCIRC OF AUSTRALIA: STATEMENT OF PURPOSE

The National Organisation of Circumcision Information Resource Centres of Australia (NOCIRC of Australia) was founded on August 8, 1993 as a non-profit organization to campaign against male and female circumcision, to encourage informed medical and legal debate on the subject, and to make available scientifically-based information for new parents making decisions about circumcision.

NOCIRC of Australia accepts as its *modus operandi* the tenets of the *Declaration of the First International Symposium on Circumcision* held in Anaheim, California, in March 1989.

NOCIRC of Australia is concerned that the prevalence of male circumcision in Australia, which stands today at 10%, is unacceptably high. NOCIRC of Australia is also concerned with the problem of Aboriginal circumcision and subincision, as well as the fact that female sexual mutilations continue to be practiced by traditional Aboriginal communities, certain Muslim immigrant groups, a small number of Africans, and by the medical profession. NOCIRC of Australia has clinically-verified information of two such female victims, one a parturient Anglo-Celtic woman who had a clitoridectomy and the other a thirteen-year-old who was involuntarily subjected to a labial excision. Regardless of the reasons cited to justify the surgery, NOCIRC of Australia regards all genital cutting as sexual mutilation and a violation of fundamental human rights.

2. ACTIVITIES OF NOCIRC OF AUSTRALIA

NOCIRC of Australia publishes a quarterly newsletter with interviews, commentary, historical surveys, reports of NOCIRC of Australia's activities, and updates from the pertinent legal and medical literature. The newsletter is distributed to members and to child ad-

Sexual Mutilations: A Human Tragedy, edited by Denniston and Milos
Plenum Press, New York, 1997

vocacy centers, including the New Children's Hospital, Westmead, the National Law Youth Council Centre, and EPOCH World-wide.

NOCIRC of Australia has called for specific legislation banning genital alteration of healthy male children. We have suggested specific legislation for each State against female genital mutilation. Only South Australia and New South Wales have promulgated such legislation. Victoria is soon to follow in the next sitting of Parliament. Commonwealth legislation was prepared by the Family Law Council for the Federal General in 1995 and its outcome is awaited with interest.

Additionally, NOCIRC of Australia is committed to the following aims:

- To provide an informational and educational bureau for parents, health professionals, the media, and concerned individuals
- To lobby the state and federal health authorities, Australian Family Law Council, professional medical associations, and politicians
- To conduct community surveys of circumcision practices
- To provide psychosocial support for victims and prospective parents
- To monitor the media and medical literature on all forms of sexual mutilation, including circumcision
- To build a network of fellow preservationists locally and overseas
- To conduct letter-writing campaigns to the medical and cultural organizations that perpetuate sexual mutilation on children
- To speak publicly about the sad and tragic facts of sexual mutilation of males and females
- To provide forums for interdisciplinary exchange through workshops and seminars.

3. MEDICAL ISSUES

The history of routine circumcision in Australia parallels that of the United States. In the late Nineteenth Century, physicians began employing circumcision for unfounded medical reasons, such as the cure and prevention of masturbation, epilepsy, rheumatism, tuberculosis, and insanity. After World War II, hospitals in Australia and the United States began the practice of routinely subjecting newborn boys to involuntary circumcision.

No comprehensive statistical records are kept of the complications of circumcision. In Australia, three circumcision-related deaths have been reported in recent years. One death occurred as a result of meningitis and septicemia through the circumcision wound. One circumcision death resulted from severe hemorrhage due to hemophilia. The last known circumcision-related death was the result of an overdose of lignocaine. Some infants have lost their entire penis as a result of circumcision. All circumcisions damage the penis and prevent full sexual functioning by desensitizing the penis through the removal of specialized erogenous structures, preventing the penile skin sheath from gliding over the shaft according to its design, destroying the protection of the glans and meatus, artificially externalizing the glans penis, and desensitizing the glans through chronic keratinization and abrasion.[1]

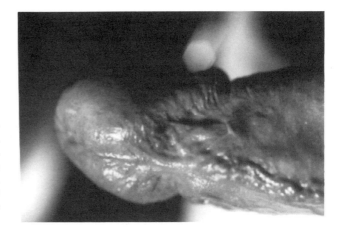

Figure 1. Ventral view of a surgically externalized glans penis of a 28-year-old American male circumcised at birth. Frenulum has been excised. Note the extensive scarring, and pitting. This man believed his penis was normal (Photograph courtesy of John A. Erickson)

4. CIRCUMCISION STATISTICS AND COSTS

Over the last ten years in Australia, there has been a significant decline in the rate of circumcision for all ages. The Australian medical colleges have been discouraging circumcision of healthy infants and the prevalence of circumcision in public hospitals remains low. Of the 20,000 annual circumcisions, 75% are performed on babies under six months.

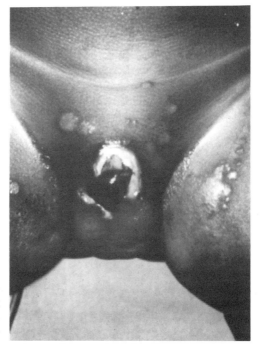

Figure 2. Total destruction of the penis of neonatally circumcised American baby from gangrene resulting from infection of circumcision wound. (Photograph by Tom Reichfelder, M.D., courtesy of John Money, M.D.)

4.1. Costs of Circumcision

Financial remuneration for circumcision by our national health insurer, Medicare, has a differential scale based on age. The following table, showing the item numbers, descriptors, and fees for circumcision, was extracted from *The Medical Benefits Schedule Book* (effective November 1995):

Item	Circumcision Procedure	Fee
30653	person under 6 months	$33.50*
306566	person between 6 and 10 months	$77.95*
30659 G	person over 10 years	$108.00*
30660 S	person over 10 years	$134.00*
30663	hemorrhage arrest requiring general anesthesia	$104.15*

*75% or 85% benefit depending on siting of operation.

Anesthetic Fees:

Item	Circumcision Procedure	Fee
30653/17705 =3BT + 2T	person under 6 months	$68.50
306566/17706=3BT + 2T	person between 6 and 10 months	$82.20
30659 G/17706=3BT + 2T	person over 10 years	$82.20
30660 S/17706=3BT + 2T	person over 10 years	$82.20
30663/17706=3BT + 2T	hemorrhage arrest requiring general anesthesia	$82.20

B and T refer to predetermined fixed basic and timed units for the anesthetic procedure. Added fees can be charged if procedure is prolonged for whatever reason.

Amputation of the tightly adherent prepuce in the young and newborn infant is technically more difficult, requires more skill, and has a higher morbidity/mortality. The Australian health insurer gives the procedure its lowest cost value. A further concern is the fact that the doctor is not bound to the charge of the scheduled fee and some charge up to $300. The parents have to pay the gap above the Medicare rebate and private insurance coverage.

4.2. Rate of Circumcision

The Australian national infant circumcision rate is calculated to be 10%. This is a slight underestimate, as not all circumcisions are claimed on *The Medical Benefits Schedule*. Aboriginal and religious ritual circumcisions, usually performed by lay persons, fall into this category.

The State of Queensland is anomalous as their rate is increasing. Victoria has the lowest rate at 7% and Queensland has a rate of 13%.

5. HUMAN RIGHTS

Involuntary, painful, and mutilative circumcision surgery of healthy children cannot be classified as therapy since the foreskin being amputated is neither diseased, deformed, nor damaged. To the contrary, circumcision is iatrogenic harm. NOCIRC of Australia has successfully lobbied various legal bodies to review the practice of subjecting children to involuntary, non-therapeutic, mutilative surgery.

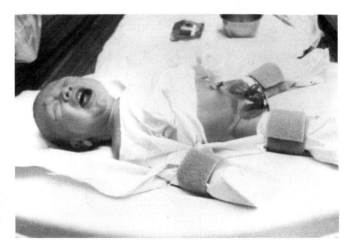

Figure 3. Baby strapped onto an immobilizing restraining board in preparation for circumcision. Penis has been swabbed with disinfectant. (Reprinted by permission of the Saturday Evening Post)

In December 1993, the Queensland Law Reform Commission made a thorough examination of the problem of circumcision. The Commission determined that circumcision could be regarded as a criminal act if the criminal code were strictly interpreted. Specifically, the Commission stated:

> The circumcision procedure is invasive, irreversible, and major. It involves the removal of an otherwise healthy organ part. It has serious attendant risks.

> As a prophylactic procedure, circumcision of neonates does not appear to be the least restrictive alternative. For a number of the adverse health conditions which have been associated with non-circumcised penises, the least restrictive preventative measure would be education of children in genital hygiene and in responsible, safe sexual practices. Circumcision as a prophylactic procedure may be appropriate for older males who have the capacity to consent to the procedure.[2]

> On a strict interpretation of the assault provisions of the Queensland Criminal Code, routine circumcision of a male infant could be regarded as a criminal act. Further, consent by parents

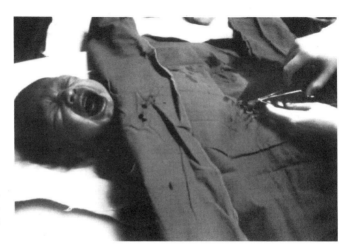

Figure 4. Baby enduring the agony of unanesthetized penile mutilation. (Reprinted by permission of the Saturday Evening Post)

to the procedure may be invalid in light of the common law's restrictions on the ability of parents to consent to the non-therapeutic treatment of children.

The findings of the Queensland Law Reform Commission have been widely published in the Australian medical press as a warning to physicians performing circumcisions that they may be liable to criminal prosecution.[3]

One of Australia's leading academics, Dr. Neville Turner, professor of Law at Monash University and president of the children's welfare group, Oz Child, has recently stated that male circumcision is a breach of human rights and has called for immediate Australia-wide legislation banning it. Dr. Turner states:

> Doctors and nurses who perform circumcision on infants, relying on the consent of the parents, are taking a grave risk. For if it is ultimately declared to be void consent, then it will have constituted an assault, and they could be civilly and criminally liable.[4]

The fundamental code of medical ethics contains the following four inherent principles:

- Autonomy: the right of the individual to make decisions on his own behalf.
- Beneficence: the duty where possible to do good.
- Non-maleficence: the duty not to harm.
- Justice: a broad principle which includes the notion of equity and fair distribution.

Circumcision of healthy children violates all four principles. As the infant and young child are not in a position to make informed decisions, the parents have a special responsibility to act in their children's best interests until they have sufficient maturity to act autonomously. They are then in a position to make a considered choice of elective surgeries, such as circumcision. The alleged health benefits of circumcision — even if they were valid — are too slight to justify involuntarily subjecting individuals to a painful, distressing, irreversible deprivation of the full and normal functions of an intact penis. These alleged benefits do not outweigh the proven risks of morbidity and mortality. Involuntarily subjecting a healthy infant to circumcision unjustifiably denies him the right to alternative treatment, more conservative treatment, or no treatment at all. The injustice is incurred by taking advantage of defenseless healthy infants. This also results in much needed health care resources (money, staff, time) being inappropriately consumed at societal expense.

Circumcision contravenes the *United Nations' Convention on the Rights of the Child,* which Australia ratified in 1990. In Article 3, Australia committed itself to ensure protection and care of children with standards established by competent authorities. Article 24 requires States parties to abolish traditional practices prejudicial to the health of children.

6. CONCLUSIONS

NOCIRC of Australia calls on the medical profession to consider the following:

- There are moral, legal, and economic reasons to call for the abolition of the involuntary circumcision of healthy children. Physicians created the social demand for the practice, and it is their duty of conscience to abolish it.
- Physicians must recognize that the male foreskin is a highly functional and specialized structure integral to the proper functioning of the penis as a whole.

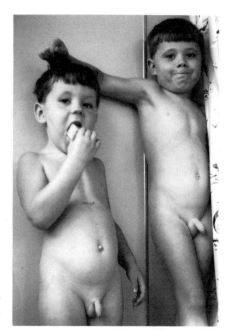

Figure 5. Normal, natural, healthy, intact penises of two hearty Australian boys. (Photography courtesy of Shaun Mather)

- Physicians have a responsibility to refuse to remove normal body parts.
- Physicians need to accept that parents do not have the right to consent to surgical removal or modification of normal male genitalia.
- Physicians need to teach hygiene, the care of normal body parts, and to explain the anatomical, physiological development, and function of the penis throughout life.
- Physicians need to incorporate safe and ethical clinical practices that respect the child's personal right to safety and bodily integrity.

7. REFERENCES

1. Warren JP, Bigelow J. The case against circumcision. British Journal of Sexual Medicine 1994:21:6–8.
2. Circumcision of Male Infants. Queensland Law Reform Commission. Q.L.R.C. R.P. December 1993
3. WN. Is there a legal risk from the foreskin? (letter)Australian Medicine, August 7, 1995:3.
4. Quigley A. Circumcise warning to parents. Herald Sun, March 13, 1996.

21

CIRCUMCISION

Are Baby Boys Entitled to the Same Protection as Baby Girls Regarding Genital Mutilation?

Zenas Baer

It is not the intent of this article to argue that female genital mutilation should be permitted, nor to judge whether female genital mutilation is worse than routine infant male circumcision. The intent of this article is to force American society, parents, insurance industry, and the medical community to address the routine mutilation of males, a procedure done for purely cultural reasons on nonconsenting babies. It is the author's position that the routine mutilation of male or female genitalia for other than medical necessity is a violation of basic human rights. A gender-specific law that does not ban male genital mutilation necessarily violates the guarantee of equal protection of law under the Federal Constitution of the United States.

1. BACKGROUND

The North Dakota Legislature was the first in the nation to pass a law banning female genital mutilation. The law became effective on August 1, 1995, and provides that "any person who knowingly separates or surgically alters normal, healthy functional genital tissue of a female minor is guilty of a Class C felony." There is an exception for the surgical alteration to correct an anatomical abnormality, or to remove diseased tissue that is an immediate threat to the health of the female minor.

North Dakota had previously not been a hot bed for the practice of female genital mutilation. Because of the international outcry and awareness of the brutality of some cultures to the genitalia of both males and females, Duane Voskuil, Ph.D., and Jody McLaughlin were successful in obtaining the passage of the first in the nation ban on female genital mutilation. The initial intent was to have a gender neutral bill enacted. Having run against political opposition to a gender neutral bill, the pair found sufficient support to pass a gender specific bill banning female genital mutilation, a rare procedure in the State of North Dakota. They then decided to challenge the gender specific law on

Sexual Mutilations: A Human Tragedy, edited by Denniston and Milos
Plenum Press, New York, 1997

Federal Constitutional equal protection grounds in United States District Court, for the District of North Dakota.

A lawsuit is currently pending against the State of North Dakota on behalf of a baby boy born after the law went into effect, arguing that the banning of female genital mutilation and not routine infant male circumcision violates the Equal Protection Clause of the Fifth and Fourteenth Amendments of the United States Constitution. Infant males suffer much more systematic and routine mutilation. The following comments will briefly describe the legal analysis under the United States Constitution regarding equal protection of laws in its application to the circumcision issue.

2. THE ISSUE — CIRCUMCISION

In the State of North Dakota, approximately 80% to 90% of all infant males are routinely circumcised. One of the Plaintiffs is an infant boy born after the passage of the female genital mutilation ban. Had the law been gender neutral, the infant boy would have had the same protection infant females have, and he would now be intact. In North Dakota, as in most of America, circumcision is done purely for social, cultural, or religious reasons on nonconsenting, incompetent babies who scream in protest. The rate of circumcision in North Dakota is alarmingly high when compared with the rate for Australia 15%, Canada 20% and Denmark 1%. In the United States alone, over 1.25 million infants annually, more than 3,300 infant males each day, one child every 26 seconds, is subjected to the unnecessary, painful mutilation without benefit of medical indication or consent for purely social or cultural reasons.

Routine male genital mutilation, i.e. "circumcision," as practiced in the United States, began in the late 19th Century to prevent masturbation which was argued to cause insanity. The rationalizations for routine infant male circumcisions have changed over the years. The current rationalizations include: to make sons resemble their circumcised fathers or peers; to improve hygiene (even though the American Academy of Pediatrics says washing is equally as effective without the inherent risks of surgery); to cure phimosis (a condition that cannot be diagnosed during infancy); to lower the incidence of male infant urinary tract infections (though females have three to four times the number of these infections as males, and no scientific studies show this to be a significant issue because this condition can easily be treated medically); to help prevent sexually transmitted diseases, including AIDS (unproven); and to prevent cancer of the penis (yet Denmark, with a male circumcision rate of less than 1%, has a lower rate of penile cancer than the United States; and as many infants die of circumcisions complications as older men die of penile cancer).

Routine circumcision continues in the United States because parents and physicians have not been given adequate information regarding the structure and function of the prepuce. Parents mistakenly believe it is a medical issue and ask physicians for advice. Physicians, who likely have been subjected to circumcision themselves, frequently wish to protect the status quo and their financial self-interest, and, therefore, cannot or do not give adequate information to parents.

Although parents have the right to consent to health care procedures for their incompetent children, they do not have the right to consent to elective surgeries on personal whims (e.g., the removal of an ear lobe would certainly be less damaging to a child and, yet, would certainly be a basis to prosecute a parent for child abuse).

The prepuce is specialized tissue, highly innervated, richly supplied with blood vessels, and uniquely endowed with stretch nerve receptors. The prepuce contributes significantly to the sexual response of the intact male, which can be especially important for sexual satisfaction in the mature male.

The amount of foreskin typically removed during a routine circumcision (more accurately called male genital mutilation), amounts to approximately 50% or more of the skin covering the average adult penile shaft. In the adult male, the foreskin equals approximately 12 to 15 square inches of highly innervated tissue.

The infant male prepuce is normally attached to the glans penis at birth, and may not become retractable until the teenage years. Infant circumcision traumatically interrupts the natural and gradual separation of the foreskin from the glans penis. Tearing the prepuce from the glans penis (forcible retraction), even when not part of an amputation, is considered child abuse by many because it is extremely painful and there is no medical reason for this painful procedure, which harms the glans penis and can introduce infection. Circumcision interferes with the natural, anatomical development of the penis (that part which is not amputated), since the circumciser tears the preputial mucosa from the glans penis as part of the amputation. This procedure scarifies, and eventually hardens and desensitizes, the glans penis.

Routine infant male circumcision is a form of genital mutilation which removes a vital, anatomical structure and functioning body part and leaves permanent scarring of the skin shaft and the glans penis. It changes the brain structure by imposing pain on a primary pleasure center. This procedure violates the physician's oath for the care of patients: First, do no harm.

The unnecessary mutilation of the genitals of females and males in the name of tradition, custom, or any other nonpathologic reason should not be accepted by conscientious health-care professionals. It breaches the fundamental code of medical ethics. Children too young to give consent must be treated as other incompetent individuals. Elective circumcision procedures should be performed only when the individual affected can give informed consent at the age of majority. Circumcisions done for medical reasons must meet the same criteria as any amputation. If there is a question of medical necessity, the circumcision should only be done upon the appointment of a guardian ad litem and with a Court's permission.

All routine childhood circumcisions, or separations of genital structures in females or males, are violations of fundamental human rights. It is the moral, and often the legal duty of all, but especially professionals, to protect the health and rights of those with little or no social power to protect themselves. A circumcision is an assault on an individual's sexuality, and a violation of his natural right to an intact body.

A law which bans female genital mutilation and allows the rampant routine mutilation of males violates the equal protection clause of the United States Constitution.

3. LEGAL ANALYSIS

Equal protection analysis often begins with the explanation offered in the classic article on the subject, Tussman and tenBroek, *The Equal Protection of the Laws*, 37 Cal L. Rev. 341 (1949). Tussman and tenBroek explained that the fundamental tension in equal protection analysis is that between the pledge of "equal laws" protecting all, and the fact that virtually every law nevertheless treats persons unequally. Nearly every statute commands that some category of persons be treated differently from others, and the equal protection principle does not forbid all legislative classification. The task of the Court is that of distinguishing legislative classifications that violate equality from those that do not.

Tussman and tenBroek famously explain as follows:

> The Court...has resolved the contradictory demands of legislative specialization and constitu-
> tional generality by a doctrine of reasonable classification...The Constitution does not require
> that things different in fact be treated in law as though they were the same. But it does require,
> in its concern for equality, that those who are similarly situated be similarly treated. The
> measure of the reasonableness of a classification is the degree of its success in treating simi-
> larly those similarly situated...[W]here are we to look for the test of similarity of situation
> which determines the reasonableness of a classification? The inescapable answer is that we
> must look beyond the classification to the purpose of the law. A reasonable classification is
> one which includes all persons who are similarly situated with respect to the purpose of the
> law...

The question of whether the legislature has denied the equal protection of the laws
cannot be answered in the abstract. The Court must always compare the reach of the classification used with the actual scope of the problem at which the law aims. And we can
only know what that problem is by examining the actual or purported purpose the law is
designed to serve. As Tussman and tenBroek put it, the question of equal protection is a
question of the degree of "fit" between the area actually occupied by the "Mischief"
aimed at, and that occupied by persons displaying the "Trait" used to define the legislative
category.

Unavoidably, however, the "fit" between the legislative classificatory means and the
substantive legislative ends, between what the legislature has aimed at and what it has hit,
will be imperfect. The Court has determined that permitting legislatures to use some classifications poses a much greater threat to the ideal of equal protection of the laws than permitting the use of others. Much of the work in deciding cases, therefore, tends to occur at
the outset of the analysis, in the course of determining what "level of scrutiny" the Court
will apply to the law. In part, this inquiry is a matter of how tight the "fit" must be between the harm and the classification before the Court will strike it down. The reason for
the adoption of the various levels of scrutiny, however, is the product of social and historical factors rather than the logical relation of means to ends.

Some classifications, for these reasons, are particularly threatening to the ideal of
equality before the law. Specifically, the desire to outlaw legal classification by race was
the obvious and explicit goal of the equal protection clause. Indeed, the Court's early
cases suggested that this was the sole import of the clause. In the *Slaughter-House Cases*,
83 U.S. (16 Wall.) 36, 81 (1873), competing butchers of the New Orleans slaughter-house
monopoly argued in part under the equal protection clause that they had been discriminated against by the grant of an exclusive monopoly to others. Justice Miller for the Court
gave that claim short shrift, and "doubt[ed]...whether any action of a State not directed by
way of discrimination against the Negroes as a class, or on account of their race, [would]
ever be held to come within the purview of the [clause]."

There has often been speculation that this limited and hostile view of equal protection was in part the result of the "floodgate" of such arguments the Court worried would
be opened by an expansive reading of the command of equal protection. That fear, speculation suggests, was in part dramatized from the Court's point of view by a troublesome
claim presented earlier that same term. In *Bradwell v. Illinois*, 83 U.S. (16 Wall.) 130
(1872), the Court faced a claim that Illinois' prohibition on the practice of law by women
violated this "equal protection" idea as well. The Court rejected the claim, and Justice
Bradley's concurrence has become famous. "Man is, or should be, woman's protector and
defender...The paramount destiny and mission of woman are to fulfill the noble and be-

nign offices of wife and mother. This is the law of the Creator." *Id.* at 151 (Bradley, J., concurring).

Although claims of sex discrimination are much more warmly welcomed under the modern equal protection clause, the Court has continued to hold that sex discrimination is different from race discrimination. This continued difference in treatment is in part based on the history of the equal protection clause, but also because the Court has felt that the real differences between the sexes make the blanket condemnation of "strict scrutiny" inappropriate. On the other hand, the dangers that legislatures may often deny equal liberty to persons of both genders based on their sex, often in the guise of granting special benefits to women, has led the Court to reject the relaxed "rational basis" test applied to equal protection claims in the economic realm.

Beginning with *Craig v. Boren*, 429 U.S. 190, 197 (1976), the Court has held that legislative classifications based on gender are subject to "intermediate scrutiny." As the Court described this approach in *Craig*, "[t]o withstand constitutional challenge...classifications by gender must serve important governmental objectives and must be substantially related to achievement of those objectives." *Id.* There is some indication that this test is undergoing some at least verbal tightening with the very recent Court decision *United States v. Virginia*, 64 U.S.L.W. 4638 (June 25, 1996). There, Justice Ginsburg for the Court stated repeatedly that "[p]arties who seek to defend gender-based government action must demonstrate an 'exceedingly persuasive justification' for the action." *United States v. Virginia*, 64 U.S.L.W. at 4640; 4642; 4643, quoting *Mississippi Univ. for Women v. Hogan*, 458 U.S. 718, 724 (1982) (O'Connor, J.). Chief Rehnquist suggested in concurrence that prior cases have only used this phrase to describe the difficulty of satisfying the intermediate scrutiny standard, and that the majority opinion seemed to make this showing an element of the test itself. *Id.* at 4640 (Rehnquist, C.J., concurring); see *United States v. Virginia*, 64 U.S.L.W. at 4643 ("we conclude that Virginia has shown no 'exceedingly persuasive justification' for excluding all women from the citizen soldier training afforded by VMI").

What the recent case also emphasizes, however, is one that must be constantly born in mind. The question is not merely whether the *law* substantially serves the important government objectives. The question is whether the *discrimination* the law engenders does so. Thus the Court repeatedly states that for a gender classification to stand, "[t]he State must show 'at least that the [challenged] classification serves important governmental objectives and *that the discriminatory means* employed are substantially related to the achievement of those objectives.'" *Virginia*, 64 U.S.L.W. at 4643, quoting *Hogan*, 458 U.S. at 724 (emphasis added). The State may not pass this test by simply showing that its law is reasonably designed to serve some important end and does so. The State must show that the discrimination itself is justified, and justified on the ground that the chosen "discriminatory means" themselves substantially serve the important interests alleged in its support.

The gender cases differ from the race cases in another way. This aspect is emphasized by Professor Tribe. *See* Lawrence Tribe *Constitutional Law* 1464–68 (2d ed. 1988). Unlike racially discriminatory laws, which are often based on simple hostility, sexually discriminatory laws are often based on or justified by a paternalistic desire to favor or "protect" women. For this reason, gender discrimination suits are often brought by men, and the goal is not to strike down the law but to *require its extension* to the plaintiffs. These cases include *Frontiero v. Richardson*, 411 U.S. 677 (1973), decided under the equal protection strand of the Fifth Amendment, in which the Court struck down a legislative presumption that all spouses of males were dependent but requiring all spouses of females to prove dependency. The plurality stated that the scheme was one of "romantic paternalism," and that it operated to "put women not on a pedestal, but in a case." The Court in *Weinberger v. Wiesenfeld*, 420 U.S. 636 (1975), threw out a section of the Social Security Act that awarded survivor's benefits to widows but not widowers responsible for dependant children. The Court found that the purpose of the law was to enable the surviving parent to remain at home to care for the child, and that in light of this objective the gender-based classification was "entirely irrational." It is no less important for a child to be cared for by its sole surviving parent when that parent is male rather than female."

And in *Stanton v. Stanton*, 421 U.S. 7 (1975), a case with interesting implications here, the Court held that Utah could not impose a parental support obligation for daughters until age 18, but for sons until age 21. "[A] child, male or female, is still a child...If a specific age of minority is required for the boy in order to assure him parental support while he attains his education and training, so, too, it is for the girl. To distinguish between the two on educational grounds is to be self-serving...[and] coincides with the role-typing society has long imposed."

In *California v. Goldfarb*, 430 U.S. 199 (1977), the Court invalidated a Social Security provision that paid survivor benefits to widowers only if they could prove substantial reliance on the deceased's income, but to widows without that proof, the Court stated that administrative convenience and sexual stereotyping were the only bases for the legislative presumption. Justice Stevens emphasized in his concurrence that unexamined and unjustified assumptions are particularly likely to be the real reason for the distinctive treatment in gender cases. "It is fair to infer that habit, rather than analysis or actual reflection, made it seem acceptable to equate the terms 'widow' and 'dependent surviving spouse.' That kind of automatic reflex is far different from...a legislative decision to favor females in order to compensate past wrongs."

Professor Tribe emphasizes that blacks were the intended beneficiaries of the equal protection clause because they were a subjugated race. He argues, however, that the fact that men are often the beneficiaries of decisions striking so-called "benign" sex discrimination "is immaterial to choosing the proper standard for evaluating legislative reinforcement of restrictive sex roles. For while our laws and institutions no longer value distinctive race roles, they still promote — with vast popular support — restrictive gender roles." Tribe, *supra* at 1569. Men in these cases can legitimately argue that these popular presumptions and prejudices burden the liberty of everyone, men as well as women, and that breaking down legislatively-reinforced gender categories offers "enhanced liberty opportunity, and power for both sexes." *Id.* at 1570.

It is, in part, the very popularity of gender-based prejudices that makes them the likely *source* of gender-biased laws. Justice Stevens has several times emphasized this, stating that it is usually "habit rather than analysis" which underlies such differential treatment of the genders. But the mere reinforcement of "habit" or prejudice is not by itself an "important governmental interest" that the State may pursue, let alone by the sort of explicit gender-based differential treatment found here. No doubt the Court in *Bradwell* thought it obvious that social habit or prejudice was sufficient to allow Illinois to prohibit women from practicing law. But that is no longer an acceptable reason for gender-based classifications.

It is the *discrimination*, not the law, that must be "substantially related" to the important interest in suit. Plainly, the State of North Dakota has a powerful interest in preventing the genital mutilation of minor females. That is not enough, however, to justify explicit gender discrimination. The discrimination itself must substantially serve the State's important interest. The discriminatory *denial* of equal protection against this procedure to infant males does nothing whatever to advance the State's interest in protecting females.

The State of North Dakota, of course, will disagree. But assuming the truth of the factual claims that the routine genital mutilation of boys has no more medical justification than it would have for girls, *all* of the State's justifications must draw support from precisely the habits and prejudices that it is the function of gender discrimination scrutiny to question. It will not do, for example, for the State to justify this discrimination on the ground that widespread popular support for the genital mutilation of boys and not girls made this law politically attractive. To allow the legislature to reinforce gender-based prejudices based on the widespread nature of gender-based prejudices is the most blatant sort of bootstrapping. See especially *Stanton v. Stanton*, 421 U.S. 7 (1975). The point of heightened scrutiny is to put such "habits" of thinking and "automatic reflexes" *themselves* under scrutiny. The fact that the discrimination here reflects and reinforces such unquestioned stereotyping is a reason to strike this law down, not to uphold it.

22

ROUTINE INFANT MALE CIRCUMCISION

Examining the Human Rights and Constitutional Issues

J. Steven Svoboda

1. INTRODUCTION

Human rights agreements—applicable either through ratification or through customary law—forbid circumcision based on such important principles as the rights of the child, the right to freedom of religion, the right to the highest attainable standard of health, and the right to protection against torture. Cultural blindness facilitates the perpetuation of many barbaric and/or egregiously discriminatory practices and conditions. The many laws against female sexual mutilation, and the discriminatory failure to outlaw and vilify male sexual mutilation, violate equal protection under both international human rights law and American legal doctrines.

1.1. Customary Law and Human Rights Agreements

Although the recent ratification of certain human rights documents has ameliorated its position somewhat, the United States has long been regarded as an outlaw by the human rights community. Among other considerations, this reputation may be attributed to tardiness and/or failure to sign and/or ratify a number of documents which have been widely accepted around the world, including the *International Covenant on Economic, Social and Cultural Rights*, the *Convention on the Rights of the Child* and until relatively recently, the *International Covenant on Civil and Political Rights*. The constitutional requirement that any ratification must be approved by the Senate has facilitated the United States' frequent failure to endorse widely-accepted human rights treaties.

Nevertheless, under well-recognized principles of international law, human rights agreements and other international laws may be widely enough observed by the community of nations to acquire the status of customary law. Customary law is applicable to all states regardless of whether they have themselves actually ratified the document in question. Therefore, the United States' failure to ratify certain human rights agreements does

Sexual Mutilations: A Human Tragedy, edited by Denniston and Milos
Plenum Press, New York, 1997

not necessarily insulate us from liability for violations of internationally recognized human rights as set forth in those documents.

2. HUMAN RIGHTS PRINCIPLES FORBID INFANT CIRCUMCISION

Well recognized human rights principles forbid circumcision, and all other forms of male sexual mutilation, as a human rights violation.

2.1. Reasons for Concern with Infant Male Circumcision

Reasons for concern with the procedure under human rights principles include a profound loss of highly specialized and sensitive sexual tissue, which also serves important protective functions, loss of bodily integrity, traumatic and highly painful disfigurement, complications with a range of severity up to and including death, and the impermissibility of any mutilation of children's sexual organs performed with neither their consent nor medical justification.

2.2. Circumcision Prohibited by Several Human Rights Documents

Several United Nations resolutions, conventions and declarations appear to forbid routine infant male circumcision. These prohibitions are based on such critical rights as the rights of the child, the right to freedom of religion, the right to the highest attainable standard of health, and the right to protection against torture.

2.2.1. Rights of the Child. The *Convention on the Rights of the Child* imposes various obligations which are violated by male sexual mutilation, including sexual abuse, torture, interference with privacy, the right to safety while under the care of a parent or guardian, and the right to health.

2.2.2. Male Sexual Mutilation Prohibited under Provisions Regarding Sexual Abuse, Torture, and Interference with Privacy. Article 34 of the *Convention on the Rights of the Child* requires states parties to protect the child from all forms of sexual exploitation and sexual abuse, and Article 36 further obliges states parties to protect the child against all other forms of exploitation prejudicial to any aspects of the child's welfare.[1] Article 37(a) of the *Convention on the Rights of the Child* forbids subjecting any child to torture or other cruel, inhuman or degrading treatment or punishment. Article 16 bars arbitrary or unlawful interference with a child's privacy, and gives children the right to the law's protection against such interference. The *Declaration of the Rights of the Child* also stipulates that children must be protected against all forms of cruelty, neglect, and exploitation.[2] Current practice of governments, such as the United States, which permit, encourage, and even arrange for circumcision are clearly and grossly in violation of all of these provisions.

2.2.3. Child's Right to Safety While under Care of Parent or Guardian Is Violated by Circumcision. Article 19.1 of the *Convention on the Rights of the Child* provides that states parties must take all measures to insure that no violence, injury, or abuse occurs while the child is under the care of a parent or legal guardian. A parent's or guardian's consent cannot justify a non-medically necessary procedure such as circumcision. Only the consent of the individual himself can permit such an operation, and no infant is capable of providing such a consent.[3]

2.2.4. Child's Right to Health Is Violated by Procedure. Article 24 of the *Convention on the Rights of the Child* addresses health issues. Section 1 obliges states parties to recognize the child's right to enjoy the highest attainable standard of health. Similarly, Section 2 of Article 24 requires states parties to pursue full implementation of the child's right to enjoy the highest attainable health standard and to take appropriate measures, *inter alia*, to diminish infant and child mortality. These guarantees are violated where a medically unnecessary and extremely painful alteration of an infant male's sexual organs is performed, subjecting the child to the risk of complications and possible death. Section 3 requires states parties to take all effective and appropriate measures with a view to abolishing traditional practices prejudicial to the health of children. Article 24.1 of the *International Covenant on Civil and Political Rights* provides that every child shall have, without any discrimination as to, *inter alia*, sex, the right to such measures of protection as are required by his status as a minor, on the part of his family, society and the state.[4]

2.3. Freedom of Religion Does Not Justify Procedure

The right of freedom of religion does not justify circumcision.

2.3.1. Children Bear Independent Right to Freedom of Religion. Children bear their own right to freedom of religion, independent of the wishes of their parents or guardians. Under Article 14.1 of the *Convention on the Rights of the Child,* children have the right to demand that states parties respect their right to freedom of thought, conscience, and religion. No infant is capable of consenting to a surgical procedure based on his own religion. Where the procedure is one based on religion, it is the parent's religion which motivates the procedure and not the religion of the person whose sexual organs are being surgically altered. Children subjected to sexual mutilation have neither asked for nor consented to the procedure. A parent's consent is therefore, again, clearly insufficient.[5]

2.3.2. Exception to Freedom of Religion Applies Here. Moreover, even if religion did somehow justify the procedure, which it clearly does not, identical language in Article 14.3 of the *Convention on the Rights of the Child*, Article 18.3 of the *International Covenant on Civil and Political Rights* and Article 12.3 of the *American Convention on Human Rights* very clearly provides that an exception to the requirement to permit freedom of conscience and religion arises where such freedom, if exercised, would result in violating the public safety, order, health, or morals, or the fundamental rights and freedoms of another human being. A traumatic disfigurement of a nonconsenting baby's sexual organs should qualify as such a violation under this exception. Therefore, human rights principles forbid the mutilation.

2.4. Treaties Prohibiting Torture Apply to Circumcision

Treaties prohibiting torture, including the *Convention Against Torture* and the *Declaration Against Torture*, also prohibit routine infant male circumcision.

2.4.1. Definition of Torture. The *Convention Against Torture* — ratified by the United States — defines torture as, *inter alia*, any act by which severe pain or suffering, physical or mental, is intentionally inflicted on a person, with the consent or acquiescence of or at the instigation of a public official.[6] The *Declaration Against Torture* holds torture to be an aggravated and deliberate form of cruel, inhuman or degrading treatment or punishment which violates the human rights and fundamental freedoms proclaimed in the *Universal Declaration of Human Rights*.[7]

2.4.2. Circumcision Constitutes Torture. Ecumenics International, which, as discussed below, is currently working closely with the United Nations to combat sexual mutilation, notes that, whether performed on male or female persons:

> Genital mutilation is a traditional practice of physiological torture and psychological trauma destroying reproductive integrity and sexual health with significant risks of death.[8]

No objective observer who has witnessed a circumcision can seriously dispute that the procedure inflicts severe pain or suffering on the child. Circumcision does constitute torture.

2.4.3. United States Routinely Violates Torture Treaties. The United States routinely violates the *Convention Against Torture* and the *Declaration Against Torture*. Article 2.1 of the *Convention Against Torture* obliges a state party to take effective legislative, administrative, judicial, or other measures to prevent acts of torture in any territory under its jurisdiction, and Article 2.2 adds that no exceptional circumstances whatsoever may justify the torture. Articles 4.1 and 4.2 of the *Convention Against Torture* state that any act of torture is a criminal offense which states parties must punish. Obviously the United States is not in compliance with these provisions: Its laws permit the procedure, and many circumcisions are initiated, promoted, allowed, and/or paid for by public health officials and/or performed in public hospitals. Furthermore, state obligations regarding circumcision extend to *all* procedures, whether or not performed with direct government participation. Article 3 of the *Declaration Against Torture* prohibits any state from permitting or tolerating torture or other cruel, inhuman and degrading treatment or punishment. The United States, by failing to take action against circumcision, as well as by subsidizing and performing the procedure, is also violating this article.

Without being explicitly defined, torture is also forbidden under Article 5 of the *Universal Declaration of Human Rights*, which we have ratified, Article 7 of the *International Covenant on Civil and Political Rights*, which the United States recently ratified, and under Article 37(a) of the *Convention on the Rights of the Child,* which we have signed but not ratified.

3. CULTURAL BLINDNESS AND CIRCUMCISION

Lawsuits and political activism play different, yet equally invaluable, roles in effecting social change. Law generally follows the current of society and does not commonly serve as the leader of dramatic social transformation. Judges rarely use their bench as a platform from which to hurl themselves into the vanguard, preferring to respond to well-established social trends. This was true, for example, with the civil rights and women's rights movements, in which activists worked for many years to lay the political groundwork, which later supported legal strategies that ultimately led to judicial acknow-ledgment of previously unimaginable rights.

Each court will naturally — almost necessarily — view all issues it addresses through a set of filters derived from that society's particular social and cultural prejudices. American judges, for instance, will base their decisions, in part, on society's almost un-conscious biases, of which ample historical and current evidence exists. Throughout the history of the United States, various horrors have been enshrined and endorsed by the laws of the United States, including slavery, "separate but equal" facilities for whites and blacks, and the disenfranchisement of all women and all non-property-owning men. Today in America, women's and men's differing socializations are reinforced by discriminatory child custody and divorce decisions.[9] This anti-male gender discrimination harms both men and women by reinforcing the presumption and perception that men's proper role is as a non-child-rearing wage-earner and women's proper role is in the home taking care of children. Such stereotypes limit the opportunities for each one of us to aspire to our full human potential.

Cultural blindness around the world has played a strong role in a broad range of body mutilations and, more specifically, sexual mutilation practices. In the United States, differing socialization and perceptions of men and women have enabled the passage of laws addressing female sexual mutilation but not male sexual mutilation. Cultural blind-ness frequently colors perceptions of human rights issues. The United States has come to tolerate altering baby boys' sexual organs in this manner. Throughout history, a broad range of body mutilation practices have been accepted, including footbinding, placing growing children in vases so that their bones would be bent to the shape of the vase, and many other forms of sexual mutilation of both sexes. As with infant male circumcision, all these practices have been carried out without the victim's consent.

4. LAWS AGAINST FEMALE SEXUAL MUTILATION, WHICH FAIL TO OUTLAW MALE SEXUAL MUTILATION, VIOLATE EQUAL PROTECTION UNDER BOTH HUMAN RIGHTS LAW AND THE UNITED STATES CONSTITUTION

Laws against female sexual mutilation that do not simultaneously prohibit male sex-ual mutilation contravene principles of equal protection enshrined in human rights law. Statutes passed by the federal government of the United States or by individual American states also violate the requirement of equal protection under the United States Constitu-tion.

4.1. Numerous Laws Forbid Only Female Sexual Mutilation

Various countries, states, and provinces have passed statutes which prohibit only fe-male sexual mutilation and do not address male sexual mutilation.

4.1.1. Federal Law in the United States. In the United States, as public and legisla-tive awareness regarding the horrors of female sexual mutilation has grown, a number of provisions regarding female sexual mutilation became law in 1995 and 1996. At the fed-eral level, a law was passed in 1996 providing that female sexual mutilation of a minor is a felony punishable by a fine of up to $250,000 and/or imprisonment for not more than five years.[10] Another new federal statute requires the Immigration and Naturalization Service to make available to all aliens who are issued immigrant or non-immigrant visas from countries where female sexual mutilation is commonly practiced information on harm caused by female sexual mutilation and information concerning potential legal consequences in the United States of performing or allowing female sexual mutilation.[11] A third federal law, passed in 1996, requires the Secretary of Health and Human Services to compile data on the number of victims of female sexual mutilation residing in the United States, including the number of minors, in order to identify communities practicing female sexual mutilation and then to carry out an outreach and education program regarding the health effects of female sexual mutilation, and to develop recommendations for education of medical students regarding female sexual mutilation.[12]

4.1.2. State Laws in the United States. This same year, California passed a law providing that female sexual mutilation of a minor is punishable by imprisonment in state prison for up to two, four, or eight years.[13] Delaware has declared female sexual mutilation of a minor a Class C felony punishable by imprisonment for up to ten years.[14] Minnesota passed a statute classifying sexual mutilation of *any* female as a felony punishable by imprisonment for more than one year.[15] California and Minnesota both enacted second laws directing their respective state departments of health services to establish and implement education, prevention, and outreach activities in communities that traditionally practice female sexual mutilation, to inform community members about the health risks and emotional trauma inflicted by this practice and informing them and the medical community of the criminal penalties.[16] North Dakota's law defines female sexual mutilation of a minor as a Class C felony punishable by up to five years imprisonment and/or a fine of up to $5,000.[17] Rhode Island passed a statute defining sexual mutilation of *any* female as felony assault, punishable by imprisonment for not more than *twenty* years, the stiffest maximum penalty in any jurisdiction.[18] Tennessee outlawed sexual mutilation of *any* female as a Class D felony punishable by not less than two nor not more than twelve years imprisonment and in addition a discretionary fine not to exceed $5,000.[19] Wisconsin created a criminal law that holds female sexual mutilation of a minor punishable by a fine of not more than $10,000 or imprisonment for not more than five years or both.[20]

4.1.3. Statutes in Other Countries. Other countries have crafted legislation to prohibit female sexual mutilation. In Egypt, the practice was banned by President Nasser in 1958.[21] Kenya banned female sexual mutilation under legislation passed in 1990.[22] New Zealand has passed a law barring and punishing by imprisonment for up to seven years the sexual mutilation of *any* female or the arranging for a child to be removed from New Zealand for the purposes of performing female sexual mutilation.[23] In the Sudan, legislation dating from 1946 bans infibulation but permits *sunnah*.[24] Sweden banned health professionals from performing female sexual mutilation in 1982.[25] The United Kingdom outlawed sexual mutilation of *any* female in 1985,[26] subsequently providing for the investigation of suspected violations and enabling the removal of a child from her home where this is the only way that her protection can be guaranteed.[27]

4.1.4. Statutes in Other Provinces. New South Wales in Australia has outlawed the sexual mutilation of *any* female and declared it punishable by imprisonment for up to seven years.[28] Although the Civil Code of Quebec does not explicitly criminalize either female sexual mutilation or male sexual mutilation, both practices should be illegal under provisions outlawing the removal of tissue from an unconsenting individual.[29] Moreover, a person who gives consent to care for another person must act in that person's sole interest, ensuring that any care for which consent is given is beneficial, advisable in the circumstances and that the risks incurred are not disproportionate to the anticipated benefit.[30] Finally, Article 19 provides that a minor incapable of giving consent may have a part of his body alienated only if that part is capable of regeneration and provided that no serious risk to his health results, both requirements which are violated by infant circumcision.[31]

4.2. Proposed Legislation Also Forbids Only Female Sexual Mutilation

A number of other countries and states have proposed legislation outlawing female sexual mutilation while not addressing male sexual mutilation. Canada's Criminal Code currently prohibits the removal of children normally resident in Canada from Canada with the intention of committing assault causing bodily harm, aggravated assault or any sexual offense.[32] While this law has a more general scope, it was passed in response to a concern that Canadian law did not contain sufficient protections against female sexual mutilation. Pending legislation would outlaw sexual mutilation of *any* female.[33] A pending bill in Illinois would classify sexual mutilation of *any* female as a Class X felony,[34] punishable by imprisonment for not less than six and not more than thirty years,[35] and by a fine of up to $10,000.[36] Legislation against female sexual mutilation has been defeated in Colorado,[37] New York,[38] South Carolina,[39] and Texas.[40]

4.3. State Laws Grant Circumcisers Special Exceptions

Other statutes actually accord circumcisers special exceptions and protections.

4.3.1. Ritual Abuse Laws Exempt Male Circumcision. Ritual abuse laws in California,[41] Idaho,[42] and Illinois[43] specifically exempt male circumcision. The need to mention circumcision and circumcisers in such statutes is certainly intriguing, to say the least. If there were no potential for male circumcision to be considered ritual abuse, then these laws would be utterly superfluous. They suggest that the legislators tacitly recognized the reasonableness — in the absence of the statutory loophole — of classifying circumcision as abusive, unethical, and/or inhuman.

4.3.2. Medical Licensing Laws Exempt Mohels Performing Male Circumcision. Medical licensing laws specifically exempt mohels for the purposes of performing male circumcision in Delaware,[44] Minnesota,[45] Montana,[46] and Wisconsin.[47] Of course, regulations and/or official tolerance permits mohels to perform the procedure in all fifty of the states, despite arguably being no more defensible under human rights or constitutional principles than are the statutory exemptions. The reprehensible double standard implicit in legislation addressing only the mutilation of one gender strikes a particular noxious note here. All three states which see fit to enshrine at the statutory level the mohels' special authorization to mutilate males have simultaneously passed laws barring female sexual mutilation.

4.4. Laws against Female Sexual Mutilation Violate Equal Protection under International Human Rights Law

No law anywhere in the world currently outlaws male sexual mutilation, either alone or in combination with a prohibition of female sexual mutilation. On the other hand, as we have seen, many statutes and proposed laws prohibit only female sexual mutilation, and others grant special protections and exceptions regarding male circumcision.

By only safeguarding females against involuntary alteration of their sexual organs, while doing nothing to protect males, laws against female sexual mutilation by definition discriminate against males. Arguably, such laws are worse than no laws at all in suggesting, through their exclusive attention to female sexual mutilation, that male sexual mutilation is a permissible and unobjectionable practice. Statutes granting special exceptions only to circumcisers of males but not to those who sexually mutilate females also clearly discriminate against males. Such laws highlight the artificiality of the culturally-based special treatment of male circumcision in the United States.

Both laws against female sexual mutilation and special statutory exceptions for male circumcision directly conflict with Article 7 of the *Universal Declaration of Human Rights*, which states:

> All are equal before the law and are entitled without any discrimination to equal protection of the law. All are entitled to equal protection against any discrimination in violation of the *Declaration* and against any incitement to such discrimination.

Therefore, a human rights violation occurs where males are discriminated against by not enjoying legal protection from sexual mutilation which is enjoyed by females. Countries, states and provinces must amend these laws, regulations, and practices to protect males as well as females from sexual mutilation.

Under Article 7 of the *Universal Declaration of Human Rights*, states cannot rest in confidence that they are violating no laws once they have amended discriminatory anti-female sexual mutilation laws to include men within their scope. Even where the state is not the mutilator, a human rights violation also occurs where males do not receive equal protection from sexual mutilation applied in a discriminatory manner, e.g., through predominant or exclusive mutilation of their gender. Worldwide, five out of six victims of sexual mutilation are male.[48] Males are entitled to equal protection against such discrimination wherever it occurs and against any incitement to such discrimination. States are thus obligated to do more than merely eliminate all their gender-specific laws against sexual mutilation. States also carry a positive obligation to apply their resources to protect males as well as females against sexual mutilation practices that are discriminatorily applied to males (or to females) and to stop anyone attempting to bring about such discriminatory sexual mutilation.

4.5. Laws against Female Sexual Mutilation Violate Equal Protection under American Law

A natural question which arises in considering the flurry of legislative activity this year against female sexual mutilation in the United States is whether the criminalization of the alteration of only female sexual organs — while not addressing male sexual mutilation — can survive Constitutional scrutiny. The answer is clearly "No." In addition to the human rights considerations discussed above, in the United States, the dramatically unequal treatment of males and females arising from the statutory prohibitions of only female sexual mutilation also violates equal protection, a basic principle enshrined in the Fifth Amendment of the *Constitution of the United States*. Since 1976, legislative classifications based on gender have been subject to an "intermediate scrutiny," which is less demanding than that accorded to classifications based on race or ethnic origin or sometimes alienage, comparable to the level of scrutiny of illegitimacy classifications, and more rigorous than the "rational basis scrutiny" attached to most other classifications. One recent Supreme Court decision suggests that the gap is narrowing between intermediate and strict scrutiny.[49] Justice Ginsburg wrote for the Court, emphasizing repeatedly that, "[P]arties who seek to defend gender-based government action must demonstrate an 'exceedingly persuasive justification' for the action."[50] The state is required to show, not only that the law substantially serves the important governmental objectives, but also that "the discriminatory means employed are substantially related to the achievement of those objectives."[51] On this basis, an equal protection lawsuit against the North Dakota female sexual mutilation law has been initiated.[52]

Unfortunately, due in part to American cultural blindness, male sexual mutilation is not viewed in the same way as female sexual mutilation. North Dakota activists against female sexual mutilation and male sexual mutilation began their attempts to institute legislative change on these issues by lobbying state legislators to pass a law banning sexual mutilation of both males and females. When it became clear that insufficient support existed for this proposed bill, the activists threw their support behind a bill banning female sexual mutilation only, planning on initiating an anti-discrimination lawsuit as soon as the ink had dried on the female-only sexual mutilation legislation.

4.6. Female-Only Sexual Mutilation Legislation Is Not Justified

One frequent justification for legislation addressing only female sexual mutilation is the supposedly dramatic contrast in degree between the severity of female sexual mutilation and male sexual mutilation. Since recent research documents that circumcision removes at least half of the skin of the penis,[53] this suggestion is certainly questionable. In a widely noted article, three researchers recently found that an average circumcision removes 51% of a male's penile skin. The long-term physical, sexual and psychological harm caused by the procedure has never been investigated because of the underlying and erroneous assumptions that the procedure is benign. Political history — notably that of women — and human rights principles alike should eloquently remind us to resist any temptation to create hierarchies of rights and then to argue that we need not or cannot now address the abuses we have placed lower in our hierarchy.

5. CONCLUSION

Laws against female sexual mutilation and laws granting circumcisers special legal loopholes are clearly vulnerable under constitutional and human rights principles. Only cultural blindness has so far insulated doctors, hospitals, mohels, parents, and other responsible parties from liability under a broad range of legal theories. No basis in international human rights law or domestic law of the United States justifies the discriminatory prohibition of only female sexual mutilation.

A number of human rights documents — whether ratified or applicable under principles of customary international law — forbid routine infant male circumcision. Statutes in a number of states and countries that outlaw female sexual mutilation but not male sexual mutilation or that grant special exceptions and protections to male circumcisers violate equal protection under both international and domestic United States law.

6. REFERENCES

1. Convention on the Rights of the Child. UN GA resolution 44/25, November 20, 1989.
2. Declaration of the Rights of the Child. UN GA resolution 1386 [XIV], November 20, 1959, Principle 9.
3. Dwyer J. Parent's religion and children's welfare: debunking the doctrine of parent's rights. California Law Review 1994;82:1371–227.
4. International Covenant on Civil and Political Rights. UN GA resolution 2200 A [XXI]. December 16, 1966.
5. Dwyer J. Parent's religion and children's welfare: debunking the doctrine of parent's rights. California Law Review 1994;82:1371–227.
6. Convention Against Torture and Other Cruel, Inhuman or Degrading Treatment of Punishment. UN GA resolution 39/46, December 10, 1984, Article 1.
7. Declaration on the Protection of All Persons from Being Subjected to Torture, and Other Cruel, Inhuman or Degrading Treatment or Punishment. UN GA resolution 3452 [XXX], December 9, 1975, Articles 1.2 and 2.
8. Ecumenics International. News Release: Ad Hoc Working Group of International Experts on Violations of Genital Mutilation. Sloatsburg, New York: Ecumenics International July 1, 1995.
9. Kimbrell A. The Masculine Mystique. New York: Ballantine Books, 1995:145–7.
10. 18 United States Code §§ 116, 1, 3571 (b) (3)
11. 104th Congress, 1st Session, House of Representatives Bill 2202.
12. 104th Congress, 2nd Session, House of Representatives Bill 3019 (e) (1).
13. California Penal Code § 273.4
14. Delaware Code Title 11, §§ 1113, 4205 (b) (3) (date of enactment July 3, 1996).
15. Minnesota Statutes §§ 609.2245, 609.02.
16. California Health and Safety Code § 124170; Minnesota Criminal Code § 144.3872.
17. North Dakota Criminal Code §§ 12.1–36–01, 12.1–32–01.4.
18. Rhode Island General Laws § 11–5–2 (date of enactment July 3, 1996).
19. Tennessee Code Annotated §§ 39–13–857, 40–35–111 (b) (4).
20. 1995 Wisconsin Act 365 (date of enactment May 28, 1996).
21. Australia Family Law Council. Female Genital Mutilation: A Report to the Attorney-General Prepared by the Family Law Council. Canberra, Australia: Commonwealth of Australia, June 1994:70.
22. Australia Family Law Council. Female Genital Mutilation: A Report to the Attorney-General Prepared by the Family Law Council. Canberra, Australia: Commonwealth of Australia, June 1994:70.
23. Crimes Act 1961, as amended 1995, 204a and 204b.
24. Australia Family Law Council. Female Genital Mutilation: A Report to the Attorney-General Prepared by the Family Law Council. Canberra, Australia: Commonwealth of Australia, June 1994:70.
25. Act 316 of 1982 Prohibiting the Circumcision of Women.
26. Prohibition of Female Circumcision Act 1985
27. The Children Act 1989.
28. Crimes (female Genital Mutilation) Amendment Act 1994 (effective May 1, 1995).
29. 1991, Chapter 64 (Bill 125), Civil Code of Quebec, Article 11.
30. 1991, Chapter 64 (Bill 125), Civil Code of Quebec, Article 12.
31. 1991, Chapter 64 (Bill 125), Civil Code of Quebec, Article 19.
32. Criminal Code Section 273.3.
33. Bill C-235, reintroduced on March 12, 1996, and originally introduced as Bill C-277 on September 29, 1994.
34. Illinois 1995–96 Sessions, House Bill 3572, introduced on February 9, 1996, would create 720 Illinois Compiled Statues 5/12–34.
35. 730 Illinois Compiled Statutes § 5/5–8–1 (3)
36. 730 Illinois Compiled Statutes § 5/5–9–1 (a) (1)
37. Colorado 1996 Sessions, Senate Bill 96–31.
38. New York 1995–96 Sessions, Senate Bills 510 and 597, and Assembly Bills 690 and 788.
39. 1994 South Carolina Sessions, House Bill 4710.
40. 1995 Texas Sessions, House Bill 2442.
41. California Penal Code § 667.83.
42. Idaho Criminal Code § 18–1506A (b).
43. 720 Illinois Compiled Statutes §§ 5/12–32 and 5/12–33(2).
44. 24 Delaware Code § 1703(e)(4).

45. Minnesota Statute § 147.09(10).
46. Montana Code § 37–3–103(h).
47. Wisconsin Statute § 448.03(g).
48. Ecumenics International. News Release: Ad Hoc Working Group of International Experts on Violations of Genital Mutilation. Sloatsburg, New York: Ecumenics International July 1, 1995.
49. United States v. Virginia, 116 S.Ct. 2264, 2275 (1996).
50. United States v. Virginia, supra, 116 S.Ct. at 2274, 2275, quoting Mississippi University for Women v. Hogan, 458 U.S. 718, 724 (1982) (O' Connor, J.).
51. United States v. Virginia, supra, 116 S.Ct. at 2275, quoting Mississippi University for Women v. Hogan, supra, 458 U.S. at 724.
52. Spring P. Suit claims N.D. genital mutilation law biased. The Forum. June 7, 1996.
53. Taylor JR, Lockwood AP, Taylor AJ. The prepuce: specialised mucosa of the penis and its loss to circumcision. British Journal of Urology 1996;77:291–5.

23

THE ASHLEY MONTAGU RESOLUTION TO END THE GENITAL MUTILATION OF CHILDREN WORLDWIDE

A Petition to the World Court, the Hague

James W. Prescott

1. IN HONORIS CAUSA

On this distinguished occasion of the Fourth International Symposium on Sexual Mutilations, University of Lausanne, Lausanne, Switzerland (9–11 August 1996), we honor Professor Ashley Montagu, an internationally renowned scientist, scholar and Humanist, who has committed his life to advancing the dignity, integrity and well-being of infants and children and their mothers throughout the world and who has pioneered in documenting the power of pleasure in human touch while condemning the pain and degradation inherent in the barbaric practice of the genital mutilations of children.

In honor of a distinguished life of science for humanity by Ashley Montagu, the Institute of Humanistic Science, the Humanist Fellowship of San Diego, California, and the National Organization of Circumcision Information Resource Centers (NOCIRC) have commemorated their decade-long effort to bring the issue of the genital mutilation of children before The World Court, The Hague, by naming this effort The Ashley Montagu Resolution To End The Genital Mutilation of Children Worldwide.

The Ashley Montagu Resolution to End the Genital Mutilation of Children Worldwide will be sent to various "Heads of State" with a request that they forward this Resolution to The World Court, The Hague, for a de jure ruling that the genital mutilation of children violates the *Universal Declaration of Human Rights* and the *United Nations Convention on the Rights of the Child.*

The Montagu Resolution will also be forwarded to the Secretary General, United Nations, and the President, Amnesty International, for their support of *The Montagu Resolution*, which affirms that the genital mutilation of children violates the *Universal Declaration of Human Rights* and the *United Nations Convention on the Rights of the Child*, which state: "No(one) child shall be subjected to torture or other cruel, inhuman or degrading treatment or punishment." (Articles 2 and 37, respectively), and other Articles of these international treaties.

Sexual Mutilations: A Human Tragedy, edited by Denniston and Milos
Plenum Press, New York, 1997

2. PREAMBLE

Pursuant to the declarations on the genital mutilations of children previously passed by the unanimous votes of the General Assembly of the First International Symposium on Circumcision (March 3, 1989), and by the General Membership of the 1988 Annual Meeting of the Humanist Fellowship of San Diego, and by the International Covenant on Civil and Political Rights, and by Resolution of the Executive Board of the World Health Organization on "Maternal and Child Health and Family Planning: Current needs and future orientation," concerning traditional practices harmful to the health of women and children," which recommended to the Forty-Seventh World Health Assembly the adoption of the following resolution: "2.(2) to establish national policies and programmes that will effectively, and with legal instruments, abolish female genital mutilation, marriage and childbearing before biological and social maturity, and other harmful practices affecting the health of women and children" (25 January 1994), the following ASHLEY MONTAGU RESOLUTION TO END THE GENITAL MUTILATIONS OF CHILDREN WORLDWIDE is hereby submitted to the FOURTH INTERNATIONAL SYMPOSIUM ON SEXUAL MUTILATIONS for approval and endorsement.

WHEREAS, the genital mutilations of children violate those inalienable human rights as enumerated in the following articles of the UNITED NATIONS UNIVERSAL DECLARATION OF HUMAN RIGHTS and the United Nations CONVENTION ON THE RIGHTS OF THE CHILD. Specifically:

UNIVERSAL DECLARATION OF HUMAN RIGHTS

ARTICLE 2:

Everyone is entitled to all the rights and freedoms set forth in this declaration, without distinction of any kind, such as race, color, sex, language, religion, political or other opinion, national or social origin, property, birth or other status;

and

ARTICLE 3:

Everyone has the right to life, liberty and security of person;

and

ARTICLE 5:

No one shall be subjected to torture or to cruel, inhuman or degrading treatment or punishment;

and

United Nations CONVENTION ON THE RIGHTS OF THE CHILD

ARTICLE 19. ABUSE AND NEGLECT

1. State Parties shall take all appropriate legislative, administrative, social and educational measures to protect the child from all forms of physical or mental violence, injury or abuse,

neglect or negligent treatment, maltreatment or exploitation, including sexual abuse, while in the care of parent(s), legal guardian(s) or any other person who has the care of the child,

and

ARTICLE 24. RIGHT OF THE CHILD TO THE HIGHEST ATTAINABLE STANDARD OF HEALTH

3. States Parties shall take all effective and appropriate measures with a view to abolishing traditional practices prejudicial to the health of children.

ARTICLE 37. TORTURE, CAPITAL PUNISHMENT AND DEPRIVATION OF LIBERTY

States Parties shall ensure that:

(a) No child shall be subjected to torture or other cruel, inhuman or degrading treatment or punishment. Neither capital punishment nor life imprisonment without possibility of release shall be imposed for offenses committed by persons below 18 years of age.

(b) No child shall be deprived of his or her liberty unlawfully or arbitrarily...

(c) Every child deprived of liberty shall be treated with humanity and respect for the inherent dignity of the human person, and in a manner which takes into account the needs of persons of their age...

(d) Every child deprived of his or her liberty shall have the right to prompt access to legal and other appropriate assistance, as well as the right to challenge the legality of the deprivation of his or her liberty before a court or other competent, independent and impartial authority and to a prompt decision on any such action;

and

WHEREAS, The WORLD HEALTH ORGANIZATION (WHO) endorsement of the recommendation of the 1979 Khartoum Seminar on Traditional Practices affecting the health of women, which recommended that governments adopt clear and definitive policies for the eradication of female genital mutilation; and

THEREFORE, BE IT RESOLVED that the FOURTH INTERNATIONAL SYMPOSIUM ON SEXUAL MUTILATIONS:

AFFIRMS that the genital mutilations of children violates the human rights of children, as contained in Articles 2, 3 and 5 of the UNITED NATIONS UNIVERSAL DECLARATION OF HUMAN RIGHTS, and Articles 19, 24 and 37 of the United Nations CONVENTION ON THE RIGHTS OF THE CHILD; and

REQUESTS all national governments to petition THE WORLD COURT, THE HAGUE, to have THE WORLD COURT declare that the genital mutilations of children are in violation of the above said Articles of the UNITED NATIONS UNIVERSAL DECLARATION OF HUMAN RIGHTS and the United Nations CONVENTION ON THE RIGHTS OF THE CHILD; and

REQUESTS that all national governments pass legislation prohibiting the practice of torture, cruelty, inhuman and degrading treatment of children which is inherent in the genital mutilations of children that are conducted as a matter of socio-cultural and religious customs and are de facto violations of the UNITED NATIONS UNIVERSAL DEC-

LARATION OF HUMAN RIGHTS and the United Nations CONVENTION ON THE RIGHTS OF THE CHILD; and

REQUESTS that all national governments and their associated agencies educate health professionals, parents and the people on these issues, specifically, the medical, psychological, sexual and mental health hazards inherent in the genital mutilations of children, and to dispel the myths and superstitions which encourage the genital mutilations of children.

APPENDIX 1

DECLARATION OF GENITAL INTEGRITY

We recognize the inherent right of all human beings to an intact body. Without religious or racial prejudice, we affirm this basic human right.

We recognize that the foreskin, clitoris and labia are normal, functional body parts.

Parents and/or guardians do not have the right to consent to the surgical removal or modification of their children's normal genitalia.

Physicians and other health-care providers have a responsibility to refuse to remove or mutilate normal body parts.

The only persons who may consent to medically unnecessary procedures upon themselves are the individuals who have reached the age of consent (adulthood), and then only after being fully informed about the risks and benefits of the procedure.

We categorically state that circumcision has unrecognized victims.

In view of the serious physical and psychological consequences that we have witnessed in victims of circumcision, we hereby oppose the performance of a single additional unnecessary foreskin, clitoral, or labial amputation procedure.

We oppose any further studies which involve the performance of the circumcision procedure upon unconsenting minors. We support any further studies which involve identification of the effects of circumcision.

Physicians and other health-care providers do have a responsibility to teach hygiene and the care of normal body parts and explain their normal anatomical and physiological development and function throughout life.

We place the medical community on notice that it is being held accountable for misconstruing the scientific database available on human circumcision in the world today.

Physicians who practice routine circumcision are violating the first maxim of medical practice, "Primum Non Nocere," "First, Do No Harm," and anyone practicing genital mutilation is violating Article V of the *United Nations Universal Declaration of Human Rights*: "No one shall be subjected to torture or to cruel, inhuman or degrading treatment..."

Adopted March 3, 1989
by the General Assembly,
First International Symposium
 on Circumcision
Anaheim, California USA

APPENDIX 2

RESOURCES

Association contre la Mutilation des Enfants (A.M.E.), Boite Postale 220, 92108 Boulogne Cedex FRANCE

Circumcision Information Network, Rich Angell, 3865 Duncan Place, Palo Alto, CA 94306 USA, Tel: 415–493–2429

Circumcision Resource Center, Ron Goldman, Ph.D., P.O. Box 232, Boston, MA 02133 USA, Tel: 617–523–0088

Doctors Opposing Circumcision (D.O.C.), George Denniston, M.D., MPH, 2442 NW Market Street #42, Seattle, WA 98107 USA, Tel: 206–368–8358, Fax: 206–368–9428

(I)NTACT, Christa Müller, Johannisstraße 4, D-66111 Saarbrucken GERMANY, Tel/Fax: 681/3–2400

Inter-African Committee, Berhane Ras-Work, President, 147, rue de Lausanne, CH-1202 Geneva SWITZERLAND, Tel: 22–731–2420, Fax: 22–738–1823

Lightfoot Associates, Hanny Lightfoot-Klein, 4040 Via Del Vireo, Tucson, AZ 85718 USA, Tel: 520–529–2029, Fax: 520–529–9411

London Black Women's Health Action Project, Shamis Dirir, Cornwall Avenue Community Centre, First Floor, 1 Cornwall Avenue, London E2 0HW ENGLAND, Tel: 181–980–3503, Fax: 181–980–6314

National Organization of Circumcision Information Resource Centers, (NO-CIRC), International Headquarters, Marilyn Fayre Milos, R.N., P.O. Box 2512, San Anselmo, CA 94979–2512 USA, Tel: 415–488–9883, Fax: 415–488–9660

NOCIRC of AUSTRALIA, Dr. George Williams, The Woodlands Medical Centre, 1 Rosemary Row, Woodlands Estate, Menai 2234 NSW AUSTRALIA, Tel: 2–543–0510, Fax: 2–543–0222

Dr. Mervyn Lander , 131 Wickham Terrace, Brisbane 4000 AUSTRALIA, Tel: 07–38394742, Fax: 07–38326674

Nurses for the Rights of the Child, Mary Conant, R.N., Betty Katz Sperlich, R.N., Mary-Rose Booker, R.N., 369 Montezuma #354, Santa Fe, NM 87501, Tel: 505–989–7377

National Organization to Halt the Abuse and Routine Mutilation of Males (NO-HARMM), Tim Hammond, P.O. Box 460795, San Francisco, CA 94146–0795 USA, Tel/Fax: 415–826–9351

National Organization of Restoring Men (NORM), International Headquarters, R. Wayne Griffiths, 3205 Northwood Drive, Suite 209, Concord, CA 94520–4506 USA, Tel: 510–827–4077, Fax: 510–827–4119

NORM - UK, Dr. John P. Warren, 3 Watlington Road, Harlow, Essex CM17 0DX ENGLAND, Tel: 44–127–941–9704, Fax: 44–127–942–9771

Rainb♀, Nahid Toubia, M.D., 915 Broadway, Suite 1109, New York, NY 10010–7108 USA, Tel: 212–477–3318, Fax: 212–477–4154

Terres des Femmes, Marion Hulverscheidt, Petra Schnull, Kreuzbergring 10, D-37075 Gottingen GERMANY

UNCircumcising Information and Resources Center, UNCIRC, Jim Bigelow, Ph.D., P.O. Box 52138, Pacific Grove, CA 93950 USA, Tel/Fax: 408–375–4326

Women's International Network (WIN), Fran P. Hosken, 187 Grant Street, Lexington, MA 02173 USA, Tel: 617–862–9431

Further Reading

Circumcision: The Hidden Trauma, Ronald Goldman, Ph.D., 1996, Circumcision Information Resource Center, P.O. Box 232, Boston, MA 02133 USA

Deeper Into Circumcision, John A. Erickson, ed., 1996, 1664 Beach Blvd., #216, Biloxi, MS 39531 USA

Say No To Circumcision!, Thomas Ritter, M.D., and George Denniston, M.D., 1996, NOCIRC, P.O. Box 2512, San Anselmo, CA 94979–2512 USA

The Joy of Being A Boy!, Elizabeth Noble with Leo Sorger, M.D., New Life Images, 448 Pleasant Lake Avenue, Harwich, MA 02645 USA

The Joy of Uncircumcising!, Jim Bigelow, Ph.D., 1995, UNCIRC, P.O. Box 52138, Pacific Grove, CA 93950 USA

CONTRIBUTORS

Sami A. Aldeeb Abu-Sahlieh, an Arab Christian of Palestinian origin with Swiss nationality is a graduate in political sciences and Doctor of Law. He is the Staff Legal Adviser in charge of Arab and Islamic Law, Swiss Institute of Comparative Law, Lausanne, Switzerland. He is the author of the text, *To Mutilate in the Name of Jehovah or Allah*, published in many languages and periodicals, and of a book in French on Muslims and human rights, *Les Musulmans Face aux Droits de l'Homme*, Winkler, Bochum (1994), the first book on human rights that treats and condemns both male and female genital mutilation.

Zenas Baer, J.D., practices law in Federal and State Courts in northern Minnesota, concentrating on federal civil rights litigation. He has filed in North Dakota the first lawsuit in the nation challenging on equal protection grounds a statute that prohibits female genital mutilation.

Jeannine Parvati Baker, M.A., is an author and educator. Her publications include *Conscious Conception, Hygieia: A Woman's Herbal*, and *Prenatal Yoga & Natural Birth*. She regularly speaks at perinatal conferences and has been published in the *Pre- and Perinatal Psychology Journal*. She is co-founder of Six Directions, a non-profit educational organization devoted to family health and environmental issues.

Mary Conant, R.N., is, along with Betty Katz Sperlich, R.N., and Mary-Rose Booker, R.N., a founder of *Nurses for the Rights of the Child*, a non-profit organization dedicated to protecting the right of infants and children to genital integrity. Her work includes supporting and advising other nurses who want to stop the socially-sanctioned genital mutilation of minors. Since 1979, she has served as a maternal-child health staff nurse at St. Vincent Hospital in Santa Fe, New Mexico, and since 1992, she has been an R.N. Conscientious Objector to infant circumcision.

James DeMeo, Ph.D., earned his doctorate at the University of Kansas and has served on the Faculty of Geography at Illinois State University and the University of Miami. He is currently the Director of the Orgone Biophysical Research Laboratory and editor of the environmental journal, *Pulse of the Planet*.

George Denniston, M.D., MPH, a graduate of the Harvard School of Public Health, is the co-author of the second edition of *Say No To Circumcision!: 40 Compelling Reasons*, and is the founder and Director of D.O.C. (Doctors Opposing Circumcision), the first group of medical professionals to uphold their premier tenet, "First, do no harm," and to defend the inherent, inalienable right of infants and children to intact sexual organs.

Didier Diers, together with Xavier Valla, founded the Association contre la Mutilation des Enfants (A.M.E.) in 1989 to fight against the mutilation of children. A.M.E. was the first European organization to speak out against genital mutilations. A.M.E. offers parents alternative documentation, collaborates with other French organizations that oppose female genital mutilation, and confronts the medical community about contraindicated surgeries. A.M.E. published the first nonsurgical treatment for teenage phimosis, written by Dr. Beauge.

Pia Grassivaro Gallo, Ph.D., graduated in Biology and received her Ph.D. in Anthropology from the University of Padua. She is Associate Professor in General Biology, Faculty of Psychology at the University of Padua. Her research work for the last 25 years has been dedicated to Somali women and to the physical development of children in Somalia. She was invited by the Somali Ministry of Public Health in 1981 to take part in a scientific mission to Somaliland, and her visit was supported by Italian and international organizations operating in Somalia. Her scientific activity in Somalia has received recognition both at national and international levels.

Jenny Goodman, M.A., M.B., Ch.B., psychotherapist, appeared in Victor Schonfeld's ground-breaking documentary, *It's A Boy!*, shown on British television in September 1995. Since then, she has been challenging circumcision both within the Jewish community and in the wider world. She has appeared twice on BBC national television, spoken on several radio programs, and has had articles published in national newspapers. She has also participated in panel discussions on circumcision, and led workshop-sessions on circumcision at Jewish women's conferences.

Tim Hammond, is the co-founder, with Wayne Griffiths, of a national network of men's foreskin restoration support groups, the National Organization of Restoring Men (NORM). In 1992, Hammond founded the National Organization to Halt the Abuse and Routine Mutilation of Males (NOHARMM), a national nonviolent, direct-action organization of men opposed to infant circumcision. He has produced many educational tools relevant to male genital mutilation in the United States, including the award-winning documentary *Whose Body, Whose Rights?*

Frederick Hodges, historian, received his degree at the University of California at Berkeley. In 1993, he began the monumental project of assembling primary historical source materials relating to the introduction and spread of genital mutilation in the Western World. Hodges has published articles on various aspects of the problem of genital mutilation in the *British Medical Journal*, the *Journal of Urology*, the *Townsend Letter*, the *Journal of Pediatrics*, and others.

Mervyn Lander, M.B, B.S., Dip.Ter.Ed., Fellow of the Royal College of Surgeons, is a pediatric surgeon, clinical lecturer at the University of Queensland, an Anglican Priest, and is the Director of the NOCIRC Center in Queensland. He is an active NOCIRC campaigner and facilitates a Restoration Group.

Hanny Lightfoot-Klein, M.A., is a cross-cultural sexologist and clinical supervisor of the American Board of Sexology. She spent the greater part of six years in the Sudan doing field research on female genital mutilation and has published extensively on the subject. Her groundbreaking book, *Prisoners of Ritual: An Odyssey Into Female Genital Circumcision*, received a book award at an international sexology conference in 1991.

Marilyn Fayre Milos, R.N., together with Sheila Curran, R.N., in 1986, co-founded the National Organization of Circumcision Information Resource Centers, and she has been the Executive Director of the organization since its founding. She is the Coordinator of the International Symposia on Sexual Mutilations, and a Diplomate of the American Board of Sexology.

Christa Müller received diplomas in both Political Economics and Business Management. Her professional experience includes work with the Parliament of the State of Hessen, the Government of the State of Hessen, the Social Democratic Party of Germany and, since

1990, with the Department of Economics and Employment of the Research Institute of the Friedrich Ebert Foundation. While visiting the West African state of Benin with her husband, Oskar Lafontaine, Governor of the State of Saarland and President of the Social Democratic Party of Germany, Ms. Müller was asked by the wife of the former President to support the Benin women in their fight against female genital mutilation. She agreed. Back in Germany, she founded (I)NTACT, an organization aimed at informing German people about female genital mutilation and collecting money to support the African groups. (I)NTACT also fights against female genital mutilation of immigrant women in Germany.

Michel Odent, M.D., was born in France in 1930, and studied medicine at the University of Paris, qualifying in general surgery, obstetrics and gynecology. He headed the Department of Obstetrics and Gynecology at the world-renowned Pithiviers Hospital from 1962 to 1986. He was commissioned by the World Health Organization to report on planned home birth in the industrialized countries from 1986 to 1990. He founded the Primal Health Research Centre in London, which studies the correlations between the primal period (fetal life, perinatal period and early infancy) and health later on in life. Dr. Odent has thirty medical journal publications and has written nine books that have been translated into 19 languages.

Miriam Pollack, M.A., earned a B.A. degree in English and Judaica from the University of Iowa and a M.A. degree in English and Education from the University of Wisconsin. She has been an educator for more than twenty years, mostly in the area of Jewish education, as a principal, curriculum writer, educational consultant, teacher of Judaic studies, Hebrew, English literature, American Jewish literature and history. Her original work, "Circumcision: A Jewish Feminist Perspective," was presented at the Judaism, Feminism and Psychology Conference in Seattle in 1992 and at the Third International Symposium on Circumcision in 1994, and was published as a chapter in *Jewish Women Speak Out: Expanding the Boundaries of Psychology*, 1995 (Canopy Press).

James W. Prescott, Ph.D., is Director, Institute of Humanistic Science, a developmental neuropsychologist and a cross-cultural psychologist who has documented the developmental origins of violence and seeks to end violence against children and women worldwide, without which, human violence cannot end.

Berhane Ras-Work, M.A., earned a B.A. in Education and an M.A. in International Relations at the Institut Universitaire de Developpement, Geneva, Switzerland. She is currently the President of the Inter-African Committee (IAC) on Traditional Practices Affecting the Health of Women and Children, the program coordinator of the Ethiopian Women's Welfare Association in Addis Ababa, an advisor to the Ethiopian Ambassador to Geneva, and the coordinator of the Non-Governmental Organization (NGO) Working Group on Traditional Practices in Geneva. In 1995, she received the United Nations 1995 Population Award for her work.

Betty Katz Sperlich, R.N., is, along with Mary Conant, R.N., and Mary-Rose Booker, R.N., a founder of *Nurses for the Rights of the Child*, a non-profit organization dedicated to protecting the rights of infants and children to genital integrity. Her work includes supporting and advising other nurses who want to stop the socially-sanctioned genital mutilation of minors. Since 1981, she has served as a staff nurse primarily in maternal-child health at St. Vincent Hospital, Santa Fe, New Mexico, and since 1992 she has been an R.N. Conscientious Objector to infant circumcision. She has a Master's Degree in Philosophy from Harvard University.

J. Steven Svoboda, J.D., Attorney at Law and author, graduated cum laude from Harvard Law School in 1991 and practices law in San Francisco, principally in the areas of civil litigation and human rights.

Xavier Valla, together with Didier Diers, founded the Association contre la Mutilation des Enfants (A.M.E.) in 1989 to fight against the mutilation of children. A.M.E. was the first European organization to speak out against genital mutilations. A.M.E. offers parents alternative documentation, collaborates with other French organizations that oppose female genital mutilation, and confronts the medical community about contraindicated surgeries. A.M.E. published the first nonsurgical treatment for teenage phimosis, written by Dr. Beauge.

Robert S. Van Howe, M.D., received his Doctor of Medicine from Stritch School of Medicine, Loyola University in Chicago, is a Fellow of the American Academy of Pediatrics, and practices at Marshfield Clinic's Lakeland Center in Minocqua, Wisconsin. His work on the issue of circumcision includes "A perspective on controversies about neonatal circumcision," published in *Clinical Pediatrics* in 1995, a poster presentation at Child Health 2000 in Vancouver, British Columbia, 1995, with George C. Denniston, "The Controversy Over Circumcision, USA," and two presentations of his own research at the Strategies for Intactivists Conference, Evanston, Illinois, 1996, "Variations in Penile Appearance and Findings" and "Neonatal Circumcision: Cost-Utility Analysis."

Franco Viviani, Ph.D., graduated in Biological Sciences from the University of Padua where he is now professor of Physical Education, Cultural Anthropology and General Biology. In 1986, he directed the film "Somalian schoolgirls speak," a documentary on female genital mutilation in Somalia. In 1991, he participated in a field research project on genital mutilation. That same year, he and Professor Pia Grassivaro Gallo received honorable mention from the Royal Academy of Overseas Science (Belgium). He has organized surveys, research projects and symposia on female genital mutilation.

John Warren, M.B., BCHIR, DCH, FRCP, trained at Cambridge University and is a consultant physician specializing in internal medicine and respiratory disease. He is the founder and Director of NOCIRC of England and, in 1994, started NORM UK (the National Organization of Restoring Men), a support group for circumcised men in England.

George Williams, M.B, Ch.B., F.R.A.C.P., Consultant Pediatrician and Perinatalogist, is a childbirth and parent educator who served as the Director of Newborn Intensive Care Unit at the Children's Hospital in Sydney, where he now has a private practice. Dr. Williams has been an anti-circumcision activist for 14 years and is the founder and co-director of NOCIRC of Australia. He has appeared on national radio and television and has contributed to many media publications on circumcision. Dr. Williams is the recipient of Australia's *Parents* magazine's 1996 Award of Merit, recognizing his efforts "to make the world a better place for children."

Gérard Zwang, M.D., was born in Paris in 1930. He has made his career as a urologic surgeon and has contributed significantly to the scientific study of sexuality. In 1975, with his colleague in Montpelier, he described the arterial origin of most cases of impotence. His first publication, *Le Sexe de la Femme* (1967), denounced female sexual mutilation, and, in 1977, he participated in the first international press conference, held in Geneva, against these mutilations. Among his other works, *La Statue de Freud*, a thorough refutation of psychoanalysis, and a *Historie des Peines de Sexe*. In 1990, he was awarded the Prix du Medoc for his *Pathologie Sexuelle*, and, in 1988, he was awarded the Prix de Medecine et Culture for his life's work.

INDEX